Clinical Anatomy Cases

An integrated Approach with Physical Examination and Medical Imaging

Sagar Dugani, MD, PhD

Clinical Fellow, General Internal Medicine
St. Michael's Hospital and University of Toronto
Toronto, Ontario, Canada

Anne M. R. Agur, BSc (OT), MSc, PhD

Professor, Division of Anatomy, Department of
    Surgery, Faculty of Medicine
Division of Physical Medicine and Rehabilitation,
    Department of Medicine
Department of Physical Therapy, Department
    of Occupational Science and Occupational
    Therapy
Division of Biomedical Communications,
    Institute of Medical Science
Rehabilitation Sciences Institute, Graduate
    Department of Dentistry
University of Toronto
Toronto, Ontario, Canada

Jeffrey E. Alfonsi, BASc, MD

Clinical Fellow, Department of Medicine
Schulich School of Medicine and Dentistry
Western University
London, Ontario, Canada

Arthur F. Dalley II, PhD, FAAA

Professor, Department of Cell and
    Developmental Biology
Adjunct Professor, Department of Orthopaedic
    Surgery
Vanderbilt University School of Medicine
Adjunct Professor of Anatomy
Belmont University School of Physical Therapy
Nashville, Tennessee

. Wolters

Philadelphia
Buenos Aire

Acquisitions Editor: Crystal Taylor
Product Development Editor: Greg Nicholl
Marketing Manager: Michael McMahon
Production Project Manager: Bridgett Dougherty
Design Coordinator: Stephen Druding
Art Director: Jennifer Clements
Art Coordinator: Jonathan Dimes of JDimes Medivisual Communications
Manufacturing Coordinator: Margie Orzech
Prepress Vendor: SPi Global

Library of Congress Cataloging-in-Publication Data

Names: Dugani, Sagar, editor. | Alfonsi, Jeffrey E., editor. | Agur, A. M. R., editor. | Dalley, Arthur F., II, editor.

Title: Clinical anatomy cases : an integrated approach with physical examination and medical imaging / [edited by] Sagar Dugani, Jeffrey E. Alfonsi, Anne M.R. Agur, Arthur F. Dalley II.

Description: Philadelphia : Wolters Kluwer, [2017] | Includes index.

Identifiers: LCCN 2016010368 | ISBN 9781451193671

Subjects: | MESH: Physical Examination | Diagnostic Imaging | Anatomy, Regional—methods | Clinical Medicine—methods

Classification: LCC RC78.7.D53 | NLM WB 200 | DDC 616.07/54—dc23 LC record available at http://lccn.loc.gov/2016010368

My parents, Manda and Basavaraj Dugani, for their constant inspiration and support (Sagar Dugani)

My wife Elizabeth, thank you for your love, smiles, patience, and support (Jeffrey E. Alfonsi)

My husband Enno and my family Kristina, Erik, and Amy for their support and encouragement
(Anne M. R. Agur)

Muriel, with love and appreciation for your continued patience and support (Arthur F. Dalley II)

And...

...to the anatomical donors:

With sincere appreciation for all those who donate their bodies for anatomical study and research, without whom much anatomical study would not be possible.

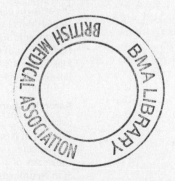

CONTRIBUTORS

Anne M. R. Agur, BSc (OT), MSc, PhD

Professor, Division of Anatomy, Department of Surgery, Faculty of Medicine

Division of Physical Medicine and Rehabilitation, Department of Medicine

Department of Physical Therapy, Department of Occupational Science and Occupational Therapy

Division of Biomedical Communications, Institute of Medical Science

Rehabilitation Sciences Institute, Graduate Department of Dentistry

University of Toronto

Toronto, Ontario, Canada

Jeffrey E. Alfonsi, BASc, MD

Clinical Fellow, Department of Medicine

Schulich School of Medicine and Dentistry

Western University

London, Ontario, Canada

Shamik Bhattacharyya, MD, MS

Clinical Fellow ·

Department of Neurology

Harvard Medical School

Neurology Resident

Department of Neurology

Massachusetts General Hospital and Brigham and Women's Hospital

Boston, Massachusetts

Nickolaus Biasutti, HBSc

MD Candidate, QMed 2018

Faculty of Health Sciences

Queen's University

Kingston, Ontario, Canada

Tanya Chawla, RCP, FRCR, FRCPC

Assistant Professor

Department of Medical Imaging

University of Toronto

Staff Radiologist

Department of Medical Imaging

Mount Sinai Hospital

Toronto, Ontario, Canada

Ernest Chiu, MD

Clinical Fellow, Division of Nephrology

Department of Medicine

University of Toronto

Toronto, Ontario, Canada

Kenneth B. Christopher, MD, SM

Assistant Professor

Department of Medicine

Harvard Medical School

Associate Physician

Division of Renal Medicine

Brigham and Women's Hospital

Boston, Massachusetts

Christine J. Chung, MD

Department of Medicine, Division of Cardiology

Columbia University Medical Center

New York City, New York

Arthur F. Dalley II, PhD, FAAA

Professor, Department of Cell and Developmental Biology

Adjunct Professor, Department of Orthopaedic Surgery

Vanderbilt University School of Medicine

Adjunct Professor of Anatomy

Belmont University School of Physical Therapy

Nashville, Tennessee

Sagar Dugani, MD, PhD

Clinical Fellow, General Internal Medicine

St. Michael's Hospital and University of Toronto

Toronto, Ontario, Canada

Sebastian Heaven, MBBCh

Postgraduate Surgical Trainee

Department of Surgery, Orthopaedic Division

McMaster University

Orthopaedic Surgery Resident

Department of Orthopaedic Surgery

Hamilton Health Sciences

Hamilton, Ontario, Canada

Marilyn Heng, MD, FRCSC

Instructor

Department of Orthopaedic Surgery

Harvard Medical School

Orthopaedic Surgeon

Department of Orthopaedic Surgery

Massachusetts General Hospital

Boston, Massachusetts

Aaron Izenberg, MD, FRCPC

Lecturer

Division of Neurology, Department of Medicine

University of Toronto

Staff Neurologist

Sunnybrook Health Sciences Centre

Toronto, Ontario, Canada

R. Phelps Kelley, AB, MD

Resident

Department of Radiology and Biomedical Imaging

University of California, San Francisco

San Francisco, California

Joshua P. Klein, MD, PhD
Associate Professor
Department of Neurology
Harvard Medical School
Chief, Division of Hospital Neurology
Department of Neurology
Brigham and Women's Hospital
Boston, Massachusetts

Kristen M. Krysko, MD, BSc
Resident Physician
Department of Neurology
University of Toronto
Toronto, Ontario, Canada

Joshua M. Liao, MD
Department of Medicine
Perelman School of Medicine
University of Pennsylvania
Philadelphia, Philadelphia

Kelsey E. Mills, MD
Obstetrician and Gynecologist
Department of Obstetrics and Gynecology
Victoria General Hospital
Victoria, British Columbia

Tri H. Nguyen, MD, MSc
Resident
Physical Medicine and Rehabilitation
University of Toronto
Toronto, Ontario, Canada

Gavin J. le Nobel, MD
Resident
Otolaryngology Head and Neck Surgery
University of Toronto
Toronto, Ontario, Canada

Sunita Sharma, MD, MPH
Associate Professor
Department of Medicine
University of Colorado School of Medicine
Aurora, Colorado

Samuel A. Silver, MD, FRCPC
University of Toronto
Toronto, Ontario, Canada

Laura E. Smith, MD
Instructor in Medicine
Harvard Medical School
Instructor in Medicine
Internal Medicine
Brigham and Women's Hospital
Boston, Massachusetts

Daniel Souza, MD, MSc
Instructor
Department of Radiology
Harvard Medical School
Staff Radiologist
Department of Radiology
Brigham and Women's Hospital
Boston, Massachusetts

Devraj Sukul, MD
Fellow, Cardiovascular Medicine
Department of Internal Medicine
University of Michigan Health System
Ann Arbor, Michigan

Piero Tartaro, MD, MScCH
Lecturer
Department of Medicine
University of Toronto
Staff Gastroenterologist
Division of Gastroenterology
Sunnybrook Health Sciences Centre
Toronto, Ontario, Canada

Sarah M. Troster, MD
Clinical Fellow, Division of Rheumatology
Department of Internal Medicine
University of Toronto
Toronto, Ontario, Canada

Janice Wong, MD, MS
Clinical Fellow
Department of Neurology
Harvard Medical School
Neurology Resident
Department of Neurology
Brigham and Women's Hospital, Massachusetts General
    Hospital
Boston, Massachusetts

Michelle J. Yu, MD, PhD
Pulmonary and Critical Care Medicine
University of California, San Francisco
San Francisco, California

Jonathan S. Zipursky, MD
Resident
Department of Medicine
St. Michael's Hospital
University of Toronto
Toronto, Ontario, Canada

Molly Zirkle, MD, MED
Assistant Professor
Department of Otolaryngology
University of Toronto
Toronto, Ontario, Canada

REVIEWERS

FACULTY

Francine Anderson, PhD, PT
Chair of Anatomy
School of Osteopathic Medicine
Campbell University
Buies Creek, North Carolina

Rebecca Brown, MPAS, PA-C
Assistant Coordinator
Le Moyne College
Syracuse, New York

Thomas R. Gest, PhD
Professor of Anatomy
Department of Medical Education
Texas Tech University Health Sciences Center
El Paso, Texas

Douglas J. Gould, PhD
Professor of Neuroscience and Vice Chair
Department of Biomedical Sciences
Oakland University William Beaumont
School of Medicine
Rochester, Michigan

Robert Hage, MD, PhD, DLO, MBA
Professor
St. George's University
St. George's, Grenada, West Indies

Jon Jackson, PhD
Visiting Professor
St. George's University
St. George's, Grenada, West Indies

Eileen Kalmar, PhD
Assistant Professor—Clinical
College of Medicine
The Ohio State University
Columbus, Ohio

H. Wayne Lambert, PhD
Professor
Department of Neurobiology and Anatomy
West Virginia University School of Medicine
Morgantown, West Virginia

Octavian Calin Lucaciu, MD, PhD
Associate Professor
Canadian Memorial Chiropractic College
Toronto, Ontario

Andrew F. Payer, PhD
Professor
Medical Education
College of Medicine
University of Central Florida
Orlando, Florida

Danielle Royer, PhD
Assistant Professor
Department of Cell and Developmental Biology
University of Colorado Denver
Denver, Colorado

Brett Szymik, PhD
Assistant Professor
Georgia Regents University/University of Georgia
Medical Partnership
Athens, Georgia

Ljubisa Terzic, MD
Associate Professor
Canadian College of Naturopathic Medicine
Toronto, Ontario

Shanna Williams, PhD
Assistant Professor
School of Medicine
University of South Carolina
Greenville, South Carolina

STUDENTS

Joshua Agranat
Boston University School of Medicine

Amier Ahmad
University of Southern Florida College of Medicine

David Ballard
Louisiana State University Health
Shreveport School of Medicine

William Blair
Lake Erie College of Osteopathic Medicine

Lucas Carlson
University of Maryland School of Medicine

William Gentry
Oceania University of Medicine

Benjamin Heyen
University of Kansas Medical School

Christopher Jacob
Becker Professional Education
Ross University School of Medicine

Christen Johnson
Wright State University Boonshoft School of Medicine

Zuhal Kadhim
University of Toronto

Bryan Klosky
Shenendoah University School of Pharmacy

Porcha Leggett
Ross University School of Medicine

Jason Lipof
George Washington University School of Medicine

Julianne Matthews
Northeastern Ohio Medical University

Francesca Nichols
University of Utah School of Medicine

Jennifer Townsend
UCSF School of Medicine

Samuel Windham
University of Missouri–Columbia School of Medicine

Kristen Wilde
Indiana University School of Medicine

Michael Wu
University of Hawaii, John A. Burns School of Medicine

PREFACE

Medical education is evolving. Yet, today, many topics are often taught in isolation, and trainees are presented with the daunting task of integrating various concepts in medicine. Several years ago, we experienced that three key topics—anatomy, physical examination, and medical imaging—were fragmented through different stages of medical education and that trainees lacked a single resource to integrate these topics. This fragmentation gave rise to the idea of *Clinical Anatomy Cases* as a way to amalgamate all three concepts into a single resource.

Clinical Anatomy Cases uses a highly graphical approach to describe seven anatomical regions. The introductory chapter outlines our integrated approach and provides the fundamentals of the physical examination, medical imaging modalities, and commonly used statistical concepts. The seven anatomical regions continue this integrated approach and lead the reader through several common clinical presentations and diseases. Where relevant, we also include a concise list of differential diagnoses and high-yield clinical pearls.

We decided to create this resource as it addresses a gap in our approach to education. We remain confident that this integrated resource will appeal to medical students, residents, and students in health disciplines including nursing, physical therapy, occupational therapy, dentistry, and physician assistants program. In addition to being beneficial to students, this book will also serve as a convenient resource for faculty members to include in their courses or integrated curricula. Further, the topics presented here complement the clinical focus of related Wolters Kluwer publications such as *Clinically Oriented Anatomy* and *Essential Clinical Anatomy*. We hope that this book generates additional resources that integrate various aspects of medical education.

KEY TO ICONS USED IN CLINICAL CASES

 = Family Medicine

 = Emergency Medicine

 = Obstetrics and Gynecology

 = Surgery

 = Internal Medicine

ACKNOWLEDGMENTS

Several years ago, we started out with the idea of integrating anatomy, physical examination, and medical imaging, and the creation of this first edition of *Clinical Anatomy Cases* would not have been possible without the guidance and advice of several outstanding individuals in the United States and Canada. We are extremely grateful to Dr. Joseph Loscalzo (Chairman of the Department of Medicine, and Physician-in-Chief at Brigham and Women's Hospital, Boston), Dr. Joel T. Katz (Director, Internal Medicine Residency Program, Brigham and Women's Hospital, Boston), Dr. Maria Yialamas (Associate Program Director, Internal Medicine Residency Program, Brigham and Women's Hospital, Boston), Dr. Vivian Gonzalez Mitchell (Assistant Program Director, Internal Medicine Residency Program, Brigham and Women's Hospital, Boston), and Dr. Stephen Ledbetter (Chief of Radiology at Brigham and Women's Faulkner Hospital, Boston) for their timely and generous advice in developing this book and in identifying faculty contributors. We thank Dr. Heather McDonald-Blumer (Division of Rheumatology, Mount Sinai Hospital/University Health Network and University of Toronto, Toronto) and Dr. Vincent Chien (Division of General Internal Medicine, St. Michael's Hospital and University of Toronto, Toronto) for supporting this initiative and for identifying faculty collaborators. We remain grateful to all of our authors (residents, fellows, and faculty members) at Brigham and Women's Hospital (Boston), University of Toronto (Toronto), and other hospitals in the United States and Canada, who took time out of their busy clinical and nonclinical schedules to be part of this project and help bring our idea to fruition.

Ultimately, this book would have remained an *idea* without the able leadership of Crystal Taylor and Greg Nicholl at Wolters Kluwer, who have remained dedicated to this book. Thank you Greg for your patience, collaboration, advice, and for steering us through the development of this book. Finally, we are grateful to Jonathan Dimes for his assistance with the art development and for crucial editing provided by Kelly Horvath.

CONTENTS

FIGURE CREDITS

CHAPTER 1 • Integrated Approach to Clinical Encounters

Bickley LS. *Bates' Guide to Physical Examination and History Taking*, 11th ed. Baltimore, MD: Wolters Kluwer Health, 2013. **Figure 1.1.**

Moore KL, Dalley AF, Agur AMR. *Clinically Oriented Anatomy*, 7th ed. Baltimore, MD: Lippincott Williams & Wilkins, 2014. **Figures 1.2–1.11 and 1.15.**

Daffner RH, Hartman MS. *Clinical Radiology*, 4th ed. Baltimore, MD: Lippincott Williams & Wilkins, 2014. **Figure 1.13.**

Smith WL, Farrell TA. *Radiology 101*, 4th ed. Philadelphia, PA: Lippincott Williams & Wilkins, 2013. **Figure 1.14.**

CHAPTER 2 • Thorax

Moore KL, Dalley AF, Agur AMR. *Clinically Oriented Anatomy*, 7th ed. Baltimore, MD: Lippincott Williams & Wilkins, 2014. **Figures 2.1–2.3, 2.23.**

Bickley LS. *Bates' Guide to Physical Examination and History Taking*, 11th ed. Baltimore, MD: Wolters Kluwer Health, 2013. **Figures 2.4, 2.5, 2.8–2.14, 2.41.**

Daffner RH, Hartman MS. *Clinical Radiology*, 4th ed. Baltimore, MD: Lippincott Williams & Wilkins, 2014. **Figure 2.6.**

Daffner RH, Hartman MS. *Clinical Radiology*, 4th ed. Baltimore, MD: Lippincott Williams & Wilkins, 2014. **Figures 2.7, 2.15–2.22, 2.24–2.26, 2.28–2.38, 2.42–2.45, 2.47–2.54.**

Moore KL, Agur AMR, Dalley AF. *Essential Clinical Anatomy*, 5th ed. Baltimore, MD: Lippincott Williams & Wilkins, 2015. **Figure 2.27.**

Agur AMR, Dalley AF. *Grant's Atlas of Anatomy*, 13th ed. Baltimore, MD: Wolters Kluwer Health, 2013. **Figure 2.39.**

Moore KL, Dalley AF, Agur AMR. *Clinically Oriented Anatomy*, 7th ed. Baltimore, MD: Lippincott Williams & Wilkins, 2013. **Figures 2.40, 2.46.**

CHAPTER 3 • Abdomen

Moore KL, Dalley AF, Agur AMR. *Clinically Oriented Anatomy*, 7th ed. Baltimore, MD: Lippincott Williams & Wilkins, 2014. **Figures 3.1–3.3, 3.4B, 3.5, 3.9, 3.10A, 3.12A,B, 3.13, 3.14A, 3.18, 3.19, 3.22, 3.25A, 3.28, 3.35C, 3.38, 3.41, 3.48, 3.54, 3.57, 3.59, 3.60.**

Bickley LS. *Bates' Guide to Physical Examination and History Taking*, 11th ed. Baltimore, MD: Wolters Kluwer Health, 2013. **Figures 3.4A, 3.10B, 3.11, 3.15, 3.16, 3.23, 3.26, 3.29, 3.35A,B, 3.36, 3.46, 3.49, 3.62.**

Daffner RH, Hartman MS. *Clinical Radiology*, 4th ed. Baltimore, MD: Lippincott Williams & Wilkins, 2014. **Figures 3.6–3.8, 3.14B, 3.17B, 3.20, 3.21, 3.24A, 3.27, 3.30, 3.31, 3.33, 3.39, 3.40, 3.42–3.44, 3.47, 3.50–3.53, 3.55, 3.56, 3.58, 3.61, 3.63, 3.64.**

Agur AMR, Dalley AF. *Grant's Atlas of Anatomy*, 13th ed. Baltimore, MD: Wolters Kluwer Health, 2013. **Figures 3.12C, 3.17A, 3.24B.**

Moore KL, Agur AMR, Dalley AF. *Essential Clinical Anatomy*, 5th ed. Baltimore, MD: Lippincott Williams & Wilkins, 2015. **Figures 3.25B, 3.34, 3.45.**

Madden ME. *Introduction to Sectional Anatomy*, 3rd ed. Baltimore, MD: Lippincott Williams & Wilkins, 2013. **Figure 3.32.**

Provenzale JM, Nelson RC, Vinson, EN. *Duke Radiology Case Review*, 2nd ed. Philadelphia, PA: Lippincott Williams & Wilkins, 2012. **Figure 3.37.**

CHAPTER 4 • Pelvis

Moore KL, Dalley AF, Agur AMR. *Clinically Oriented Anatomy*, 7th ed. Baltimore, MD: Lippincott Williams & Wilkins, 2014. **Figures 4.1–4.3, 4.6–4.14, 4.17, 4.24.**

Bickley LS. *Bates' Guide to Physical Examination and History Taking*, 11th ed. Baltimore, MD: Wolters Kluwer Health, 2013. **Figures 4.4, 4.5, 4.15, 4.16.**

Daffner RH, Hartman MS. *Clinical Radiology*, 4th ed. Baltimore, MD: Lippincott Williams & Wilkins, 2014. **Figures 4.18–4.23, 4.25–4.33.**

CHAPTER 5 • Back

Moore KL, Dalley AF, Agur AMR. *Clinically Oriented Anatomy*, 7th ed. Baltimore, MD: Lippincott Williams & Wilkins, 2014. **Figures 5.1–5.3, 5.4A, 5.6, 5.10–5.12, 5.14–5.21, 5.23.**

Bickley LS. *Bates' Guide to Physical Examination and History Taking*, 11th ed. Baltimore, MD: Wolters Kluwer Health, 2013. **Figure 5.4B.**

Agur AMR, Dalley AF. *Grant's Atlas of Anatomy*, 13th ed. Baltimore, MD: Wolters Kluwer Health, 2013. **Figure 5.5.**

Brant WE, Helms CA. *Fundamentals of Diagnostic Radiology*, 3rd ed. Philadelphia, PA: Lippincott Williams & Wilkins, 2007. **Figure 5.7A.**

Smith WL, Farrell TA. *Radiology 101*, 4th ed. Philadelphia, PA: Lippincott Williams & Wilkins, 2014. **Figures 5.7B, 5.8.**

Schwartz ED, Flanders AE. *Spinal Trauma*. Philadelphia, PA: Lippincott Williams & Wilkins, 2007. **Figure 5.9.**

Daffner RH, Hartman MS. *Clinical Radiology*, 4th ed. Baltimore, MD: Lippincott Williams & Wilkins, 2014. **Figures 5.22, 5.24–5.27, 5.29–5.31.**

Berquist TH. *MRI of the Musculoskeletal System*, 6th ed. Philadelphia, PA: Lippincott Williams & Wilkins, 2013. **Figure 5.28.**

CHAPTER 6 • Upper and Lower Extremities

Moore KL, Dalley AF, Agur AMR. *Clinically Oriented Anatomy*, 7th ed. Baltimore, MD: Lippincott Williams & Wilkins, 2014. **Figures 6.1, 6.2, 6.4–6.10, 6.12–6.14, 6.15A, 6.16, 6.17, 6.19–6.22, 6.24, 6.25, 6.28, 6.36, 6.41, 6.43, 6.45, 6.47, 6.49, 6.51–6.53, 6.55, and 6.58.**

Carter PJ. *Lippincott Textbook for Nursing Assistants*. Philadelphia, PA: Wolters Kluwer, 2016. **Figure 6.3.**

Nath JL. *Using Medical Terminology*, 2nd ed. Baltimore, MD: Lippincott Williams & Wilkins, 2013. **Figure 6.11.**

Smith WL, Farrell TA. *Radiology 101*, 4th ed. Philadelphia, PA: Lippincott Williams & Wilkins, 2014. **Figures 6.15B and 6.18B.**

Greenspan A, Beltran J. *Orthopedic Imaging*, 6th ed. Philadelphia, PA: Wolters Kluwer Health, 2015. **Figure 15C.**

Dudek RW, Louis TM. *High-Yield: Gross Anatomy*, 5th ed. Baltimore, MD: Lippincott Williams & Wilkins, 2015. **Figure 6.18A.**

Bickley LS. *Bates' Guide to Physical Examination and History Taking*, 11th ed. Baltimore, MD: Wolters Kluwer Health, 2013. **Figures 6.23, 6.26, 6.30, 6.33, and 6.59.**

Pope TL, Harris JH. *The Radiology of Emergency Medicine*, 5th ed. Philadelphia, PA: Lippincott Williams & Wilkins, 2013. **Figure 6.27.**

Erkonen WE, Smith WL. *Radiology 101*, 3rd ed. Philadelphia, PA: Wolters Kluwer, 2010. **Figure 6.29.**

Daffner RH, Hartman MS. *Clinical Radiology*, 4th ed. Baltimore, MD: Lippincott Williams & Wilkins, 2014. **Figures 6.31, 6.34, 6.35, 6.39, 6.40, 6.44, and 6.46.**

Barker LR, et al. *Principles of Ambulatory Medicine*, 7th ed. Philadelphia, PA: Lippincott Williams & Wilkins, 2007. **Figure 6.32.**

Chew FS. *Skeletal Radiology*, 3rd ed. Philadelphia, PA: Lippincott Williams & Wilkins, 2010. **Figure 6.37.**

Boulware DW, Heudebert GR. *Lippincott's Primary Care Rheumatology*. Philadelphia, PA: Lippincott Williams & Wilkins, 2011. **Figure 6.38.**

Brant WE, Helms CA. *Fundamentals of Diagnostic Radiology*. Philadelphia, PA: Lippincott Williams & Wilkins, 2007. **Figure 6.50.**

Berquist TH. *MRI of the Musculoskeletal System*, 6th ed. Philadelphia, PA: Lippincott Williams & Wilkins, 2013. **Figure 5.54.**

Geschwind JH, Dake MD. *Abrams' Angiography*, 3rd ed. Philadelphia, PA: Lippincott Williams & Wilkins, 2014. **Figure 6.56.**

CHAPTER 7 • Head and Neck

Moore KL, Dalley AF, Agur AMR. *Clinically Oriented Anatomy*, 7th ed. Baltimore, MD: Lippincott Williams & Wilkins, 2014. **Figures 7.1, 7.2, 7.4, 7.6–7.8, 7.16–7.19, 7.22, 7.23, 7.26, 7.27, 7.29–7.31, 7.33, 7.36, 7.37, 7.46.**

Daffner RH, Hartman MS. *Clinical Radiology*, 4th ed. Baltimore, MD: Lippincott Williams & Wilkins, 2014. **Figures 7.3, 7.5, 7.11, 7.15, 7.24, 7.35, 7.38, 7.39, 7.41, 7.42, 7.44, 7.48–7.54.**

Bickley LS. *Bates' Guide to Physical Examination and History Taking*, 11th ed. Baltimore, MD: Wolters Kluwer Health, 2013. **Figures 7.9, 7.10, 7.12–7.14, 7.20, 7.21, 7.25, 7.32, 7.34, 7.40, 7.43, 7.45.**

Harrison LB, Sessions RB, Kies MS. *Head and Neck Cancer*, 4th ed. Philadelphia, PA: Lippincott Williams & Wilkins, 2014. **Figure 7.28.**

Integrated Approach to Clinical Encounters

JEFFREY E. ALFONSI • SAGAR DUGANI •
ANNE M. R. AGUR • ARTHUR F. DALLEY II

1

INTRODUCTION TO AN INTEGRATED APPROACH TO MEDICINE

The practice of medicine is the art and science of evaluating and optimizing the health of a patient. According to the World Health Organization, health is "a state of complete physical, mental and social well-being and not merely the absence of disease or infirmity" and is determined by biologic, psychological, and social factors. To evaluate a patient's health, the clinician must integrate knowledge in anatomy, physical examination, biochemistry, and medical imaging to characterize the etiology of the presenting symptoms. During undergraduate and postgraduate education, many of these concepts are often taught in isolation. This book aims to facilitate the process of thinking clinically and critically by integrating the fundamentals of anatomy, physical examination, and medical imaging into the clinical evaluation of a patient. We begin this chapter with the clinical case of Mr. John Smith.

> *Mr. Smith is a 30-year-old male who visits his primary care provider with a chief complaint of right knee pain. Four days prior, he developed sudden-onset knee pain that has made it difficult to ambulate. Mr. Smith has also experienced abdominal discomfort and diarrhea over the last week. He has not taken any medications and does not have drug allergies. As his primary care provider, you are aware that Mr. Smith has experienced intermittent episodes of abdominal pain and diarrhea in the past that have resolved without intervention. As his provider, you consider if the two presenting symptoms—right knee pain and abdominal discomfort with diarrhea—are related or independent of each other.*

How should the clinician approach this situation?

INITIAL EVALUATION

Based on the chief complaint, the clinician develops a *differential diagnosis* and, throughout the history, physical examination, and interpretation of tests (also called *investigations*), attempts to narrow the differential diagnosis to arrive at the most likely etiology. In medical emergencies, the clinician may obtain a brief history, stabilize the patient, and then obtain additional information from the patient or collateral sources such as family members, witnesses, and emergency responders.

The initial evaluation begins with the clinician observing the patient and focuses on four components: general appearance and grooming, greeting, behavior and expression, and posture and gait.

The general appearance and grooming provide information on the patient's overall health.

1. Does the patient appear well or sick? If the patient appears sick, does this reflect an acute change or is this consistent with the patient's chronic illnesses?
2. Does the patient's appearance match his or her stated age?
3. Does the patient look malnourished, or is there an obvious change (increase or decrease) in weight? Is this change uniform, or is it restricted to a specific part of the body?
4. Is the patient wearing appropriate clothing and footwear, or is there a risk of weather-related injuries?
5. Are the patient's hair, nails, and skin well groomed? Does the patient have body odor, which along with other factors may suggest inadequate self-care and hygiene?

During the greeting, the clinician assesses the appropriateness of the patient's initial interaction.

1. Does the patient make appropriate eye contact?
2. When the patient shakes hands, do the hands feel warm or cool/clammy?
3. Do the patient's facial gestures match his or her verbal expressions, or is there discordance?

The third component is evaluation of the patient's behavior and expression, which provides information on the overall physical and psychological state.

1. Does the patient appear to be breathing normally, or is it labored?
2. Does the patient appear to be in obvious distress or pain?
3. Does the patient maintain appropriate eye contact throughout the interview?
4. Does the patient appear to have involuntary movements, tremors, or facial twitching?

The final component is the evaluation of posture and gait, which helps identify possible impairment in the neurological, musculoskeletal, or endocrine systems.

1. Does the patient have normal gait? (Chapter 6)
2. Does the patient swing his or her arms while ambulating, or are the arms locked in a particular position?
3. Does the patient maintain normal posture while ambulating and while sitting?

Returning to the case, the initial evaluation revealed that Mr. Smith was well groomed and appropriately dressed. He appeared his stated age, but was frail, and his facial expression showed he was in discomfort. Despite his discomfort, he greeted the clinician pleasantly. While walking into the examination room, Mr. Smith maintained a normal posture, but had difficulty bearing weight on his right leg.

■ DETAILED EVALUATION

The detailed evaluation involves obtaining a detailed history, performing a physical examination, and ordering laboratory tests and imaging. History taking will not be covered in this book, and we will begin with the physical examination.

■ PHYSICAL EXAMINATION

A complete physical examination involves evaluation of the following components, most of which will be addressed in the relevant chapters:

- General appearance, behavior, and vital signs (Chapter 1)
- Cardiovascular examination (Chapter 2)
- Respiratory examination (Chapter 2)
- Abdominal and retroperitoneal examination (Chapter 3)
- Peripheral vascular examination (Chapter 6)
- Musculoskeletal examination (Chapter 6)
- Neurologic examination (Chapters 5, 6, and 7)
- Head and neck examination (Chapter 7)

In special circumstances, dermatologic, gynecologic (Chapter 4), urologic (Chapter 4), psychiatric, ophthalmologic, and otolaryngologic examinations may also be performed.

The clinician should obtain consent prior to performing a physical examination. Exact definitions of consent vary based on the state, province, or country of practice, but, in general, it involves informing the patient or his or her substitute decision maker about the planned examination/intervention, the benefits and risks of the examination/intervention, and available reasonable alternatives. Consent is intervention specific and, in emergency situations, can be overridden as long as the patient's interests and wishes are kept in mind.

Here is one approach to preparing a patient for an examination (although several are possible):

- *Positioning and Appropriate Lighting*: It is important that the patient be positioned appropriately, for example, sitting upright in an examination chair or lying supine on an examination table. Further, ensuring that there is appropriate lighting to examine the relevant system(s) is also important.
- *Supervision and Draping*: The clinician should perform maneuvers that are within his or her scope of practice and expertise and ensure appropriate supervision, when necessary. Further, the clinician should clarify the patient's preference for having a chaperone in the room during the examination. For example, a patient may prefer to have a female chaperone in the room during a breast or pelvic examination. Finally, the patient should be appropriately draped such that only

essential areas are exposed. For example, while performing an abdominal examination, a drape is placed over the pelvic area and lower extremities; while performing a breast examination, only the breast being examined is exposed, while the other breast should be covered with a drape.

■ *Equipment*: The clinician should have all necessary equipment (e.g., stethoscope, reflex hammer, eye chart) for the physical examination.

Vital Signs

After performing an initial evaluation, the clinician obtains vital signs. Vital signs provide essential information on the stability of the patient. There are four vital signs: body temperature, blood pressure (BP), heart rate (HR), and respiratory rate (RR). Abnormalities in these signs may occur when one or more anatomic systems are affected by disease, trauma, or medications. In some instances, the following parameters are also measured and reported with vital signs: arterial oxygen saturation (O_2 sat), height, weight, body-mass index (BMI), and pain index; however, these are not classically regarded as "vital signs."

Temperature

There are at least four approaches to measuring temperature: oral, aural (tympanic membrane), axillary, and rectal. The average oral temperature is 98.6°F (37°C) and fluctuates from 96.4°F (35.8°C) in the morning (usually at 6:00 AM) to 99.1°F (37.3°C) in the afternoon or evening (usually between 4 and 6 PM).

● **CLINICAL PEARL**

Compared to oral temperature:

Rectal temperature is higher by 0.4°C–0.5°C.
Aural temperature is higher by 0.8°C–1°C.
Axillary temperature is lower by 1°C.

Body temperature is regulated by the hypothalamus, which, in turn, is affected by several intrinsic and extrinsic factors. Temperatures within the normal range are considered *normothermia*, temperatures below 95.0°F (35°C) are considered *hypothermia*, and temperatures above 98.9°F (37.3°C) or an afternoon temperature above 99.9°F (37.7°C) fall into one of three pathologic groups: fever, hyperthermia, or hyperpyrexia. The presence of fever suggests an underlying infection, inflammatory process, autoimmune condition, malignancy, hemolysis, venous thrombosis, or medication side effect, among other etiologies. Fever may also result from alterations in the hypothalamus' *set point;* as a result, there is a central drive to raise the body's temperature. *Hyperthermia* increases body temperature without altering the hypothalamus' set point. This usually occurs in the presence of extrinsic factors such as heat stroke, use of stimulants such as cocaine, or as a side effect of medications (resulting in neuroleptic malignant syndrome [NMS] or malignant hyperthermia). Hyperpyrexia is characterized by temperatures above 106°F (41.1°C) and can result from CNS hemorrhage, underlying infection, or as a side effect of medications (namely, NMS or malignant hyperthermia). Hyperpyrexia requires urgent attention as it can be life threatening.

● **CLINICAL PEARL**

NMS is a combination of hyperthermia, rigidity, and autonomic dysregulation and is a possible side effect of antipsychotic medications. Malignant hyperthermia is hypermetabolism of skeletal muscle that occurs in susceptible patients after exposure to certain inhaled anesthetic medications and muscle relaxant medications such as succinylcholine.

Serotonin syndrome is caused by excessive serotonin in the body from illicit drugs such as ecstasy or from polypharmacy. Patients may be hyperthermic with associated rigidity, hyperreflexia, myoclonus, confusion, diaphoresis, and autonomic instability.

Blood Pressure

BP is a functional measure of the circulatory system and is affected by the volume of fluid in the circulatory system, ability of the heart to effectively pump blood to the body, systemic inflammation associated with infections, and the ability of the nervous system to relax or constrict blood vessels. In addition, the patient's age, sex, medical comorbidities, medications, and social stressors can affect BP.

BP fluctuates throughout the day. The goal is to obtain numerous measurements to approximate the true BP, and there are various methods to do so:

- *Ambulatory BP monitoring* requires a patient to wear a BP cuff for 24–48 hours. The patient's BP is automatically measured every 15–20 minutes during the day and every 30–60 minutes at night. Ambulatory monitoring has several advantages: it normalizes natural physiologic BP variation that might incidentally be captured during a clinic visit, it eliminates "white coat hypertension" associated with clinic settings, it can uncover "masked hypertension," and it reduces the number of clinic visits a patient has to make. Although ambulatory monitoring requires a patient to wear a BP cuff for 24–48 hours and is considered to be cumbersome, it is regarded as the reference standard to diagnose hypertension.

- *Home blood pressure monitoring* requires a patient to check his or her BP 10–15 times over a 1-week period in order to estimate the average BP. This approach has similar advantages to the ambulatory monitoring approach.

- *Office blood pressure monitoring* requires one or more BP measurements to be taken during a single office visit. Office measurements are more likely to vary from the patient's true BP compared to ambulatory or home monitoring. **Figure 1.1** summarizes the technique of obtaining a BP manually.

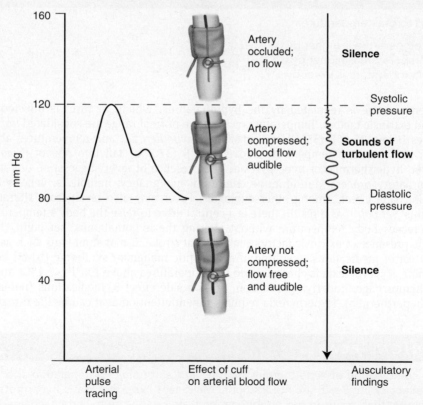

FIGURE 1.1. Measuring blood pressure. An appropriately sized blood pressure cuff is inflated around the arm of the patient to compress and occlude arterial blood flow. Next, the cuff is deflated while auscultating for Korotkoff sounds, and the first instance of this marks the systolic pressure. As the cuff is further deflated, sounds of turbulent blood flow remain audible, until they become inaudible. The first instance of this marks the diastolic blood pressure.

TABLE 1.1. Pulse pressure (PP) and asymmetry in measurement of blood pressure (BP)	
Definition	Causes
Wide PP is a PP > 50% of the systolic pressure.	Hyperdynamic states such as hyperthyroidism, aortic insufficiency (or regurgitation), fever, anemia, and pregnancy
Narrow PP is a PP < 25% of the systolic pressure.	Cardiac tamponade, constrictive pericarditis, aortic stenosis, and shock
Asymmetric BP is a difference of more than 10 mm Hg in the systolic pressure between the right and left extremities.	Aortic dissection, peripheral artery disease, subclavian stenosis, and errors in measurement

PP is the difference between the systolic and diastolic BP. Blood pressure should be measured in both arms, and the readings are normally within 5–10 mm Hg of each other. Several conditions are associated with asymmetric BP measurements as described in **Table 1.1** and in Chapter 2.

Several factors can complicate BP readings, including the presence of weak Korotkoff sounds; body habitus of the patient, particularly if the wrong type/size of cuff is used; type of equipment used (manual vs. automatic); and arrhythmias.

Heart Rate and Rhythm

HR and rhythm are important signs related to the circulatory system and are affected by the respiratory, endocrine, and nervous systems as well as by drugs and fever, among other etiologies. In addition to the HR, the clinician documents if the heart rhythm is regular or irregular and if the arterial pulse is weak or bounding.

Normal hearts have a regular HR of 60–100 beats per minute (bpm). HRs below 60 bpm are termed *bradycardia*, and HRs above 100 bpm are termed *tachycardia*. The differential diagnosis for bradycardia and tachycardia is presented below.

Sinus Bradycardia	Sinus Tachycardia
Normal finding in some athletes	Hyperthyroidism
Acute myocardial ischemia	Acute myocardial ischemia
Increased intracranial pressure	Fever, volume depletion, and sepsis
Hypothyroidism	Stimulants including caffeine, toxins, anxiety, recreational drugs, and exercise
Sick sinus syndrome	Anemia, hypoxia, and chronic obstructive pulmonary disease (COPD)
Medication side effect	Heart failure Pulmonary embolism

Orthostatic Vital Signs

When the clinician suspects blood loss or dehydration, and the patient's resting BP is within the normal range, orthostatic vital signs should be measured. With the patient supine, the clinician measures the BP and HR. The patient is then asked to stand for 2–3 minutes, following which the BP and HR are again measured. A symptomatic patient or a drop in diastolic BP of 10 mm Hg or more, drop in systolic BP of 20 mm Hg or more, or an increase in HR of 30 bpm or more is indicative of orthostatic changes and suggests low circulating blood volume.

Respiratory Rate

The RR is an important vital sign affected by the respiratory, circulatory, renal, and nervous systems. The normal adult RR is 12–18 breaths per minute. The clinician assesses if the patient's breathing pattern is normal and quiet or if it is labored and requires the use of accessory respiratory muscles. The clinician also monitors the breathing pattern for the presence of respiratory pauses and for the duration of the expiratory phase, as these can be altered in conditions such as asthma and COPD.

Oxygen Saturation

Arterial O_2 sat is a measure of arterial oxygenation and is normally 95% or higher on room air (or *ambient air*, in which O_2 concentration is 21%). O_2 sat was initially measured using arterial puncture and chemical analysis, but now it can be calculated noninvasively using pulse oximetry. Pulse oximetry may be unreliable in the presence of hemoglobin-based abnormalities such as sickle cell anemia, carbon monoxide poisoning, or anemia. In such cases, co-oximetry can be performed in the laboratory to determine the true O_2 sat.

Body Mass Index

$$BMI = [weight, measured\ in\ kg]/[height, measured\ in\ meters]^2$$

Different cutoff points may be used for different ethnicities:

<18.5 kg/m²	underweight
18.5–24.9 kg/m²	normal
25.0–29.9 kg/m²	overweight
≥30.0 kg/m²	obese

Vital Signs in an Anatomic Context

As described above, vital signs are affected by numerous anatomic systems. Many of these systems are interrelated, such that changes in one can affect the others. Here, we describe how the circulatory, respiratory, renal, nervous, and endocrine systems interact to alter the vital signs.

The *circulatory system* consists of the cardiovascular and lymphatic systems, which serve to transport blood and lymph in the body. The cardiovascular system comprises the *pulmonary* and *systemic circulations* (**Fig. 1.2**). BP and HR are direct measures of the circulatory system. The

FIGURE 1.2. The circulatory system. Schematic representation of right and left heart pumping blood to the pulmonary and systemic circulation systems, respectively. *RA,* right atrium; *LA,* left atrium; *RV,* right ventricle; *LV,* left ventricle.

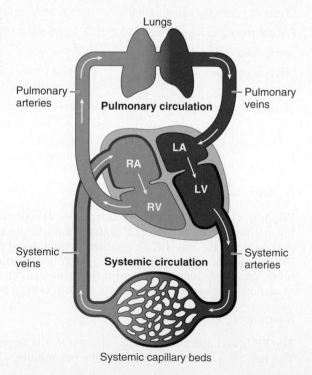

circulatory system also regulates temperature by increasing blood flow to dilated vessels near the skin where heat can be exchanged with the environment. If the circulatory system fails to adequately pump blood (e.g., in the setting of heart failure), then fluid accumulates in the lungs causing an increase in RR and a decrease in arterial O_2 sat. HR can be regulated by the nervous system via the vagal nerve and BP via the autonomic nervous system.

The *lymphatic system* is closely related to the circulatory system. During a 24-hour period, ~20 L of plasma is filtered out of the circulatory system into the interstitial space. Approximately 17 L is reabsorbed into the circulatory system, leaving 3 L in the interstitial space that is transported to the circulatory system via the lymphatic system (**Fig. 1.3**). In addition to its circulatory function, the lymphatic system is important to the body's immune system. As shown in **Figure 1.3**, several superficial lymphatic vessels track along the venous system and eventually drain into deep lymphatic vessels, which, in turn, drain into the right lymphatic duct or the thoracic duct. The right lymphatic duct drains lymph from the right side of the head, neck, thorax, and right upper limb into the venous circulation at the junction of the right internal jugular vein and the right subclavian vein (blue shaded area in **Fig. 1.3**). The thoracic duct receives lymph from the rest of the body and empties it in the venous circulation at the junction (also known as *left venous angle*) of the left internal jugular vein and left subclavian veins.

The *respiratory* (or *pulmonary*) *system* comprises airways, lungs, and the diaphragm (innervated by the phrenic nerve) and is responsible for transporting and exchanging oxygen and carbon dioxide between the environmental air and the circulating blood (**Fig. 1.4**). The respiratory system directly impacts O_2 sat. The respiratory system works in conjunction with the renal system to regulate blood pH. The circulatory system delivers blood to the kidneys where it passes through *nephrons* and undergoes filtration to remove waste material and excess electrolytes that are subsequently expelled in urine through the ureters, bladder, and urethra. The kidney is also responsible for the regulation of fluids (BP), pH, calcium, and electrolytes and for the production of erythropoietin to stimulate red blood cell (RBC) production. As a result, the renal and respiratory systems can affect RR. The renal system also helps regulate BP.

In addition to being affected by the circulatory, respiratory, and renal systems, vital signs are also affected by hormones. The *endocrine system* consists of structures that produce and secrete hormones into the bloodstream that then exert a physiologic or pathologic response throughout the body. For example, in hyperthyroidism, the thyroid gland produces an excess of thyroid hormone (triiodothyronine [T_3] and thyroxine [T_4]), which, in turn, can increase the HR, body temperature, BP, and RR.

Returning to the case, Mr. Smith's vital signs were assessed and recorded as follows:

Aural temperature: 97.2°F
Blood Pressure: 125/85 (right arm) and 130/90 (left arm)
Heart Rate: 72 bpm and regular rhythm
Respiratory Rate: 14 breaths per minute and without pauses or evidence of distress
Oxygen saturation: 98% on room air (ambient air, and not using supplemental oxygen)
BMI: 28.1 kg/m², calculated at a visit 1 month ago, and was not repeated

Focused Physical Examination

After recording Mr. Smith's vital signs, the clinician next performs a focused physical examination while keeping in mind the underlying anatomy. One approach for performing an examination is based on the IPPA method: inspection, palpation, percussion, and auscultation. The IPPA method is a general framework and has some notable exceptions. One, during an abdominal examination, the clinician first auscultates the abdomen as palpation and percussion can affect bowel sounds. Two, during a musculoskeletal examination (e.g., of the knee or hip), percussion and auscultation are not necessary. Finally, in addition to IPPA, some physical examinations include maneuvers specific to an anatomic region. For example, the knee examination will include assessment of gait, range of motion (ROM), motor power, and joint stability. The details on how to perform a specific physical examination along with special tests or maneuvers are described in the relevant chapter.

During inspection and palpation, the first organ system to be encountered is the *integumentary system*. The integumentary system consists of the skin (epidermis and dermis), hair, nails, and the

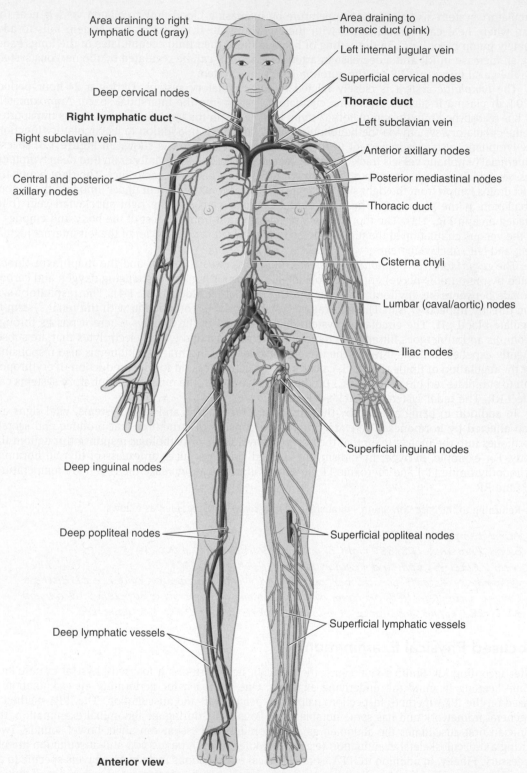

Area draining to right lymphatic duct (gray)

Area draining to thoracic duct (pink)

Left internal jugular vein

Superficial cervical nodes

Deep cervical nodes

Thoracic duct

Right lymphatic duct

Left subclavian vein

Right subclavian vein

Anterior axillary nodes

Central and posterior axillary nodes

Posterior mediastinal nodes

Thoracic duct

Cisterna chyli

Lumbar (caval/aortic) nodes

Iliac nodes

Superficial inguinal nodes

Deep inguinal nodes

Deep popliteal nodes

Superficial popliteal nodes

Superficial lymphatic vessels

Deep lymphatic vessels

Anterior view

FIGURE 1.3. The lymphoid system. Pattern of lymphatic drainage. The right superior quadrant (depicted in *gray*) drains to the right venous angle, usually via the right lymphatic duct. The rest of the body (depicted in *pink*) ultimately drains into the left venous angle via the thoracic duct.

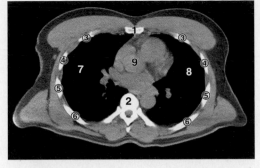

Transverse CT scan
1 Sternum
2 Vertebral body
3–6 Ribs
7 Right pulmonary cavity
8 Left pulmonary cavity
9 Mediastinum

(A) Inferior view

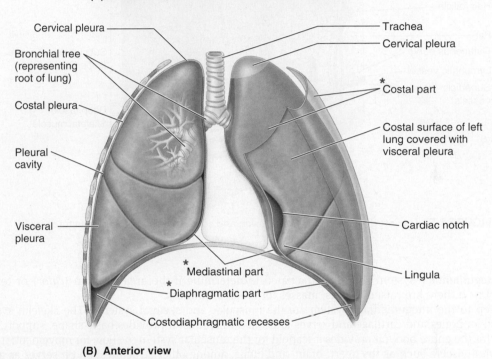

(B) Anterior view

FIGURE 1.4. The thoracic cavity. **A.** CT scan of transverse cross-sectional view of the thoracic cavity. **B.** Coronal cross section of the thoracic cavity. The lung invaginates a continuous membranous pleural sac; the visceral pleura covers the lungs, and the parietal pleura lines the thoracic cavity. The *asterisks* denotes that these structures are part of the parietal pleura.

subcutaneous tissue just beneath it. The integumentary system protects the viscera from the external environment, stores fat, regulates temperature, and synthesizes vitamin D. The *epidermis* is a *keratinized epithelium* composed of a tough *superficial* epithelial layer overlying a deep, *basal* layer that is pigmented and has regenerative potential. The epidermis is devoid of blood vessels and lymphatics and relies on the underlying, vascularized dermis for nutrition. As shown in **Figure 1.5**, the *dermis* has vascular and lymphatic beds and nerve terminals that convey sensory information including pain and temperature. Although the vast majority of nerve fibers terminate in the dermis, a few also penetrate the epidermis. The dermis is composed of a dense layer of collagen and elastic fibers. Below the dermis is *subcutaneous tissue* (superficial fascia), which is composed of loose connective tissue, fat, sweat glands, superficial blood and lymphatic vessels, and cutaneous nerves. Subcutaneous tissue is the primary site where body fat is stored; therefore, the thickness of this layer varies from person to person and among different body parts in the same person.

The integumentary system is inspected for swelling (*tumor*), redness (*rubor*), scars and lesions, dryness, hair loss, and pigmentation and color changes such as pallor, cyanosis, and jaundice. Next,

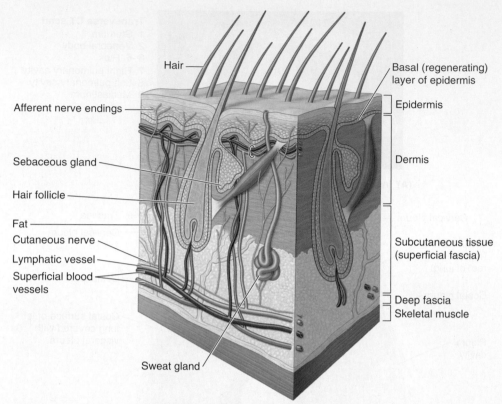

Hair

Basal (regenerating) layer of epidermis

Epidermis

Afferent nerve endings

Dermis

Sebaceous gland

Hair follicle

Fat

Subcutaneous tissue (superficial fascia)

Cutaneous nerve

Lymphatic vessel

Superficial blood vessels

Deep fascia

Skeletal muscle

Sweat gland

FIGURE 1.5. The integumentary system. The skin and some of its specialized structures.

the integumentary system should be palpated to determine if the area is warm (*calor*) or tender (*dolor)* or if there are raised lesions, masses, or areas of fullness.

Deep to the integumentary system are the muscular and skeletal systems. The skeletal system consists of bones and cartilage and serves four main functions: It provides basic shape, support, and frame for the entire body; it provides a scaffold for the muscular system to allow for movement; it protects vital viscera such as the heart, brain, and lungs, among other structures; and it serves as a site where hematologic cells are produced. The skeletal system is illustrated in **Figure 1.6** and is further discussed in the Back (Chapter 5) and Upper and Lower Extremity (Chapter 6) chapters.

Closely related to the skeletal system is the *articular system*, which consists of joints and ligaments. The articular system serves to connect bones of the skeletal system, thereby promoting flexibility and ROM to the skeletal system. The three main types of joints can be affected by infection, trauma, or inflammation, thereby impairing mobility and ROM. For physical examination purposes, the synovial joint can be best assessed. Synovial joints can be inspected for swelling and erythema, palpated for the presence of fluid and crepitus, and tested through different ROM.

While evaluating joint movement, it is important to consider the *muscular* and *nervous* systems. There are three types of muscle tissues: The first is *skeletal striated muscle tissue*, which is composed of voluntary, striated, somatic muscles that make up the gross skeletal muscles. These muscles can be inspected for signs of trauma, palpated for masses, and tested for strength. The second is *cardiac striated muscle tissue*, which is composed of involuntary, striated muscles that form the myocardium. The third is *smooth unstriated muscle tissue*, which is composed of involuntary, unstriated visceral muscles that form most of the muscular layer of hollow organs and tunica media of blood vessels.

The *nervous system* works in conjunction with the muscular system. The nervous system is responsible for perceiving the external environment, activating muscles and glands, and regulating the body's interactions with the external environment. It is also involved in cognition, movement, sensation, coordination, posture, and gait. The nervous system can be divided into the *central nervous system* (*CNS*) and *peripheral nervous system* (*PNS*), as shown in **Figure 1.7**.

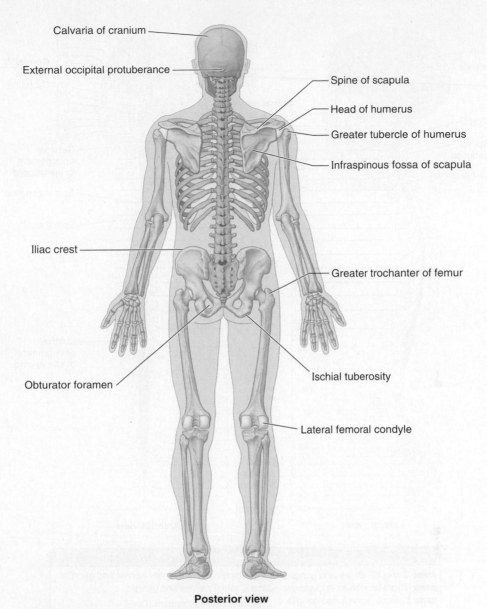

Calvaria of cranium

External occipital protuberance

Spine of scapula

Head of humerus

Greater tubercle of humerus

Infraspinous fossa of scapula

Iliac crest

Greater trochanter of femur

Obturator foramen

Ischial tuberosity

Lateral femoral condyle

Posterior view

FIGURE 1.6. The skeletal system. Bone markings and formations.

After the muscular, skeletal, articular, and nervous systems are examined, attention is shifted to the viscera, which are located beneath the muscles and bones. Viscera are essential components of the circulatory, respiratory, renal, and urinary systems. Viscera can also be part of the digestive system, which is discussed in the chapters on the Thorax (Chapter 2) and Abdomen (Chapter 3).

Documenting and Communicating Findings from the Physical Examination

At the end of the physical examination, the clinician documents the findings that can then be communicated with the patient and other practitioners. In all instances, it is important to document and communicate physical examination findings using appropriate terminology for anatomical terms, planes, and movements. The terminology in this book conforms to the *International Anatomical Terminology*; the official terms can be found on the Web site of the International Federation of Associations of Anatomists (IFAA) at *www.unifr.ch/ifaa* and are summarized in **Figures 1.8 and 1.9**.

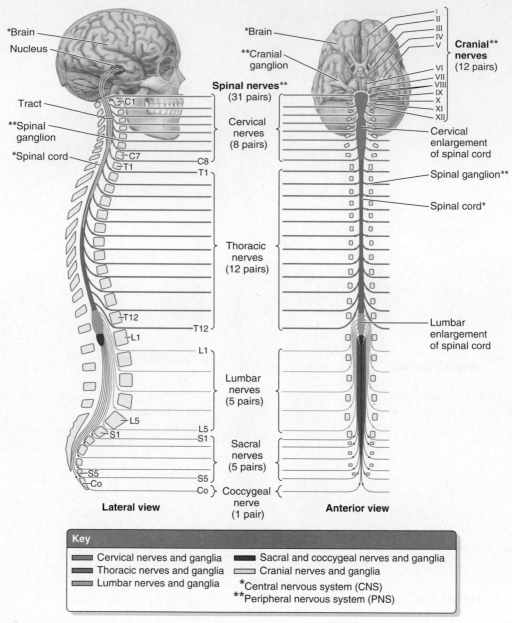

FIGURE 1.7. Basic organization of the nervous system. The CNS consists of the brain and spinal cord, and the PNS consists of nerves and ganglia.

The terminology used by the IFAA is based on the anatomic position. As patients can be examined in various positions, for example, while lying on the back (*supine*) or the chest (*prone*), it is important to develop standard anatomic positions to communicate physical examination findings. The accepted internationally convention to define all anatomic positions involves the person standing upright, as illustrated in **Figure 1.8**, with:

■ Head, eyes, and feet directed forward (anteriorly)
■ Arms at the side with the palms facing forward (anteriorly)
■ Lower limbs close together, with the toes pointing forward (anteriorly)

Regardless of the patient's position, the patient should be visualized as being in the anatomic position, and all movements should be described accordingly. The important exception is that the

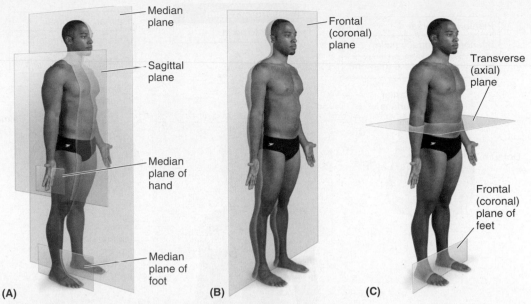

FIGURE 1.8. Anatomical planes.

majority of patients are examined while supine, which affects the location of organs. Therefore, the location of organs should be described with the patient in the supine position instead of the anatomic position.

Four anatomical planes dissect the body in the anatomic position and are also used to describe radiological findings, as shown in **Figure 1.9**.

Returning to the case, a complete physical examination was performed on Mr. Smith. Given his chief complaint of abdominal pain and knee swelling, attention was focused on these systems, and the following findings were documented:

- *General examination: The patient appeared thin and in mild distress, but was well groomed and appeared his stated age.*
- *Vital signs: T, 97.2°F; BP, 125/85 (left); HR, 72 bpm, regular; RR, 14 breaths per minute, O_2 sat, 98% on ambient air; and BMI 28.1.*
- *Head and neck: Eyes, ears, and nose examination was normal. The lips, gums, and teeth were normal, but the oropharynx revealed an ulcer on the inner right cheek.*
- *Cardiac: On inspection, there were no scars; on palpation, there were no heaves or thrills, and the apex was palpated in the fifth intercostal space along the left midclavicular line. On auscultation, heart sounds were normal without audible murmurs.*
- *Lymphatic: On palpation, no abnormal lymph nodes were identified in the neck, axillae, or groin.*
- *Respiratory: On inspection, the patient was not in respiratory distress. On palpation, the trachea was midline. The chest was resonant to percussion in all lung fields. On auscultation, breath sounds were normal without crackles, wheezes, or rubs.*
- *Abdominal: On inspection, there were no scars, masses, or bulging flanks. On auscultation, bowel sounds were increased. Deep palpation revealed mild tenderness throughout the abdomen. The liver edge was smooth, and the liver span was estimated to be 10 cm. The spleen was not palpated. There was no evidence of hernias. A rectal examination revealed a skin tag. The sphincter tone was normal, the prostate was smooth and not enlarged, and there was light brown stool in the rectal vault. Analysis of the stool revealed evidence of occult blood.*
- *Vascular: On palpation, the abdominal aorta was not enlarged, and on auscultation, bruits were not heard. On palpation, pulses were equal and symmetric in the femoral, popliteal, and pedal arteries. There was no edema or varicose veins.*

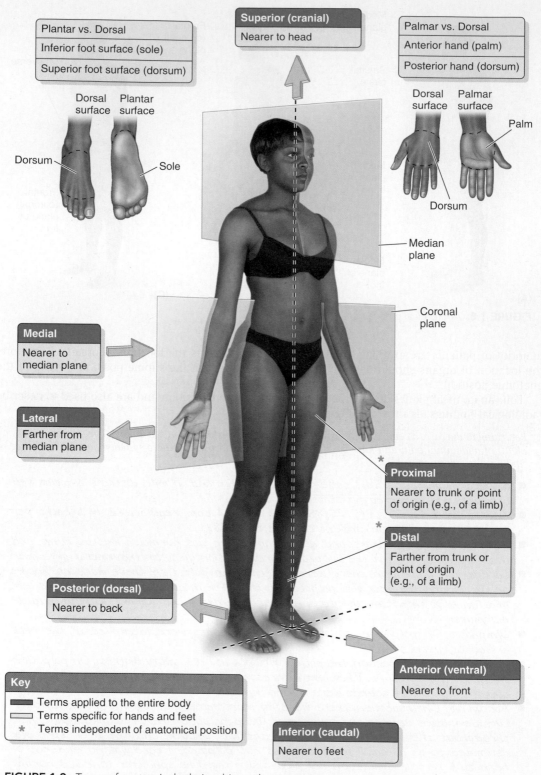

Plantar vs. Dorsal

Inferior foot surface (sole)

Superior foot surface (dorsum)

Dorsal surface   Plantar surface

Dorsum

Sole

Superior (cranial)

Nearer to head

Palmar vs. Dorsal

Anterior hand (palm)

Posterior hand (dorsum)

Dorsal surface   Palmar surface

Palm

Dorsum

Median plane

Coronal plane

Medial

Nearer to median plane

Lateral

Farther from median plane

* **Proximal**

Nearer to trunk or point of origin (e.g., of a limb)

* **Distal**

Farther from trunk or point of origin (e.g., of a limb)

Posterior (dorsal)

Nearer to back

Key

⬛ Terms applied to the entire body

☐ Terms specific for hands and feet

* Terms independent of anatomical position

Anterior (ventral)

Nearer to front

Inferior (caudal)

Nearer to feet

FIGURE 1.9. Terms of anatomical relationship and comparison.

- *Neurologic:* Mental status and cognition were normal. Cranial nerves II–XII were intact. Motor examination revealed weakness in knee flexion and extension on the right side, likely secondary to significant pain. Otherwise, motor strength was equal, symmetric, and rated 5/5. Reflexes were equal, symmetric, and rated 2+. Sensation to touch, temperature, vibration, and proprioception was intact.
- *Dermatologic:* On inspection, there were no rashes, lesions, or ulcers.
- *Musculoskeletal:* Normal posture, antalgic gait.
  - *Right knee:* Normal alignment, was larger than the left knee, and was erythematous without scars or muscle atrophy; on palpation, it was warm and swollen. There was mild joint line tenderness. There was no crepitus. ROM—both flexion and extension—was reduced. All ligaments were intact, and the joint was stable.
  - *Left knee:* Normal alignment and no scars or muscle atrophy. On palpation, there were no masses, tenderness, or crepitus. ROM was normal. All ligaments were intact, and the joint was stable.
  - Both hips and ankles were normal.

LABORATORY TESTS

Laboratory investigations can complement the physical examination. One method of categorizing laboratory tests is as follows:

1. Complete blood count (CBC) and differential quantifies the number of RBCs, white blood cells (WBCs), and platelets. A low RBC count is called *anemia*, and the mean corpuscular volume (MCV) can help distinguish different causes, whereas a high RBC count is called *polycythemia*. A low WBC count is *leukopenia*, and a high count is *leukocytosis*. Lastly, a low platelet count is called *thrombocytopenia*, and a high count is called *thrombocytosis*. A CBC can also quantify the number of subtypes of WBCs such as neutrophils and lymphocytes. In dehydrated patients, all three cell lines may be elevated indicating hemoconcentration.
2. Metabolic panel includes a wide range of tests that can assess electrolytes, namely, sodium (hyponatremia and hypernatremia), potassium (hypokalemia and hyperkalemia), chloride (hypochloremia and hyperchloremia), bicarbonate (metabolic acidosis and metabolic alkalosis), magnesium (hypomagnesemia and hypermagnesemia), phosphate (hypophosphatemia and hyperphosphatemia), and calcium (hypocalcemia and hypercalcemia). Other metabolic tests include liver enzymes, bilirubin, amylase and lipase for abdominal pathology, creatinine and urea (BUN) for kidney function, cholesterol, glucose, hemoglobin A1c, lactate, and endocrine function such as thyroid-stimulating hormone (TSH), follicle-stimulating hormone (FSH), and parathyroid hormone level.
3. Coagulation panel includes an assessment of blood clotting. The international normalized ratio (INR or PT) and the partial thromboplastin time (PTT) measure the function of the extrinsic and intrinsic coagulation system, respectively.
4. Urine can be tested for electrolytes and osmolality. Urinalysis can indicate the pH; presence of protein in renal failure; ketones and glucose in diabetes; RBCs in trauma, cancer, or renal disease; and WBCs, nitrites, and leukocyte esterase in urinary tract infections. Urine can also be tested for toxins and drugs.
5. Microbiology assesses fluid (e.g., blood, urine, sputum, cerebrospinal fluid [CSF]) or skin for the presence of bacteria, fungus, and parasites. Polymerase chain reaction (PCR) may be used to detect viral genetic material in the fluid.
6. A wide range of other investigations exists, including cancer markers (e.g., CA-125 and prostate-stimulating antigen [PSA]), inflammatory markers (C-reactive protein [CRP] and erythrocyte sedimentation rate [ESR]), gene testing, biopsies, and viral serology.

MEDICAL IMAGING

Medical imaging can augment the physical examination by producing visual representations of the patient's anatomy. Additionally, medical images can be used to guide procedures such as sampling tissue (biopsies), restoring arterial patency and perfusion (revascularization), placing tubes into the stomach or intestine to deliver nutrition/medication (gastrostomy tube placement), and removing stones or rerouting obstructions from ducts in the biliary tree or ureters. When radiology is used for guiding procedures, it is termed *interventional radiology*.

Depending on the modality used for diagnostic or interventional purposes, the principle of creating medical images may involve exposing tissue to radiation, which can be an energy participle (e.g., photons) or a waveform (e.g., sound waves). Tissues differentially absorb or reflect energy, and a sensor detects how the radiation was altered by the tissue it passed through.

The radiation used to generate images can be categorized as ionizing or nonionizing radiation. Ionizing radiation, such as x-rays, can damage DNA or create free radicals in cells; they may be unsafe in pregnancy and carry a potential risk of malignancy. Nonionizing radiation does not carry sufficient energy to create ions, and examples include radio waves, microwaves, and light waves. Magnetic resonance imaging (MRI) utilizes radio waves, and ultrasonography (US) uses high-frequency sound waves to create images. MRI and US do not cause cellular damage and are safer in pregnancy.

One of the key principles of medical imaging is related to attenuation. Attenuation is the loss of energy of a beam of radiant, ultrasound, or other energy because of absorption, scattering, beam divergence, and other causes as the beam propagates through a medium. Different tissues attenuate energy differently, and this principle can be applied to generate medical images.

Given the risk of ionizing radiation, radiation exposure is regulated by a number of organizations, one of which is the International Commission on Radiation Protection (ICRP). **Table 1.2** presents the exposures from various imaging modalities and compares them to background radiation.

● CLINICAL PEARL

In pregnancy, the radiation risk depends on the stage of pregnancy. During preimplantation (the first or second postconceptus week), damage is considered to be an *all-or-none* phenomenon. Absorbed radiation dosage is the amount of radiation absorbed per unit of mass, and is measured in the unit gray (Gy). A fetal radiation dose of 50–100 mGy may cause the failure of blastocyst implantation and result in spontaneous abortion. If the embryo successfully implants, no long-term consequences are expected because the cells of the blastocyst are omnipotent and can replace damaged cells during this period. During weeks 1–8, a phase marked by organogenesis, exposures to implanted embryos can cause physical growth retardation. The developing fetus is most vulnerable to radiation damage between weeks 8 and 15. During this period, exposures between 100 and 200 mGy are associated with intrauterine growth retardation (IUGR) as well as CNS effects such as microcephaly and mental retardation. There is no safe radiation exposure, but defects in physical growth and brain development tend to occur at exposures of 100 mGy or higher.

TABLE 1.2. Radiation exposure associated with various medical imaging modalities

Investigation	Effective Radiation Dose (mSv)	Natural Background Equivalent
Bone density	0.01	1 d
Chest x-ray	0.1	10 d
Mammography	0.7	3 mo
X-ray (upper GI series)	2	8 mo
Cardiac CT scan (calcium score)	2	8 mo
CT scan of the head	2	8 mo
CT colonography	5	20 mo
CT scan of the chest	8	3 y
CT scan of the abdomen	10	3 y
CT scan of the spine	10	3 y

Adapted from the Canadian Association of Radiologists.

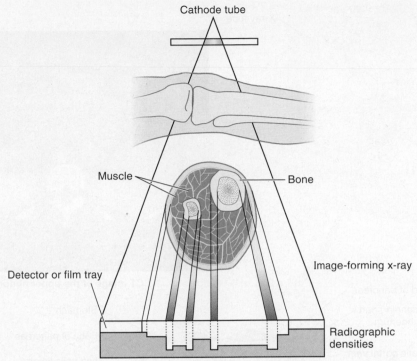

FIGURE 1.10. Principles of x-ray image formation. The x-ray beam passes through tissue and is attenuated—scattered or absorbed—to varying degrees depending on the characteristics of the tissue it encounters prior to striking the detector.

X-Rays

X-rays use electromagnetic radiation to generate images. Traditionally, the film used to detect x-ray attenuation is composed of silver bromide and silver iodine. When the film is exposed to x-rays, it turns black. Digital sensors have largely replaced film in modern imaging modalities; however, the principle stays the same (**Fig. 1.10**). To produce an x-ray image, ionizing radiation in the form of an x-ray beam is directed through the anatomical region of interest, and the beam is attenuated by the patient's tissue. X-rays passing through air (e.g., in the lungs) experience minimal attenuation, and most of the beam passes through unaltered, striking the film and changing the color to black. Therefore, air is termed *radiolucent*. On the other hand, more dense tissues such as bone substantially attenuate the x-ray beam, which decreases the number of photons that pass through. Bone is termed *radiopaque* and appears white on x-ray film. Intermediate tissues like fat cause some attenuation and appear gray.

The skeletal system is largely studied clinically via x-rays. Although bones are usually readily apparent in radiographic images, cartilage elements may not be, and their presence is often "inferred" by the distance (*radiographic joint space*) between articulating bones, thereby providing important information regarding joint health and integrity.

Fluoroscopy is a form of x-ray imaging that can sequentially detect incoming radiation and create a series of real-time moving images. Fluoroscopy is used in interventional radiology to visualize coronary arteries, assess bone alignment during orthopedic surgeries, evaluate the patency and function of the gastrointestinal (GI) tract, and perform joint injections. Fluoroscopy can also be used to assist interventional procedure such as lung biopsies as well as to guide the safe placement of catheters and stents, for instance.

Computed Tomography

Computed tomography, also called *CT* or *CAT scans*, is based on the same principle as x-ray. A CT scanner consists of an x-ray tube that rotates around the patient in a spiral pattern, taking hundreds to thousands of x-ray images at different angles and rungs of the spiral to create 2- and

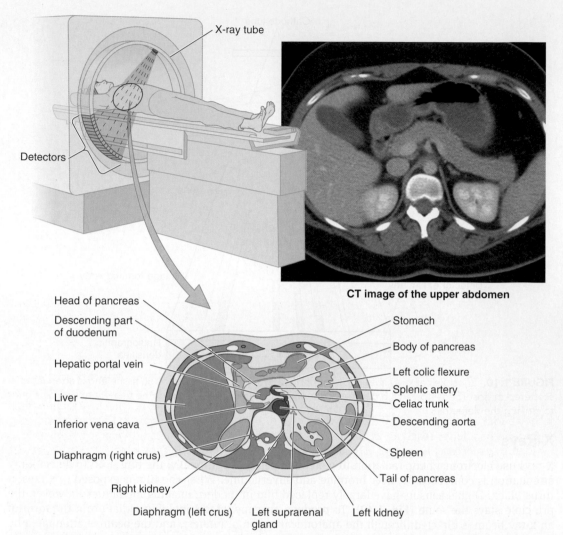

CT image of the upper abdomen

FIGURE 1.11. Technique for producing a CT scan. The x-ray tube rotates around the supine person, and a beam of x-rays passes through from a variety of angles. X-ray detectors on the opposite side of the body measure the amount of radiation that passes through a horizontal section. A computer reconstructs images from several scans, and a CT scan is produced.

3-dimensional images (**Fig. 1.11**). The scanner also has arrays of digital detectors that can detect x-rays and measure the extent of the x-ray beam attenuation. Instead of just black, white, or gray pixels, digital detectors can detect a more precise level of attenuation, reported in Hounsfield units (HU). The most attenuated or radiopaque tissues appear white and have an HU of 1,000, as seen in bone. The least attenuated or radiolucent tissues like the aerated lung have an HU of − 1,000 and appear black (**Table 1.3**). When CT images are viewed, a window, or range, of HU centered on a specified value is displayed. For example, default CT images display HU 1,000 to − 1,000 (a range of 2,000) centered at 0. To focus on specific regions of the body, the window "we look through" can be optimized. For example, to visualize images of the abdomen, a window range of 350 centered at 50 is used. A CT scan is useful to visualize CNS tumors and hemorrhage, visceral neoplasms, intra-abdominal or intrathoracic pathology, and musculoskeletal injuries and to stage cancers. The major drawback of a CT scan is the amount of radiation exposure.

Radiocontrast

Radiocontrast can be used to distinguish tissues and organs that are in close proximity or to assess function (described below). Because x-rays, fluoroscopy, and CT scans are all based on x-rays,

TABLE 1.3. Tissue types and their Hounsfield units

Tissue	Hounsfield Units
Bone	1,000
Liver	40–60
Brain, white matter	20–30
Brain, gray matter	37–45
Blood	40
Cerebrospinal fluid	15
Water	0
Fat	−50 to −100
Air	−1,000

similar radiocontrast agents can be used. The contrast agents are radiopaque and appear white. The two main radiocontrast agents used are barium sulfate and iodine.

Barium sulfate (or barium) is a contrast agent used to assess the digestive system. When barium is swallowed, it lines the GI tract and can be helpful in assessing the mucosa and lumen for defects (e.g., restrictions, polyps, or ulcers) or dysfunction (e.g., dysmotility or reflux). Theoretically, barium can exacerbate a high-grade obstruction by impacting and worsening the severity of the obstruction. In practice, however, dilute iodinated contrast or barium is often helpful in identifying the level and etiology of an obstruction on a CT scan. For suspected bowel perforation, iodinated contrast or dilute barium can help identify the location of perforation. Barium spillage should be avoided if possible in the case of a GI tract perforation, as there is a theoretical risk of causing inflammation of the abdominal lining called the *peritoneum* (*peritonitis*). Barium can cause hypokalemia that can lead to a mild allergic reaction, abdominal pain, diarrhea, renal damage, and fatal arrhythmias.

Iodine-based contrast agents are water soluble and can be ingested or injected to enhance CT scans and fluoroscopy imaging. Iodinated contrast agents can be used in suspected GI tract perforation or obstructions because the body more readily absorbs them. Adverse effects of iodine contrast include allergic-/anaphylactic-type reactions as well as skin necrosis, chemical pneumonitis, contrast-induced nephropathy (CIN), and pulmonary edema. CIN usually occurs within 48–72 hours of exposure. Hydrating the patient before and after contrast is given and minimizing the amount of contrast used reduces the risk of CIN, while the use of *N*-acetylcysteine (NAC) has limited effectiveness. The risk of CIN can be estimated with various clinical calculators that take into account age, kidney function, diabetes, sepsis or hypovolemia, heart failure, amount of contrast used, and anemia. Finally, contrast agents can produce allergic reactions. Pretreatment with an established protocol and using drugs such as prednisone and diphenhydramine has been shown to reduce allergic reactions.

Nuclear Medicine

In nuclear medicine, radioactive isotopes are incorporated into biological molecules and then injected into or inhaled by the patient (**Table 1.4**). Once inside the body, certain cell types preferentially absorb these isotopes, thereby providing a mechanism to selectively label particular cell types. These radioactive isotopes undergo natural decay and emit gamma rays that are detected by a camera to generate images (**Fig. 1.12**). Nuclear medicine can be used to scan bones to detect metastases; thyroid tissue for cancer, goiters, or hyperthyroidism; heart for perfusion, function, and viability; lungs for ventilation/perfusion mismatches; and the liver for cholestasis and hemangiomas.

Positron emission tomography (PET) is a type of nuclear imaging that utilizes isotopes with short half-lives. In this approach, biological molecules (e.g., glucose, water, ammonia, or molecules that bind to receptors of interest) with radioactive isotopes are injected into the patient's circulatory system. Cells that are more metabolically active will take up most of this radioactive material. Typical radioactive isotopes used are fluorine 18 (^{18}F; $t_{1/2}$ 110 minutes), nitrogen 13 (^{13}N; $t_{1/2}$ 10 minutes), carbon 11 (^{11}C; $t_{1/2}$ 20 minutes), oxygen 15, and rubidium 82. When these isotopes undergo natural decay, they emit positrons and gamma rays, the latter of which are detected by a sensor.

TABLE 1.4. Common isotopes and organ targets

Isotope	Organ
Chromium 51	GI tract (bleed)
Iodine 131	Thyroid, liver, kidney
Technetium 99	Skeleton, heart muscle, lung, thyroid, liver, gallbladder, kidney
Xenon 133	Lung
Thallium	Heart

Adapted from World Nuclear Association.

Using this approach, metabolically active areas such as sites of infection, inflammation, and neoplasms can be detected. As a result, PET imaging can be used to stage cancer; image the brain and heart; and, when combined with MRI, can provide superior anatomical images.

Magnetic Resonance Imaging

MRI is based on the principle of magnetic fields and radiofrequency (RF) waves. MRI is the best imaging modality for soft tissue assessment and characterization. It can be used to assess the articular and muscular systems that are not seen well on traditional x-ray, as well as intracranial, intraspinal, musculoskeletal, and cardiac pathology (**Table 1.5**). To enhance MRI images, gadolinium is used as a contrast agent to highlight vessels and soft tissue. Major reactions to gadolinium include anaphylaxis and nephrogenic systemic fibrosis, the latter of which is a serious but rare condition affecting those with preexisting renal dysfunction or on renal dialysis.

FIGURE 1.12. Anterior and posterior views of a normal full body bone scan. Note the injection site where the radiolabeled technetium 99m is injected. The technetium accumulates in bone that is more metabolically active. *Darker* color implies that more technetium has accumulated and that that area of bone has more bone growth or repair. It may be normal for increased technetium to be deposited in bone such as the vertebrae, pelvic bones, and sternum, especially if the deposits are symmetric. (Courtesy of Joel A. Vilensky.)

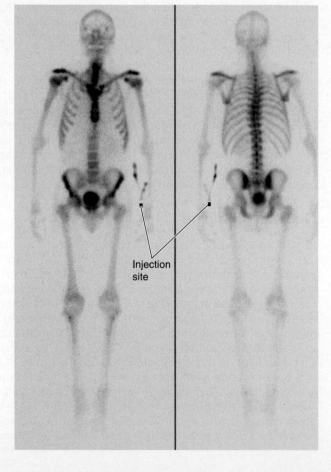

Injection site

TABLE 1.5. Common MRI pulse sequences and their applications	
Sequence Name	**Application**
DWI (diffusion-weighted imaging)	Measures passive diffusion of water, or edema in stroke, MS plaques, HSV encephalitis, myocarditis
FLAIR (fluid attenuated inversion recovery)	CSF suppression for infarction, MS, head injury, SAH
BOLD (blood oxygen level–dependent imaging)	Functional MRI
T2* (star)	Depict hemorrhage, calcification, and iron deposition

To generate images using MRI, patients are placed inside a strong magnetic field (usually 1.5–3 tesla). Atoms with an odd mass number such as ^{1}H (hydrogen), ^{19}F (fluorine), ^{31}P (phosphorus), and ^{13}C (carbon) will align with the main magnetic field (also called the *longitudinal field*). Next, the MRI machine emits pulses of RF waves perpendicular to the main magnetic field at specific resonant frequencies that differ based on the nuclei of interest (e.g., hydrogen). The RF pulses are absorbed by the aligned nuclei causing them to become excited. Excited nuclei begin to rotate—or precess—in phase with each other at a higher energy level and align in the plane of the RF pulse—called the *transverse plane*—instead of with the main magnetic field. When the RF pulse is switched off, the nuclei cannot maintain this higher energy state and realign with the main magnetic field. As the nuclei realign with the main magnetic field, they emit energy that is detected and amplified by an RF receiver. Based on the location and intensity of the detected signal, images are created (**Fig. 1.13**).

MRI takes advantage of different concentrations of hydrogen protons (or *proton density*) in different tissue types. The greater the proton density, the higher the RF signal detected by the MRI, and the *whiter* the tissue appears. Additionally, two time constants help further differentiate tissue

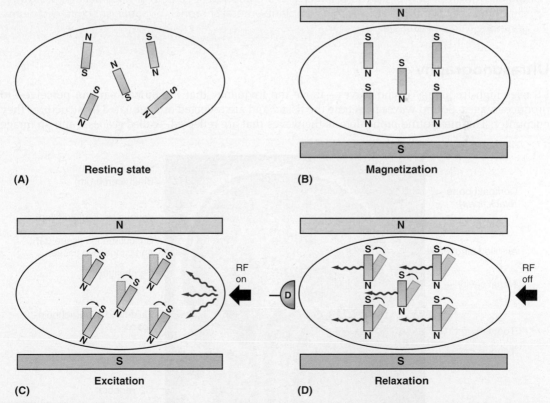

FIGURE 1.13. Principles of magnetic resonance imaging. **A.** Nuclei in their random, resting state. **B.** Nuclei aligned in the main magnetic field (longitudinal plane) of the MRI. **C.** Nuclei after being excited by an RF pulse into a higher energy state, which causes nuclei to rotate or precess in phase with each other and align in a transverse plane. **D.** Nuclei returning to steady state and emitting RF signal once the RF pulse is turned off.

types. The first is T1, or the *longitudinal relaxation time*, which measures how quickly nuclei in a tissue realign with the longitudinal magnetic field after an RF pulse is turned off. The second is T2, or the *transverse relaxation time*, which measures the decay of the transverse magnetic field after the RF signal is turned off due to interactions between spinning nuclei in a tissue. The more nuclei that exists in a tissue (or the more dense a tissue is), the more the nuclei interfere with each other, and the faster the transverse signal decays. For instance, fatty tissue has fixed collections of dense protons. As a result, fatty tissue can quickly realign with the main magnetic field (short T1). Moreover, fat has many protons that can interfere with each other after RF pulses are switched off, and the transverse magnetization decays quickly (short T2). Water and blood are less dense than fat, so nuclei take longer to realign with the main magnetic field (long T1). Similarly, adjacent nuclei in water and blood are more spaced out, so there is less interference between adjacent nuclei compared to fat. As a result, there is a slower decay of the transverse magnetization (long T2).

T1 and T2 can be used to highlight different tissues. In T1-weighted images, tissues with shorter T1 times such as fatty tissue appear bright. On the other hand, the slow realignment of water with the longitudinal field results in a lower signal, such that water appears dark on T1-weighted images (**Fig. 1.14**). T1-weighted images are good for highlighting anatomy. In T2-weighted images, tissues with longer T2 times appear bright. T2-weighted images cause water-based media such as CSF to appear bright and fat to appear dark. T2-weighted images are good for depiction of pathology such as edema, infarction, inflammation, and acute hemorrhage. T2 images are also used to detect deoxyhemoglobin in functional MRI.

● CLINICAL PEARL

Patients must be screened for the presence of metal objects prior to obtaining an MRI. If there is concern of metal objects/shrapnel in the eyes or in other parts of the body, orbital x-rays are obtained. Medical records and surgical reports are needed to screen for pacemakers, orthopedic implants, cochlear implants, surgical implants, metal shrapnel, or aneurysm clips. Titanium is generally MRI compatible.

Ultrasonography

US uses high-frequency sound waves—above the frequency that the human ear can perceive—to produce images. Sound waves penetrate the tissue and are reflected or attenuated by structures they encounter. The ultrasound probe detects the waves that are reflected—called *echoes*—and an image

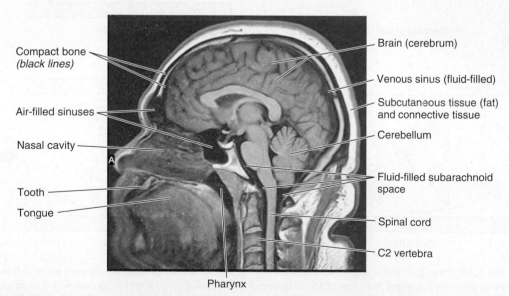

FIGURE 1.14. Sagittal T1-weighted MRI of the head. The *black* low-signal areas superior to the anterior and posterior aspects of the nasal cavity are the air-filled frontal and sphenoidal sinuses.

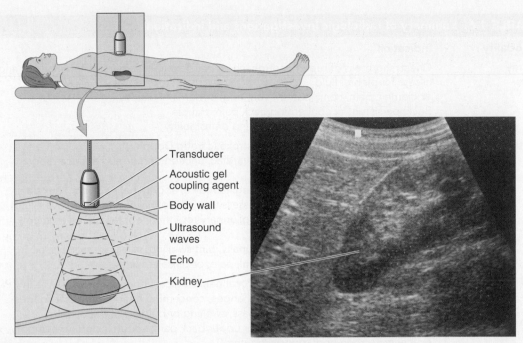

FIGURE 1.15. Technique for producing an ultrasound image of the upper abdomen. The image results from the "echo" of ultrasound waves bouncing off of abdominal structures. The image of the right kidney is displayed on a monitor.

is constructed (**Fig. 1.15**). The x-axis of the image is based on where the echo physically strikes the probe, while the y-axis, or depth, is determined by the timing of when the echo arrives at the probe.

Structures are considered *hyperechoic* if they produce strong echoes and typically appear bright on ultrasound. Examples of hyperechoic material include needle tips and bones, and such material prevents sound waves from passing through them. As a result, structures deep to a hyperechoic structure (such as bone) may appear black because all of the sound waves are reflected off the hyperechoic material and limited signal can pass through. The dark region below a hyperechoic structure is called a *shadow*. Tissues such as fluid that attenuates incoming ultrasound waves do not produce an echo and are called *anechoic*. Anechoic tissues appear black and may provide an "acoustic window," which is helpful for assessment of structures that lie deep to them. For instance, the urinary bladder can help in evaluating the genitourinary organs when it is full. Hypoechoic structures such as aerated lung have partial echo production.

A US probe is used to generate images. The probe is composed of a piezoelectric material, which has a unique chemical structure that allows for the interconversion of pressure and electrical energy. When electrical energy is passed through the piezoelectric material, pressure is created that then generates sound waves. Linear probes are used for superficial structures such as blood vessels. Phased probes are pie shaped and better for deeper imaging such as cardiac, abdominal, and thoracic imaging.

The depth of the US image is determined by the frequency of the sound wave. Lower frequency waves penetrate deeper structures but with lower resolution, whereas higher frequency waves penetrate tissues more superficially, but with higher resolution. *Gain* is a measure of pixel intensity. A higher gain implies brighter pixels and vice versa.

US has three main modes, each of which can provide different types of information about the underlying anatomy. B-mode, or *brightness mode*, measures different echo strengths based on the tissue type and displays anatomical information. M-mode, or *motion mode*, looks at one area as it changes over time. M-mode is used in echocardiography, for example, to quantify blood flow through a heart valve. Finally, *Doppler mode* highlights flow to or away from the probe by detecting the mean velocity of sound waves parallel to flow. Doppler is good for valvular pathology and arterial or venous disease.

US as an imaging modality is used for fetal monitoring, trauma (focused assessment with sonography for trauma, or FAST), assessment of viscera and vascular structures, and musculoskeletal pathology.

Table 1.6 presents a summary of radiological investigations.

TABLE 1.6. Summary of radiologic investigations and indications

Modality	Indication
X-ray	Chest: shortness of breath, cough, chest pain, trauma, screen for tuberculosis and assess for pleural fluid Abdomen: pain, constipation, vomiting, abdominal distension Back: persistent or concerning back pain, trauma Extremity: trauma, joint pain, swelling or instability
Ultrasound	Neck: thyroid nodule, neck mass, stroke (carotid Doppler) Chest: shortness of breath, assess cardiac function or murmur (echocardiogram), breast mass or pain Abdomen: abdominal pain, vomiting, jaundice, abdominal swelling, flank pain, renal failure, trauma (FAST scan), assess volume status (inferior vena cava filling) Pelvis: pelvic pain, vaginal bleeding, urinary retention, obstetrical assessment, testicular pain or mass Extremity: soft tissue mass, occasionally joint swelling, swelling, redness, or warmth in an extremity, cold, painful, pale, or pulseless limb
CT scan	Head: stroke evaluation, seizures, focal neurological abnormalities, change in level of consciousness, cognitive changes, concerning headache, nasal congestion with pain and anosmia, oral mass, swelling or bulging of the eye, trauma Chest: shortness of breath, chest or upper back pain, cough including hemoptysis, cancer screen or diagnosis, trauma Abdomen: pain, suspected down perforation or obstruction, renal colic, cancer screen or diagnosis, trauma, symptoms of liver failure, fever of unknown origin, jaundice, abdominal swelling Back: pain, trauma, neurological symptoms Pelvis: pain, trauma, vaginal bleeding Extremity: trauma, suspected fractures not seen on x-ray, bone pain, mass, swelling of an extremity, cold, painful, pale, or pulseless limb
MRI	Head: stroke evaluation (more sensitive and specific), tumors, focal neurological symptoms, symptoms concerning for multiple sclerosis such as optic neuritis or unilateral weakness, seizures, hearing changes (sensorineural), concerning headache, cognitive changes, endocrine symptoms or vision changes concerning for pituitary adenoma Chest: assess cardiac function, breast mass Abdomen: jaundice, fever with right upper quadrant pain, assess liver, pancreas or biliary system for malignancy Pelvis: malignancy assessment (especially cervical, prostate, and rectal), assessment of placenta position Back: urinary retention with fecal incontinence and lower extremity weakness (cauda equina syndrome), back pain especially if recent infection or trauma; chronic or radiating leg pain Extremity: masses or pain, deep ulcers (osteomyelitis)
Nuclear imaging	Table 1.4

Returning to the case, the clinician needs to choose which imaging modality will be helpful in establishing a diagnosis, bearing in mind the cost of medical imaging procedures and the radiation dose that the patient will be exposed to. To guide the clinician, guidelines and algorithms have been developed.

For Mr. Smith, the clinician has two primary conditions on the differential diagnosis: septic arthritis and Crohn disease. To evaluate the patient's knee, the clinician ordered an arthrocentesis to assess for joint infection and an x-ray to assess bone integrity. As there was no evidence of joint laxity on physical examination, an MRI to assess the soft tissue around the knee was not indicated. US can confirm the presence of a joint effusion; however, this would not have changed management and, therefore, was not performed. A CT scan and nuclear imaging of the knee would likewise have no role. To evaluate for Crohn disease, the clinician ordered an abdominal CT scan. Double contrast barium enema, MRI, US, and nuclear imaging could have also been ordered to assess for Crohn disease; however, these modalities may not be available everywhere.

■ APPLYING THE CLINICAL FINDINGS

One final concept to consider is the reliability of physical examination maneuvers and investigations such as medical imaging. After performing these tests, the clinician is often faced with several important questions:

1. What proportion of patients with a given disease will have a positive physical examination finding?
2. If the patient has a negative physical examination finding, does it mean that the patient does not have the disease under consideration?
3. If the patient has a positive physical examination finding, does it mean that he or she has the disease, or is this a false finding?

These questions are important as they determine if the clinician will order additional diagnostic tests to investigate whether a patient has a disease, or if the clinician has a low level of clinical suspicion and decides to watch how the patient's symptoms progress. These questions also reflect that physical examination maneuvers and investigations have characteristics that make them *more likely* or *less likely* to predict the presence of disease. Here, we provide an introduction to key terms that will help the clinician interpret physical examination maneuvers and investigations.

Sensitivity and Specificity

Sensitivity is the proportion of people with disease who test positive (the test could be a physical examination maneuver or a laboratory test). *Specificity* is the proportion of people without disease who test negative. Sensitivity and specificity are test characteristics that suggest that there is a *gold standard* technique to confirm the presence of disease and that all other tests would be compared with the gold standard. This is further illustrated in **Table 1.7**.

Sensitivity = proportion of people with a given disease who test positive for it

$$= \frac{\text{true positive}}{\text{true positve} + \text{false negative}}$$

Specificity = proportion of people without disease and who test negative for it

$$= \frac{\text{true negative}}{\text{true negative} + \text{false positive}}$$

In the above example, the gold standard technique to diagnose a knee infection is to perform an arthrocentesis and assess the synovial fluid for the presence of bacteria by staining the cell wall (Gram stain) or by growth in culture medium. Several studies have reported the incidence of different signs and symptoms in the setting of confirmed knee infection and are summarized in a study by Margaretten and colleagues. In this article, joint *pain* had a sensitivity of 85% and *fever* had a sensitivity of 57%, which means that of all people with a confirmed knee infection (using a gold standard technique), 85% had joint pain and 57% had fever. Therefore, knowing the sensitivity and specificity of a test can be helpful in ruling in or ruling out a disease. For example, a positive finding on a test with a high specificity is helpful in *ruling in* disease, insofar as the vast majority without disease is not expected to test positive on that particular test. Similarly, a negative finding on a test with a high sensitivity is helpful in *ruling out* disease, as the vast majority with disease is expected to test positive on that particular test.

TABLE 1.7. **Sensitivity and specificity**		
	Disease *Present* (based on gold standard)	**Disease *Absent* (based on gold standard)**
Test result *positive*	True positive (TP)	False positive (FP)
Test result *negative*	False negative (FN)	True negative (TN)

> **● CLINICAL PEARL**
>
> The clinical value of sensitivity and specificity can be usually remembered by:
>
> SPin: **s**pecific test, **p**ositive finding, rule **in**
> SNout: **s**ensitive test, **n**egative finding, rule **out**

Likelihood Ratios

Although sensitivity and specificity are important test characteristics helpful in ruling in or ruling out disease, when the clinician obtains a positive or negative test result, he or she is faced with another question: Does the presence of a positive test result mean that the patient has a disease?

In our case, since Mr. Smith complains of right knee pain, does it mean that he has septic arthritis?

To answer this question, the clinician can rely on calculating positive (LR +) or negative (LR −) likelihood ratios.

Positive likelihood ratio is defined as:

$$LR+ = \frac{\text{probability of having positive test result in the setting of disease}}{\text{probability of having positive test result in the absence of disease}}$$

$$= \frac{\text{sensitivity}}{1 - \text{specificity}}$$

Similarly, *negative likelihood ratio* can be defined as:

$$LR- = \frac{\text{probability of having negative test result in the setting of disease}}{\text{probability of having negative test result in the absence of disease}}$$

$$= \frac{1 - \text{sensitivity}}{\text{specificity}}$$

For a patient presenting with a painful and swollen knee, the LR + and LR − for various risk factors for an infected or septic joint are available to the clinician. For example, presence of knee *prosthesis* has an LR + of 3.1, and presence of a skin infection has an LR + of 2.8. Therefore, if a patient presents with a painful knee, the history and physical examination should involve exploring these risk factors, as these are associated with a higher likelihood of having a septic joint.

Returning to the case, an arthrocentesis was performed, and Mr. Smith had normal synovial fluid without evidence of infection. An x-ray of the knee showed mild soft tissue swelling. Unfortunately, the abdominal CT scan revealed evidence of inflammation of the bowel, which, along with oropharynx ulcer on examination, would be consistent with Crohn disease (Chapter 3). Mr. Smith was referred to a gastroenterologist for further evaluation and management.

■ CONCLUSION

This chapter has illustrated how clinicians need to integrate knowledge of anatomy, physical examination maneuvers, investigations, and medical imaging to assess patients and make diagnoses. This approach will be continued through the textbook that is organized by anatomical region. Each chapter begins by reviewing the major anatomy, physical examination maneuvers, and common laboratory and medical imaging investigations relevant to the viscera within that region. Following this introduction are a series of common cases that will help the reader to identify the disease etiologies, signs, symptoms, physical examination findings, laboratory results, and imaging abnormalities. These cases will help highlight the importance of applying an integrated approach to the practice of clinical medicine.

Thorax

CHRISTINE J. CHUNG • DEVRAJ SUKUL • MICHELLE J. YU
• SAGAR DUGANI • DANIEL SOUZA • SUNITA SHARMA

2

The thorax, bordered by the neck and abdomen, is divided into structures of the thoracic wall and the viscera contained within its cavity. The thoracic wall consists of ribs of the thoracic cage, intercostal muscles, fascia, muscles, subcutaneous tissues, and skin overlying its surface. The structures present on the posterior surface of the thorax are discussed in Chapter 5.

The thoracic cage is composed of 12 thoracic vertebrae posteriorly, with 12 pairs of ribs and associated cartilage (**Fig. 2.1**). The cartilage of ribs 1 through 7 helps attach the ribs to the sternum and allows the rib cage to move synchronously with the diaphragm during respiration. The cartilage of ribs 8 to 10 connects to form a single attachment to the sternum, whereas ribs 11 and 12 do not attach to the sternum and are considered floating ribs. Between each pair of ribs lies the intercostal space, which is occupied by intercostal muscles. The intercostal arteries, veins, and nerves are located just below the inferior margin of each rib. The sternum is composed of three parts: manubrium, body, and xiphoid process. The joint where the manubrium and the body fuse is called the *sternal angle* and is an important landmark when measuring the jugular venous pressure (JVP) (**Fig. 2.1**).

The thoracic cavity is divided into the mediastinum, a central compartment that contains the heart and major blood vessels of the cardiovascular system, and the right and left pulmonary cavities that contain the lungs. In addition to the lungs, the components of the respiratory system contained in the thorax include the trachea and the bronchi and are separated from the abdomen by the diaphragm (**Fig. 2.2**). The esophagus is the only organ of the gastrointestinal (GI) system contained within the thorax.

■ INITIAL EVALUATION AND ASSESSMENT

Thoracic diseases typically manifest with chest pain, and a differential diagnosis can be developed based on organ(s) most likely to be involved (**Table 2.1**). Another important presenting symptom is dyspnea, and the presence of labored respiration with use of accessory muscles, breathlessness, inability to speak in complete sentences, pallor, cyanosis, or diaphoresis should be noted. The differential diagnosis for dyspnea is broad and may relate to different organ systems (**Table 2.2**).

General Thoracic Examination

To evaluate thoracic pathology, a physical examination is performed with the patient supine or seated with arms by the side. The chest is exposed and a drape placed across the abdomen and below. The anterior chest wall differs in males and females, who typically have more mammary and fat tissue (**Fig. 2.3**; see Chapter 4 for anatomy, physical examination, and pathology of the breast). A systematic physical examination involves inspection, palpation, percussion, and auscultation.

The clinician stands in front of the patient and inspects the skin for scars suggestive of prior procedures or surgeries (e.g., vertical midsternal scar may indicate a major cardiac surgery, such as coronary artery bypass grafting or aortic valve replacement; visible bulge in the upper anterior chest wall may indicate presence of a cardiac pacemaker or defibrillator). The shape of the chest wall is inspected for barrel chest (increased anteroposterior diameter), pectus excavatum (concave appearance of anterior chest wall), and pectus carinatum (convex appearance of anterior chest wall) (**Fig. 2.4**). The chest wall is inspected throughout the respiratory cycle. Paradoxical inward movement of the lower rib cage during inspiration may be observed in moderate to severe chronic obstructive pulmonary disease (COPD).

Following inspection, the chest is palpated in areas with reported pain to determine tenderness in underlying muscles and bones or the presence of masses or nodules. With the patient in the left lateral decubitus position, the point of maximal impulse (PMI) is palpated at the junction of the

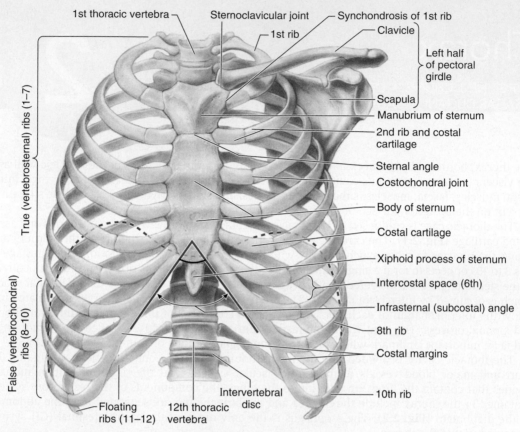

FIGURE 2.1. The thoracic cage consists of 12 thoracic vertebrae and 12 pairs of ribs. The sternal angle is the joint where the manubrium and body of the sternum fuse.

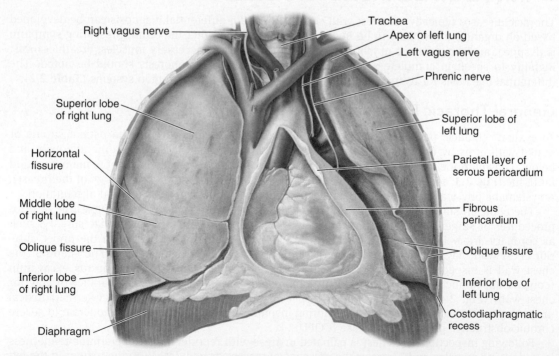

FIGURE 2.2. Contents of the thoracic cage. The heart is contained within the fibrous pericardium. The right lung has three lobes, and the left lung has two lobes.

TABLE 2.1. Causes of chest pain categorized by organ system

Organ System	Symptom (Chest Pain)
Cardiac	Acute coronary syndrome, cardiac tamponade, congestive heart failure, pericarditis, myocarditis, Takotsubo cardiomyopathy
Pulmonary	Pneumothorax, pneumonia, empyema, hemothorax, malignancy, sarcoidosis
Vascular	Aortic dissection, pulmonary embolism
Mediastinal	Pneumomediastinum
Gastrointestinal	Esophageal rupture, diffuse esophageal spasm, gastroesophageal reflux disease, pancreatitis, cholecystitis, peptic ulcer disease
Cutaneous/musculoskeletal	Trauma, costochondritis, shingles

TABLE 2.2. Causes of dyspnea categorized by organ system

Organ System	Symptom (Dyspnea)
Cardiac	Congestive heart failure, myocardial ischemia, cardiac tamponade, arrhythmia, valvular disease
Pulmonary	Asthma, chronic obstructive pulmonary disease, pneumonia, interstitial lung disease, pneumothorax, pulmonary embolism, pleural effusion, empyema, hemothorax, noncardiogenic pulmonary edema
Other	Chest wall muscle weakness, paralysis, anemia, anxiety, sepsis

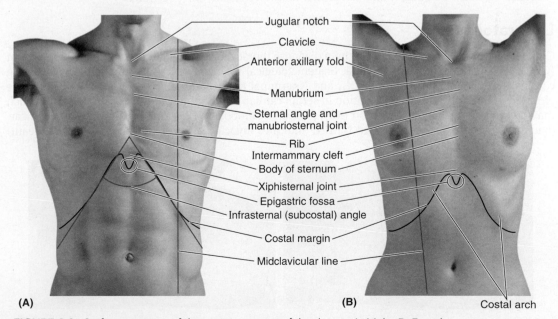

Jugular notch
Clavicle
Anterior axillary fold
Manubrium
Sternal angle and manubriosternal joint
Rib
Intermammary cleft
Body of sternum
Xiphisternal joint
Epigastric fossa
Infrasternal (subcostal) angle
Costal margin
Midclavicular line

(A)   **(B)**   Costal arch

FIGURE 2.3. Surface anatomy of the anterior aspect of the thorax. **A.** Male. **B.** Female.

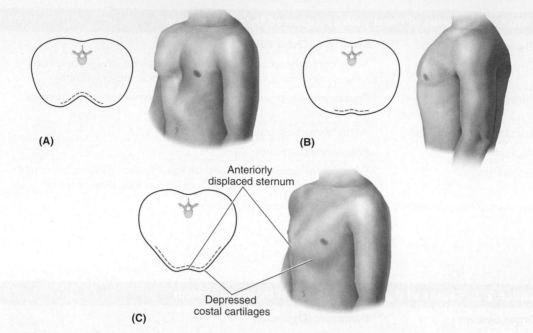

(A)

(B)

Anteriorly
displaced sternum

Depressed
costal cartilages

(C)

FIGURE 2.4. Deformities of the thoracic wall. **A.** Funnel chest (*pectus excavatum*). **B.** Barrel chest. **C.** Pigeon chest (*pectus carinatum*).

left midclavicular line and fifth intercostal space (**Fig. 2.5**). Following palpation, the chest wall is percussed, and a dull sound is audible over the heart. Percussion over the lung fields generates a hollow (resonant) sound; however, the presence of a dull sound may be suggestive of underlying fluid, mass, or consolidation. Following this, the chest wall is auscultated to identify cardiac S_1 and S_2 sounds and cardiac murmurs; this is further discussed in the Heart section. As with palpation of lung fields, auscultation typically reveals breath sounds that can be diminished in the presence of underlying fluid or masses. Further, additional respiratory sounds such as crackles and expiratory wheezes may also be audible and are further discussed in the Lung section.

Laboratory Tests

Common laboratory investigations to help diagnose thoracic diseases include a complete blood count (CBC) to diagnose infections, anemia, or hematological malignancy. Cardiac biomarkers, including cardiac troponin, creatine kinase (CK), and N-terminal brain natriuretic peptide (NT-BNP), may be elevated in cardiac disease. An elevation in serum cardiac troponin indicates myocardial death, which may be seen in myocardial infarction (MI), pulmonary embolism (PE), and cardiac infiltrative or cardiac inflammatory disease. Elevated NT-BNP indicates myocardial stress (and not myocardial death)

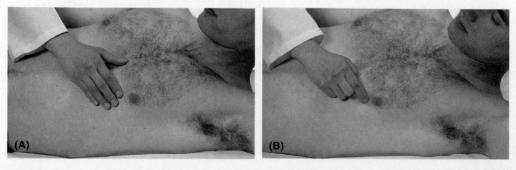

(A)

(B)

FIGURE 2.5. Palpation of the point of maximal impulse (PMI). **A.** With the patient in the left lateral decubitus position, the junction of the midclavicular line and fifth intercostal space is identified. **B.** Once the PMI is located, finer assessments are made using one finger to determine the location, amplitude, size, and intensity of the impulse.

and may be elevated in PE or exacerbations of congestive heart failure (CHF). Notably, baseline NT-BNP levels increase with age and may be falsely lowered in obese individuals, which should be considered when interpreting serum NT-BNP levels. Serum electrolytes (sodium, potassium) and renal function (creatinine, bicarbonate, and blood urea nitrogen [BUN]) can also be measured to characterize renal function that can be impaired in cardiac and respiratory disease; this is discussed in the Clinical Cases. Pleural fluid contributing to respiratory disease can also be assessed for presence of infectious exudates, bacteria, and malignant cells and is further discussed in the Clinical Cases.

Thoracic Imaging

Typical imaging modalities include x-rays, computed tomography (CT), magnetic resonance imaging (MRI), and ultrasonography. In certain instances, nuclear imaging (e.g., ventilation/perfusion [V/Q] scans to diagnose PE or positron emission tomography [PET] to assess areas of increased metabolic activity seen in inflammation or malignancy) may be performed.

Chest x-rays are a typical initial investigation to assess thoracic disease. The standard x-ray is performed with the patient upright and the anterior chest against the film. The x-ray beam enters from behind the patient and exits through the front, resulting in a posterior–anterior (PA) x-ray. On a properly exposed x-ray, the thoracic vertebrae should be barely discernible through the heart (**Fig. 2.6**).

Portable chest x-rays are typically performed on critically ill patients for whom obtaining upright PA films may be unsafe. In portable x-rays, the x-ray beam enters from the front and exits through the back to generate an anteroposterior (AP) x-ray that is characterized by a larger appearance of the heart, shallow lung volumes, and higher position of the clavicles. Portable exams were designed to confirm appropriate positioning of central intravenous (IV) lines, endotracheal tubes, nasogastric tubes, and other invasive equipment used in intensive care settings. If a chest x-ray is required for evaluation of lung or cardiac disease, upright PA and lateral films should be performed when possible. One approach to reading x-rays is as follows:

1. Determine the x-ray orientation (e.g., AP, PA, or lateral decubitus).
2. Assess respiratory structures including the position (or possible deviation) of the trachea, mediastinum, lungs and pleura, and costophrenic angles. Lung markings are generated by pulmonary arteries and veins (**Fig. 2.7**) and not by air-filled bronchi, which have thin walls that do not provide significant contrast to the aerated lungs. Nipple shadows may be mistaken for lung nodules, but can be distinguished by their characteristic symmetric location across the lower thorax.
3. Assess bony structures for fractures or joint space disease.
4. Assess the cardiac border and size and the presence of calcification.
5. Assess the diaphragm and abdomen. Occasionally, free air may be visualized inferior to the diaphragm.

CT scans generate high-resolution images of pulmonary, chest wall, mediastinal, and cardiovascular structures. CT scans can also be used for image-guided percutaneous biopsy. MRI scans are typically used to stage cancers, such as thymoma, mesothelioma, or Pancoast tumor of the lung apex. MRI scans also assess myocardial function and viability, and valvular heart disease. MRI

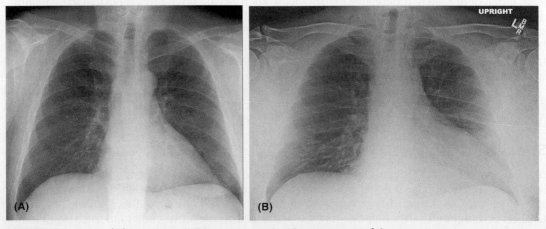

FIGURE 2.6. Normal chest x-rays. **A.** PA erect x-ray. **B.** AP erect image of the same patient.

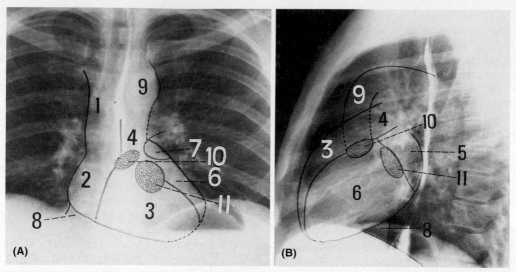

FIGURE 2.7. Identification of cardiac structures and great vessels. **A.** PA. **B.** Lateral. *1,* superior vena cava; *2,* right atrium; *3,* right ventricle; *4,* pulmonary outflow tract; *5,* left atrium; *6,* left ventricle; *7,* left atrial appendage; *8,* inferior vena cava; *9,* ascending aorta and aortic arch; *10,* aortic valve; *11,* mitral valve.

and PET scans are used to distinguish nonviable, infarcted myocardium from chronically ischemic, hibernating myocardium that may still be viable. MRI scans have better spatial resolution than do PET scans, allowing for assessment of both transmural disease and subendocardial disease. Thus, they are more sensitive in detecting earlier stages of ischemic disease. Magnetic resonance angiography (MRA) can be used to evaluate vascular aneurysms or stenoses.

Nuclear imaging may also be used to evaluate thoracic diseases. V/Q scans use inhaled radiolabeled gas for ventilation imaging, followed by IV injection of radiolabeled macroaggregated albumin particles for perfusion imaging, and can be used to diagnose PE. V/Q scans are used for those with a contraindication to administration of IV contrast. Radioisotope studies using thallium 201 and technetium 99m sestamibi are used to evaluate cardiac perfusion and function. Perfusion images are usually obtained during rest and stress, induced either with exercise on a treadmill or injection of a pharmacologic agent like adenosine that simulates the effects of exercise. Ischemic disease can be detected as a perfusion defect induced by stress that reverses with rest. Notably, V/Q scans are often indeterminate in those with underlying lung disease and have been largely replaced by CT angiography.

PET scans are frequently used in oncologic diagnosis and staging. Fludeoxyglucose (18F-FDG) PET scans can evaluate qualitative and quantitative uptake of glucose by tissues and are used as a marker of metabolic activity. Due to rapid proliferation, more aggressive cancer cells generally have higher activity and uptake than do normal cells. PET scans of the whole body are used to stage thoracic cancers, including those of the lung, esophagus, and breast, as well as lymphomas. However, indolent or slowly progressive malignancies, such as carcinoid, bronchioloalveolar carcinoma, and certain types of lymphoma, can be negative on PET studies. In addition, PET studies with a radiolabeled form of glucose can be used to distinguish infarcted myocardial tissue from chronically ischemic or hibernating myocardium, as the latter can demonstrate metabolic activity following restoration of adequate blood flow. Thus, both PET and MRI viability studies play an important role in predicting the benefit of coronary revascularization.

Ultrasonography can be used to assess for the presence of fluid in the pleural and pericardial spaces. It can also be used to perform a transthoracic echocardiography (TTE) and assess cardiac function and contractility (e.g., cardiac ejection fraction) and cardiac valvular function.

Special Tests

In some instances, a TTE may not provide adequate views of the aortic and mitral valves. In these instances, transesophageal echocardiography (TEE) may be done to better visualize these valves as well as the left atrium. Imaging related to the GI system is discussed in Clinical Cases and in Chapter 3. Lung and heart biopsies may be performed to diagnose conditions such as interstitial lung disease and cardiac amyloid, respectively.

SYSTEMS OVERVIEW

■ LUNGS

Overview

The thoracic cavity contains the lungs, pleurae (membranes that line the lungs), and a central mediastinum that contains the heart and parts of the trachea and esophagus. The mediastinum separates the two lungs. The right lung consists of three lobes (superior, middle, and inferior), whereas the left lung consists of two lobes (superior and inferior). At the level of the sternal angle, the trachea bifurcates into two main bronchi that enter each lung. These bronchi divide into multiple segments to ultimately generate pulmonary alveoli, which represent the most basic structural units of gas exchange in the lung.

The respiratory system consists of the lungs and airways that bring oxygen into the body and alveoli that enable gas exchange for cellular metabolism and eliminate carbon dioxide. The flow of air through the respiratory system is controlled by the larynx and diaphragm.

Physical Examination

Examination begins with inspecting the skin for cyanosis. The neck is inspected for use of accessory respiratory muscles (including the sternocleidomastoid [SCM], scalene, trapezius, pectoralis minor, and intercostal muscles), if the trachea is midline and if chest wall movement during respiration is symmetric (**Table 2.3**).

In addition, the nails are inspected for evidence of clubbing (**Fig. 2.8**), which is painless enlargement of the terminal phalanges of the digits seen in numerous medical conditions including those

TABLE 2.3. **Muscles of respiration**			
		Inspiration	**Expiration**
Normal (quiet)	Major	Diaphragm (active contraction)	Passive (elastic) recoil of lungs and thoracic cage
	Minor	*Tonic contraction* of external intercostals and interchondral portion of internal intercostals to resist negative pressure	*Tonic contraction* of muscles of anterolateral abdominal walls (rectus abdominis, external and internal obliques, transversus abdominis) to antagonize diaphragm by maintaining intra-abdominal pressure
Active (forced)		In addition to the above, *active contraction* of sternocleidomastoid, descending (superior) trapezius, pectoralis minor, and scalenes, to elevate and fix upper rib cage	In addition to the above, *active contraction* of muscles of anterolateral abdominal wall (antagonizing diaphragm by increasing intra-abdominal pressure and by pulling inferiorly and fixing inferior costal margin): rectus abdominis, external and internal obliques, and transversus abdominis
		External intercostals, interchondral portion of internal intercostals, subcostales, levatores costarum, and serratus posterior superior[a] to elevate ribs	Internal intercostal (interosseous part) and serratus posterior inferior[a] to depress ribs

[a]Recent studies indicate that the serratus posterior superior and inferior muscles may serve primarily as organs of proprioception rather than motion.

Source: Agur AMR, Dalley AF. *Grant's Atlas of Anatomy*, 13th ed. Baltimore, MD: Lippincott Williams & Wilkins, 2013.

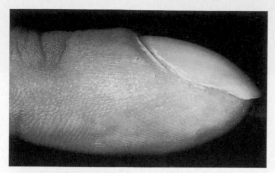

FIGURE 2.8. Clubbing of the nails evident by swelling of soft tissue at the nail base. The normal angle between the nail and proximal fold is lost, and the angle increases to 180° with the nail bed appearing spongy.

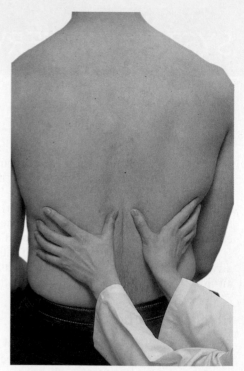

FIGURE 2.9. Assessment of chest expansion. If movement of rib cage is symmetric and normal, then the thumbs will move an equal distance apart with each breath.

with chronic hypoxemia. COPD is one exception, which does not present with clubbing. Clubbing is detected by holding the nail beds of two fingers of opposite hands in apposition and looking for the absence of a diamond window (Schamroth sign).

After inspection, areas of reported pain are palpated to identify underlying soft tissue or musculoskeletal pathology. To assess chest expansion, both hands are placed at the level of the 10th rib, a loose ridge of skin is raised over the spine between the thumbs, and the patient is instructed to take a deep breath. If the movement of the rib cage is symmetric and normal, the thumbs will move an equal distance apart with each breath (**Fig. 2.9**). To examine for tactile fremitus (palpable vibrations transmitted through the bronchopulmonary system to the chest wall), the lateral ulnar surface of both hands is placed on the posterior chest and the patient is asked to repeat the word "ninety-nine" (**Fig. 2.10**). A difference in vibration between the two sides is considered abnormal. Decreased tactile fremitus is seen in pleural effusions, pneumothorax, or neoplasm due to impaired transmission of low-frequency sounds; increased tactile fremitus is seen in pneumonia due to enhanced transmission through consolidated tissue.

During percussion (**Fig. 2.11**), the following notes may be audible: normal resonance, associated with normal lung tissue; hyperresonance, associated with lung tissue superior to an area of pleural effusion (typically, the area below the pleural effusion is dull to percussion); dullness, associated with lobar consolidation; tympany, associated with a large pneumothorax; and resonance in the lung apex (Kronig isthmus) that may be decreased in conditions such as tuberculosis and Pancoast tumor.

Auscultation of the lungs is the primary method to detect diseases of the respiratory system. Bronchial sounds are best heard over the manubrium, but can be detected over more distal portions of the lungs when air is replaced by material such as fluid, pus, or blood. Vesicular sounds are decreased in COPD and diseases with impaired ventilation. Crackles are audible with pulmonary edema, atelectasis, and interstitial fibrosis, among other pathologies. Wheezes are high-pitched, musical sounds generated by turbulent airflow through narrowed airways and are audible during

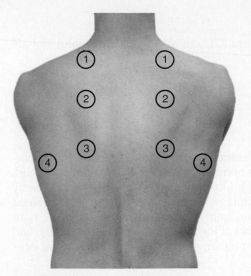

FIGURE 2.10. Locations for assessing tactile fremitus.

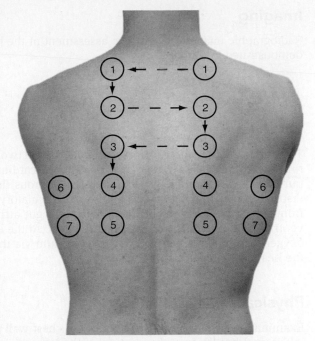

FIGURE 2.11. Locations for percussion and auscultation of lung fields using a systematic "ladder" pattern.

expiration in COPD, asthma, and cardiogenic pulmonary edema. Stridor is a high-frequency sound that indicates upper airway obstruction and often occurs during inspiration. Rhonchi are low-pitched sounds that suggest increased secretions in large airways. Rubs are grating, creaky sounds often associated with pleural disease.

In addition, transmission of the patient's spoken or whispered voice through the chest wall may be distorted. Increased transmission suggests that air has been replaced by solid or fluid (e.g., inflammatory cells and bacteria in lobar pneumonia, fluid in pulmonary edema, or blood in alveolar hemorrhage). When auscultation of spoken words is louder than usual, this is called *bronchophony*. Whispered pectoriloquy occurs when whispered words that are normally faint and indistinct are heard louder and clearer. Distortion of words, in which "E" sounds like "A" (E-to-A change), is referred to as *egophony* and occurs with lobar consolidation such as pneumonia (**Fig. 2.12**).

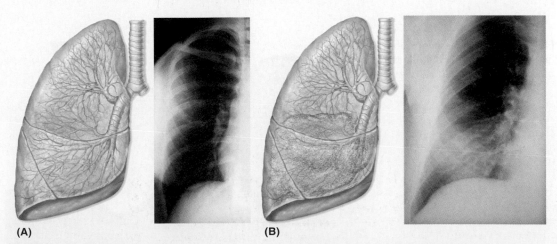

(A)   **(B)**

FIGURE 2.12. Anatomy and corresponding radiograph in (A) normal and (B) disease state (lobar pneumonia).

Imaging

Radiographic images can enhance assessment of the lungs. CT and MRI scans are helpful and are demonstrated in Clinical Cases.

■ HEART

Overview

The heart consists of four chambers (two atria and two ventricles) and is contained within a fibroserous membrane called the *pericardium*. The pericardium normally contains a small amount of fluid, but can be filled with larger amounts (e.g., serous fluid, blood, or malignant effusions), thereby restricting cardiac function and resulting in circulatory collapse and, possibly, death. Venous blood from the body enters the heart through the right atrium, from where it travels through the right ventricle and pulmonary artery into the lungs. At the level of the alveoli, gas exchange occurs, and oxygen-rich blood is returned to the left atrium via the pulmonary veins. Oxygen-rich blood exits the heart via the aorta.

Physical Examination

Examination begins with inspection of the chest wall anatomy for visible "cardiac lifts," along the left sternal border or at the junction of the left anterior axillary line and fifth intercostal space for evidence of right and left ventricle hypertrophy, respectively. Following this, the JVP should be assessed. The JVP reflects filling pressure of the right atrium and is best assessed using pulsations in the right internal jugular vein. To assess the JVP, the head of the examination table is elevated to ~30°. Using tangential lighting, pulsations of the right external jugular vein are identified. Scanning the region of the SCM muscle, reflected pulsations of the internal jugular vein are identified, noting the highest point of pulsations (**Fig. 2.13**) and measuring the vertical distance from this point to the sternal angle (e.g., 5 cm). To this distance, 4 cm (distance between sternal angle and middle of right atrium) is added. This represents the distance from the sternal angle to the middle of the right atrium, giving a JVP of 9 cm.

Following inspection, the heart is palpated. With the patient in the left lateral decubitus position, the PMI is palpated at the junction of the left midclavicular line and fifth intercostal space (see **Fig. 2.5**). A laterally displaced PMI suggests cardiomegaly, and a sustained, high-intensity PMI suggests cardiac hypertrophy. A retracted PMI, in which the impulse retracts during systole, is associated with severe tricuspid regurgitation and constrictive pericarditis. Right or left ventricular enlargement can also result in a PMI that is diffusely palpable across the left

FIGURE 2.13. Estimation of JVP. The highest point of oscillation in the internal carotid artery marks the level of the JVP.

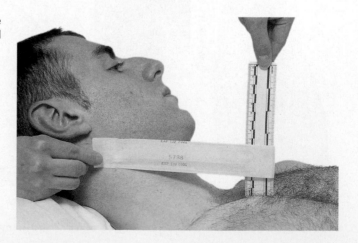

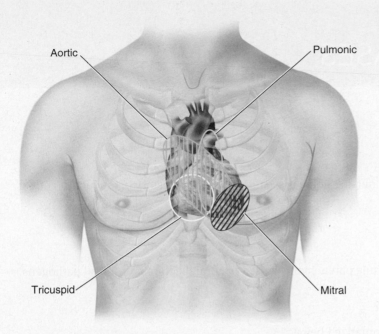

FIGURE 2.14. Location for auscultation of cardiac murmurs.

Aortic

Pulmonic

Tricuspid

Mitral

chest wall. Right ventricular enlargement may also result in a palpable parasternal right ventricular heave.

In general, percussion over the heart generates a dull sound. Dullness that extends beyond 10.5 cm from the midsternal or midclavicular line can be seen in cardiomegaly. Following percussion, the heart is auscultated to identify S_1 and S_2 heart sounds and abnormal murmurs (**Fig. 2.14**). Murmurs are attributed to turbulent blood flow and may reflect underlying valvular heart disease. Valvular stenosis (e.g., aortic stenosis) refers to an abnormally narrowed valvular orifice that impedes blood flow, whereas valve regurgitation (e.g., mitral regurgitation) refers to valve leaflets that fail to fully close, thereby allowing blood to travel in a retrograde direction. Auscultation of heart sounds and simultaneous palpation of carotid pulsation can help determine the timing of the murmur during the cardiac cycle. Murmurs that coincide with upstroke of the carotid pulse are systolic. Systolic murmurs can be a normal finding, but all diastolic murmurs are abnormal and usually indicate valvular disease.

Imaging

Radiographic images can enhance assessment of the heart. Ultrasound, CT, and MRI scans are helpful and are demonstrated in Clinical Cases.

■ ESOPHAGUS

Overview

The esophagus is the main structure of the GI system present in the thorax. No specific physical examination maneuvers exist for the esophagus, but diseases related to the esophagus are described in the Clinical Cases.

Imaging

Radiographic images can enhance assessment of the esophagus. CT scans can be helpful and are demonstrated in Clinical Cases.

CLINICAL CASES

 PNEUMONIA

Presentation

A 70-year-old female residing at a nursing home presents with a 1-day history of productive cough, tachypnea, and confusion.

Definition

Pneumonia is an infection of the lung parenchyma caused by viral, bacterial, or fungal pathogens.

What are common causes?

The most common causes are summarized below.

Bacteria	The most common pathogens for community-acquired pneumonia (CAP) are *Streptococcus pneumoniae*, *Mycoplasma pneumoniae*, and *Chlamydia pneumoniae*. *Staphylococcus aureus* can present as bilateral nodular infiltrates with central cavitations and thin-walled cavities called *pneumatoceles*, bronchopleural fistulas, and empyema. Bacteria common in aspiration pneumonia include *Klebsiella pneumonia*; *Escherichia coli*; *Pseudomonas aeruginosa*; and *Peptostreptococcus, Actinomyces, Bacteroides, Fusobacterium, Proteus, Serratia,* and *Prevotella* species. *Legionella pneumophila* is an atypical cause of pneumonia from contaminated water.
Fungi	Histoplasmosis, coccidiomycosis, blastomycosis, aspergillosis, mucormycosis, cryptococcosis, *Pneumocystis jirovecii* pneumonia, and sporotrichosis
Parasites	Hydatid disease, paragonimiasis, and amebiasis

> ● **CLINICAL PEARL**
>
> Viral infections may predispose a patient to a superimposed bacterial infection.

What is the differential diagnoses?

Dyspnea and cough: The differential diagnosis includes pneumonia (infection), aspiration, CHF, PE, COPD exacerbation, and mucus plug, as listed in **Table 2.2**.

What symptoms might be observed?

Symptoms include cough, dyspnea, and pleuritic chest pain.

What are the possible findings on examination?

Vital signs: Fever, tachycardia, tachypnea, and hypoxia.
Inspection: Use of accessory muscles of respiration and asymmetric chest wall expansion may be observed.
Palpation: Tactile fremitus, rales, and egophony.

Percussion: Dullness over affected lung fields.

Auscultation: Decreased or bronchial breath sounds (Sp 0.96) and whisper pectoriloquy/bronchophony over affected lung fields.

What tests should be ordered?

Laboratory tests: CBC (leukocytosis, thrombocytopenia suggests infection) and metabolic panel (BUN: Cr > 20:1 suggests hypovolemia). If thrombocytopenia, consider disseminated intravascular coagulation (DIC) and check coagulation panel (elevated international normalized ratio [INR], elevated partial thromboplastin time [PTT], reduced fibrinogen) and peripheral blood smear (schistocytes). Microbiology (sputum and blood cultures, pharyngeal cultures [influenza A and B, respiratory syncytial virus]) and urine studies (legionella, histoplasma, and pneumococcus antigens).

Imaging: Chest x-ray (focal consolidation or infiltrate is consistent with bacterial pneumonia; interstitial pattern is consistent with atypical bacterial or viral pneumonias); bilateral patchy opacities suggest multifocal pneumonia or emerging acute respiratory distress syndrome (ARDS). CT scans without contrast can identify an abscess, cavitation, or empyema (**Figs. 2.15 to 2.18**).

Diagnostic Scores

PSI: The Pneumonia Severity Index (PSI) score was derived as part of the Pneumonia Patient Outcome Research Team (PORT) study and uses medical history, presenting x-ray, and laboratory test results to calculate a score that helps to predict 30-day mortality. Several online calculators can aid in this calculation.

CURB-65: Uses patient variables (confusion, blood **u**rea levels, **r**espiratory rate, **b**lood pressure, and age) to calculate 30-day mortality. As with PSI, online calculators can aid in the calculation of the CURB-65 score.

> ● **CLINICAL PEARL**
>
> Other risk calculators include SMART-COP and the SCAP (severe CAP) score.

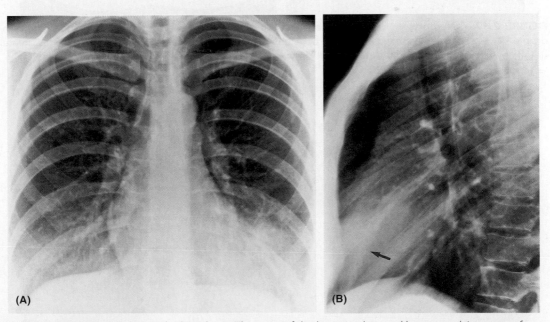

(A)   **(B)**

FIGURE 2.15. Consolidation in the lingula. **A.** The apex of the heart is obscured by an overlying area of consolidation in this frontal x-ray. **B.** Lateral x-ray clearly demonstrates the anterior location of the consolidation (*arrow*).

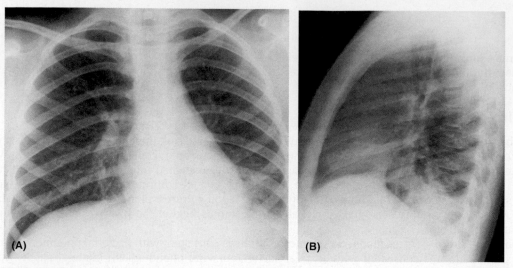

FIGURE 2.16. Left lower lobe pneumonia. **A.** The left costodiaphragmatic angle is obscured in this frontal x-ray due to focal consolidation in the left lower lobe. **B.** Lateral x-ray reveals the posterior location of the consolidation.

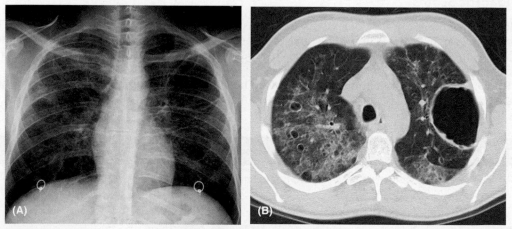

FIGURE 2.17. *Pneumocystis jirovecii* edema pattern in a patient with an acquired immunodeficiency syndrome. **A.** X-ray shows bilateral groundglass opacities and pneumatoceles. **B.** CT scan demonstrates greater detail of changes in lung architecture.

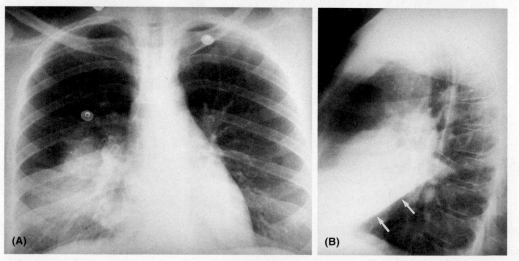

FIGURE 2.18. Right middle lobe pneumonia. **A.** PA x-ray revealing obliteration of the right cardiac silhouette. **B.** Lateral x-ray shows the consolidation involves the middle lobe. Note the sharp definition of the major fissure (*arrows*) on the right side.

CHRONIC OBSTRUCTIVE PULMONARY DISEASE

Presentation

A 52-year-old male with a 100-pack-year smoking history presents with acute on chronic dyspnea, cough, and sputum production worsening over 3 days, particularly in the morning.

Definition

COPD is characterized by progressive airflow obstruction and is associated with emphysema and chronic bronchitis. Emphysema is structural enlargement of terminal bronchiole airspaces due to destruction of airspace walls, and chronic bronchitis is chronic productive cough ≥3 months in each of 2 successive years and without other causes.

What are common causes?

The most common risk factors include exposure to cigarette smoke, fumes, or inorganic dusts as well as genetic predisposition.

> ● **CLINICAL PEARL**
>
> Although the dose–response curve of COPD development due to cigarette smoke is individualized, smoking less than 10–15 pack-years is unlikely to cause COPD, whereas ≥40 pack-years has a positive likelihood ratio of 12. However, for patients aged 55–80 years with >30-pack-year history and currently smoking or having quit in the previous 15 years, COPD screening is not indicated. Instead, an annual low-dose chest CT scan is indicated for lung cancer screening and can often detect emphysematous changes. If patients are symptomatic for COPD, then pulmonary function tests (PFTs) are the first-line evaluation.

What is the differential diagnosis?

Dyspnea and cough: The differential diagnosis includes pneumonia (infection), aspiration, CHF, PE, COPD exacerbation, and mucus plug, as listed in **Table 2.2**.

What symptoms might be observed?

Symptoms include chronic cough, sputum production, dyspnea on exertion, and chest tightness.

What are the possible findings on examination?

Vital signs: Tachypnea and hypoxia.
Inspection: Tripod breathing, use of accessory muscles, pursed-lip breathing, cyanosis, and distended jugular veins due to increased intrathoracic pressure during expiration. Extremities may show asterixis due to hypercapnia. Clubbing is not typical in COPD and warrants evaluation for malignancy, interstitial lung disease, or bronchiectasis.
Percussion: Hyperinflation and increased resonance.
Auscultation: Decreased breath sounds, wheezes, basilar rales, distant heart sounds, increased anteroposterior diameter, depressed diaphragm, Hoover sign (paradoxical retraction of the lower interspaces during inspiration), and prominent cardiac P_2.

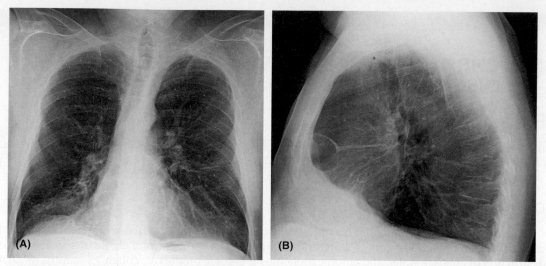

FIGURE 2.19. Chronic obstructive pulmonary disease (COPD). Frontal **(A)** and lateral **(B)** x-rays reveal hyper-inflated lungs, resulting in flattening of the hemidiaphragms.

What tests should be ordered?

Laboratory tests: CBC (leukocytosis if infection, anemia), metabolic panel (elevated bicarbonate if chronic respiratory acidosis, elevated BNP), and arterial blood gas ([ABG] hypercapnia, hypox-emia, and acidemia). Consider serum α-1-antitrypsin deficiency (AATD) testing if family history, age ≤ 45 years, or minimal tobacco exposure; and, microbiology (sputum cultures if an adequate sample is obtained).

Imaging: Chest x-ray may show hyperinflated lungs, flattened diaphragm (or hemidiaphragm), increased retrosternal airspace, bullae, prominent vascular opacities, "vascular pruning," or rap-idly tapered vessel calibers (**Fig. 2.19**). Chest CT scans may reveal centrilobular emphysema (upper lobe involvement), panacinar emphysema (lung bases, more common in AATD), and paraseptal emphysema (subpleural air trapping at periphery), or a combination of these patterns (**Fig. 2.20**).

Special Tests

PFTs: Spirometry pre- and postbronchodilator administration; partial or irreversible obstruction is consistent with COPD, and reversible obstruction is consistent with asthma. $FEV_1/FVC \leq 0.70$

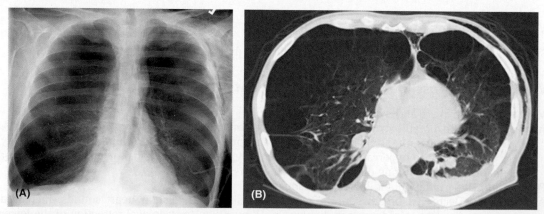

FIGURE 2.20. Bullous emphysema. **A.** Frontal x-ray reveals large bullae resulting in absence of lung markings in bilateral upper lobes and in the periphery of the lower lobes. **B.** CT image of the large cystic bullae resulting in compression of the normal lung tissue, otherwise known as *vanishing lung disease*.

or < 5th percentile of the lower limit of age-adjusted normal is diagnostic of obstruction. FEV1 represents the forced expiratory volume in one second, which is the volume of air exhaled in the first second during maximal effort; FVC represents the forced vital capacity, which is the total volume exhaled during the duration of the test. Decreased inspiratory capacity and vital capacity, increased total lung capacity, functional residual capacity (FRC), and residual volume suggest hyperinflation, which reflects gas trapping in the alveoli seen in COPD.

Diagnostic Scores

Staging is based on the Global Initiative for Chronic Obstructive Lung Disease (GOLD) guidelines, which combine symptoms, history of exacerbation, and forced expiratory volume (FEV_1) to assess exacerbation risk. GOLD stage 1 or 2, which confers low risk, has mild–moderate airflow obstruction with 0–1 exacerbations per year. GOLD stage 3 or 4, which confers high risk, has severe to very severe airflow obstruction and ≥2 exacerbations per year. Questionnaires such as the modified Medical Research Council scale and the COPD assessment test exist to help assess symptoms.

> ● **CLINICAL PEARL**
>
> Precipitants for COPD exacerbations are often viral or bacterial (e.g., *Haemophilus influenzae, Moraxella catarrhalis, S. pneumoniae*, and *P. aeruginosa*), and respiratory infections with atypical bacteria are an uncommon cause. The single best predictor of exacerbations is a history of exacerbations irrespective of COPD severity as assessed by the GOLD staging.

PLEURAL EMPYEMA

Presentation

A 56-year-old male, who was in a recent snowmobile accident, presents with fever, dyspnea, sputum production, and pleuritic chest pain that is worsening despite 7 days of antibiotic therapy.

Definition

Pleural empyema is the presence of infected pleural fluid, characterized by a positive Gram stain or by aspiration of purulence.

What are common causes?

See Pneumonia, Clinical Cases.

What is the differential diagnosis?

Pleuritic chest pain: The differential diagnosis includes flail chest, PE, aspiration, pneumonia, and asthma exacerbation.
Dyspnea and cough: The differential diagnosis include pneumonia (infection), aspiration, CHF, PE, COPD exacerbation, and mucus plug, as listed in **Table 2.2**.

What symptoms might be observed?

Symptoms include cough, pleuritic chest pain, and fever. The fever may not resolve despite antibiotics.

What are the possible findings on examination?

Vital signs: Fever, tachycardia, tachypnea, hypoxia, and hypotension due to septic shock.

Inspection: Labored breathing and asymmetric chest wall expansion.

Palpation: Decreased tactile fremitus over affected lung fields. Skin overlying an empyema is typically warm.

Percussion: Dullness over affected lung fields.

Auscultation: Decreased breath sounds, pleural friction rub, or egophony over affected lung fields.

Clubbing: Raises concern for malignant effusion and empyema.

Chest mass: An undrained empyema can present as a soft, fluctuant mass, which may elicit cough upon palpation due to connection between the mass and the pleural cavity. A cutaneous fistula may develop with spontaneous drainage.

What tests should be ordered?

Laboratory tests: CBC (leukocytosis and predominance of neutrophils or bands with infection) and metabolic panel (elevated serum lactic acid with hypotension or infection and elevated lactate dehydrogenase [LDH]). Sputum culture may reveal presence of bacteria. Influenza (A and B) tests can be done to rule out viral upper respiratory tract infection.

Imaging: Ultrasound can distinguish fluid (vs. pneumonia or solid masses) and free pleural effusions (vs. loculated) (**Figs. 2.21 and 2.22**). Contrast-enhanced chest CT scans provide optimal evaluation of an empyema by revealing loculations, thickened parietal pleura, and air with pleural fluid.

Special Tests

Thoracentesis: Recommended if at least one of the following is present: free-flowing but fluid layer > 1.0 cm on lateral decubitus; loculated, thickened parietal pleura seen on CT scan; and pleural

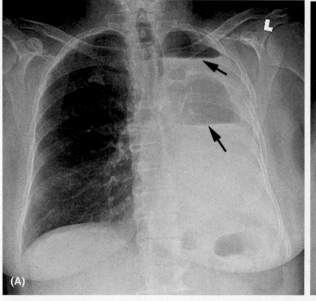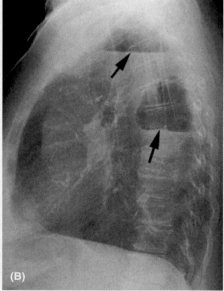

FIGURE 2.21. Complications from a left pneumonectomy. Frontal (**A**) and lateral (**B**) films reveal air–fluid levels (*arrows*) in the cavity left behind after pneumonectomy in a patient with fever and elevated WBCs. This indicates loculation of the fluid collection, which is suspicious for an empyema.

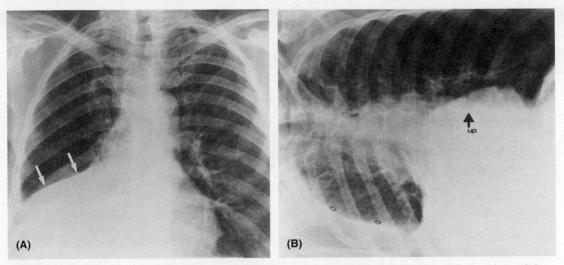

(A)

(B)

FIGURE 2.22. Right pleural effusion. **A.** Frontal x-ray reveals atelectasis of the right middle and lower lobes, with a suspected right pleural effusion (*arrows*). **B.** Most of the fluid layers out with the patient in the right lateral decubitus position, indicating the fluid is unlikely to be loculated (*open arrows*).

fluid clearly delineated by ultrasound. Investigations of pleural fluid include Gram stain and culture, pH, glucose, LDH, total protein, cell count, and differential. Foul odor is diagnostic of anaerobic infection. If diagnostic thoracentesis is performed first (**Fig. 2.23**), the following criteria indicate need for complete drainage of the pleural space via chest tube insertion: pH < 7.20, glucose < 60 mg/dL, LDH > 1,000 IU/dL, white blood cells (WBCs) > 25–100 K/µL polymorphonuclear leukocytes (PMNs), or red blood cells (RBCs) < 5,000/mm^3.

Light criteria: An exudative effusion is suggested by the presence of at least one of the following criteria: total protein$_{effusion}$:total protein$_{serum}$ > 0.5, LDH$_{effusion}$:LDH$_{serum}$ > 0.6, or LDH$_{effusion}$ > 2/3 upper limit of normal of LDH$_{serum}$.

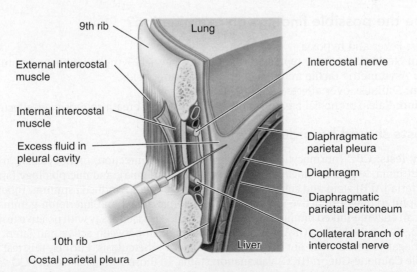

9th rib

Lung

External intercostal muscle

Intercostal nerve

Internal intercostal muscle

Excess fluid in pleural cavity

Diaphragmatic parietal pleura

Diaphragm

Diaphragmatic parietal peritoneum

10th rib

Liver

Collateral branch of intercostal nerve

Costal parietal pleura

FIGURE 2.23. Technique for midaxillary thoracentesis. The needle is inserted superior to the rib toward the middle of the intercostal space to avoid the intercostal arterial and venous branches.

PULMONARY TUBERCULOSIS

Presentation

A 25-year-old healthy male who recently returned from an extended work project in India presents with a 3-week history of fever, night sweats, dull interscapular pain, nocturnal cough, and hemoptysis. He is found to have a positive purified protein derivative (PPD) skin test and a chest x-ray showing a right upper lobe cavity.

Definition

Pulmonary tuberculosis is a mycobacterial infection of the airways, including the larynx, bronchi, and parenchyma.

What are common causes?

Common pathogens that cause cavitary lesions: atypical mycobacteria such as *Mycobacterium kanasii* and *Mycobacterium xenopi*, *Klebsiella* species, *S. pneumoniae*, *S. aureus*, *H. influenzae*, *P. aeruginosa*, fungi, and *P. jirovecii*. Lung cancers such as squamous cell carcinoma, Kaposi sarcoma, and some lymphomas can form cavitary lesions.

What is the differential diagnosis?

Dyspnea and cough: The differential diagnosis includes pneumonia (infection), aspiration, CHF, PE, COPD exacerbation, and mucus plug, as listed in **Table 2.2**.
Pleuritic chest pain: The differential includes flail chest, PE, aspiration, pneumonia, and asthma exacerbation.

What symptoms might be observed?

Symptoms include cough, pleuritic chest pain, diurnal fever peaking in the late afternoon or evening, hemoptysis, and night sweats.

What are the possible findings on examination?

Vital signs: Fever and hypoxia.
Inspection: Neck masses may represent tuberculous cervical lymphadenitis or scrofula.
Palpation: Asymmetric tactile fremitus over affected lung fields.
Percussion: Dullness over affected lung fields.
Auscultation: Rales, bronchial breath sounds, and amphoric breath sounds over affected lung fields.

What tests should be ordered?

Laboratory tests: CBC (normocytic anemia, leukocytosis if infection, monocytosis), metabolic panel (hyponatremia, hypoalbuminemia, hypergammaglobulinemia), and microbiology (sputum for acid-fast bacteria [AFB] stain and culture based on three samples of induced sputum, tuberculin skin test [not helpful to diagnose active tuberculosis in endemic areas] and interferon-gamma release assay [IGRA], an enzyme-linked immunosorbent assay [ELISA]-based assay with positive test $> 0.34\,\text{IU/mL}$ [Sn 0.92, Sp > 0.99]). The IGRA test does not distinguish between active and latent disease; however, a negative result rules out both active and latent tuberculosis. Further, this test is not affected by bacille Calmette-Guérin (BCG) vaccination status. In those with a history of BCG vaccination and who are not at increased risk for poor outcome if infected, a tuberculosis skin test result $< 15\,\text{mm}$ may be regarded as a false positive if the IGRA result is negative.

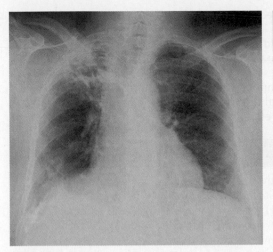

FIGURE 2.24. Old tuberculous infection. Right upper lobe consolidation, scarring, and ipsilateral tracheal and mediastinal shift, characteristic of both active and prior granulomatous infection. Comparison to previous x-rays is helpful when determining onset of disease.

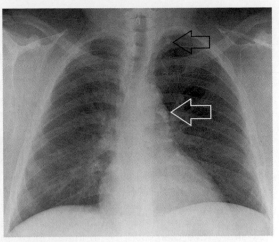

FIGURE 2.25. Ranke complex. Frontal view with calcified left upper lobe pulmonary nodule (*black arrow*) at site of initial infection and subsequent spread of disease to the ipsilateral hilar lymph node (*white arrow*).

Imaging: Chest x-ray may be normal in active pulmonary tuberculosis. Primary tuberculosis is typically associated with hilar adenopathy, right middle lung collapse, and middle or lower lung involvement, whereas reactivation tuberculosis is typically associated with upper lobe infiltrates. Other findings seen in reactivation tuberculosis include fibronodular or "miliary" lesions, tuberculomas, and cavitation. CT scans are more sensitive than chest x-rays to detect small apical lesions. Findings in both reactivation and primary tuberculosis include fibrotic lesions, pleural effusions, cavities, infiltrates, traction bronchiectasis, centrilobular nodules, and branching linear lesions (**Figs. 2.24 to 2.26**).

Special Tests

Bronchoscopy: In endobronchial tuberculosis, lesions include erythematous, vascular, ulcerated tissue, granulation tissue, hilar node rupture, perforation of a node into the bronchus, or caseous

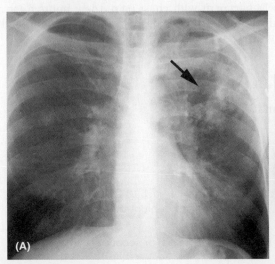

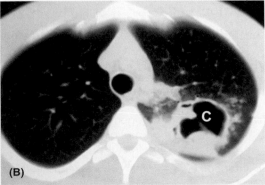

FIGURE 2.26. Tuberculosis involving the left upper lobe. **A.** Frontal x-ray shows consolidation and cavitary disease (*black arrow*). **B.** Axial CT scan further characterizes the abscess cavity. *C, cavity.*

or calcific material. Brushings and bronchoalveolar lavage with AFB stains and cultures are helpful, but not required for diagnosis.

Thoracentesis: Tuberculosis pleural effusion should be considered in those with an undiagnosed exudative effusion. These effusions are exudative in nature and are lymphocyte predominant. Of note, these effusions are associated with scant mesothelial cells in the pleural fluid. Although AFB smears of pleural fluid are rarely positive, a lymphocytic exudate confirms a clinical suspicion for tuberculosis and warrants treatment. A pleural fluid adenosine deaminase level above 40 U/L supports the possibility of a tuberculosis pleural effusion.

> ● CLINICAL PEARL
>
> Negative pressure isolation is indicated in active pulmonary tuberculosis; however, most extrapulmonary tuberculosis does not warrant isolation. During hospitalization, isolation is required until one of the following is achieved: (1) three negative sputum AFB smears, (2) one negative sputum nucleic acid amplification test + two negative AFB smears, (3) establishment of alternative diagnosis, or (4) initiation of antimycobacterial therapy with three subsequent negative sputum AFB smears. All cases of tuberculosis should be reported to the Department of Health.

> ● CLINICAL PEARL
>
> In healthy patients with a single positive tuberculosis skin test or IGRA result, the test should be repeated as it most likely represents a false-positive result. If the patient is symptomatic or is at risk for infection, progression, and a poor outcome (e.g., immunocompromised and children age <5 years), then treatment should be initiated based on the single positive result.

 # PNEUMOTHORAX

Presentation

A 34-year-old female presents to the Emergency Department with chest pain a few hours after a motor vehicle accident in which she was a restrained passenger. She describes shortness of breath and right-sided anterior chest pain that is worse with deep inspiration.

Definition

A pneumothorax is the presence of air in the pleural space.

What are common causes?

The most common causes are summarized below.

Traumatic	Iatrogenic (i.e., due to a procedure in the hospital, such as CT guided lung biopsy) or non-iatrogenic (e.g., a gunshot wound or blunt thoracic trauma with rib fractures)
Spontaneous	Primary spontaneous (in those without lung disease) or secondary (in those with lung disease such as COPD)
	Risk factors for primary spontaneous pneumothorax include male gender, cigarette smoking, and tall/thin body habitus.

Tension	Occurs when pressure in the pleural space remains positive throughout the respiratory cycle
	Increased pressure causes compression of the lung parenchyma and surrounding mediastinal structures resulting in reduced venous return to the heart (**Fig. 2.27**).
	Can result from any cause of pneumothorax

What is the differential diagnosis?

Chest pain: The differential diagnosis includes flail chest, fracture, and hemothorax. Also see Tables 2.1 and 2.2.

What symptoms might be observed?

Symptoms of pneumothorax include dyspnea and pleuritic chest pain.

What are the possible findings on examination?

Vital signs: Tachypnea, tachycardia, and hypoxia and, in the setting of hypotension, would raise concern for tension pneumothorax.
Inspection: May be in distress. Inspection may reveal signs of trauma such as penetrating wounds, bruises, or flail chest. The jugular vein may be distended, and the trachea may be deviated away from the affected side, both of which are concerning for tension pneumothorax.
Palpation: Asymmetric chest wall expansion and subcutaneous emphysema.
Percussion: Hyperresonance over affected lung fields.
Auscultation: Decreased or absent breath sounds over affected lung fields.

What tests should be ordered?

Laboratory tests: ABG may help to evaluate the degree of impairment in oxygenation and ventilation; however, it is not required for diagnosis.
Imaging: CT imaging is the gold standard test to diagnose and estimate the size of a pneumothorax in clinically stable patients. Chest x-rays can be obtained in stable patients to confirm the diagnosis of pneumothorax. Typical findings include absence of pulmonary vessels extending to

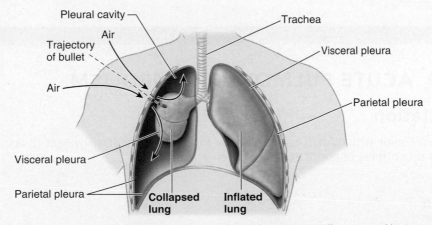

FIGURE 2.27. Pleural anatomy. The pleural cavity is a potential space normally occupied by a small amount of fluid between its visceral and parietal layers. If a sufficient amount of air enters the pleural cavity, it will disrupt the surface tension responsible for adhering the visceral to the parietal pleura and keeping the lung expanded within the walls of the thoracic cavity. The elastic recoil of the lung will lead it to collapse, resulting in atelectasis. When a lung collapses, the pleural cavity becomes a real space and may contain air (pneumothorax), blood (hemothorax), or lymphatic fluid (chylothorax).

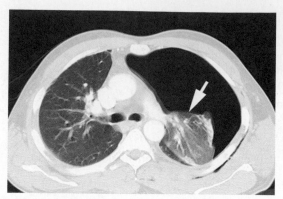

FIGURE 2.28. Tension pneumothorax on CT scan with large left-sided collection of free air, and mediastinal shift to the right. Note the collapsed lung posteriorly (*arrow*).

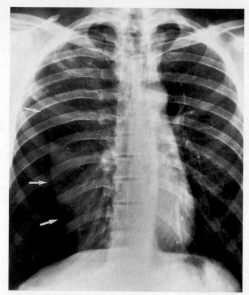

FIGURE 2.29. Tension pneumothorax on chest x-ray (*arrows*), with mediastinal displacement to the left.

the chest wall, visible pleural line that is distinctly separated from the chest wall, and increased lucency in the area of pneumothorax. In a tension pneumothorax, the mediastinal structures are shifted away from the affected side (**Figs. 2.28 and 2.29**). The use of chest ultrasound is increasing for rapid bedside diagnosis in the critically ill.

● CLINICAL PEARL

Tension pneumothorax is diagnosed clinically, and not by radiographic assessment. It is a medical emergency that requires immediate needle thoracostomy and chest tube placement.

 # ACUTE PULMONARY EMBOLISM

Presentation

A 63-year-old female with ovarian cancer presents to the Emergency Department 12 hours after the onset of acute shortness of breath and pleuritic chest pain.

Definition

PE is obstruction of one or more vessels in the pulmonary arterial vasculature by material (e.g., thrombus, air, fat, or tumor) that originated in another part of the body. Depending on the extent and location of the obstruction, significant hemodynamic instability may occur. If systolic blood pressure (BP) <90 mm Hg or drop in systolic BP of ≥40 mm Hg from baseline for >15 minutes, the PE is classified as massive. All other acute PEs are classified as submassive.

TABLE 2.4. Dichotomized Wells score	
Variable	**Points**
PE as likely as or more likely than alternative diagnosis	3
Signs and symptoms of DVT	3
Heart rate > 100 beats/min	1.5
Immobilization or surgery in previous 4 weeks	1.5
Previous DVT or PE	1.5
Hemoptysis	1.0
Cancer	1.0
Total score ≤4 >4	Category PE unlikely PE likely

PE, pulmonary embolism; DVT, deep vein thrombosis.

What are common causes?

Most arise from thrombi in deep veins of the lower extremities. However, thrombi in other venous vascular beds (e.g., upper extremity deep veins, pelvic veins, and chambers of the right heart) may embolize to the pulmonary vasculature. Therefore, risk factors associated with deep vein thrombosis (DVT) likely increase the risk of PE as well (**Table 2.4**).

What is the differential diagnosis?

Acute dyspnea: The differential diagnosis includes MI, pneumothorax, hemothorax, and aspiration. Also see **Tables 2.1 and 2.2**.

What symptoms might be observed?

Symptoms include chest pain (typically, pleuritic); dyspnea; hemoptysis; cough; palpitations; light-headedness; wheezing; nausea; vomiting; dysphagia; hematemesis; and leg swelling, pain, or warmth.

What are the possible findings on examination?

Vital signs: Hypotension with reflex tachycardia. Tachypnea and tachycardia may be present, but are nonspecific.
Inspection: Evidence of labored breathing.
Palpation: Right ventricular lift may be detected over the left parasternal border.
Percussion: Typically normal.
Auscultation: May reveal prominent P_2, indicative of pulmonary hypertension. A right-sided gallop rhythm (S_3 or S_4), along with pleural friction rub, may be present.

Special Tests

TTE: May reveal right ventricular dilation, diminished right ventricular function, and increased tricuspid regurgitation.
McConnell sign: The presence of regional wall motion abnormalities with sparing of the right ventricular apex may be seen in acute PE (Sn 0.77, Sp 0.94).

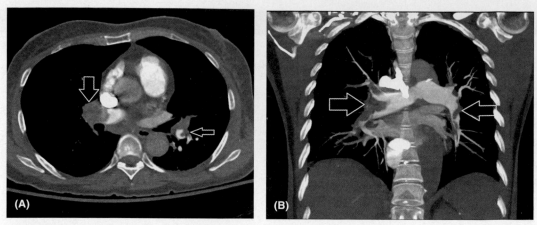

FIGURE 2.30. CT scan of large pulmonary embolism resulting in right heart strain. **A.** Axial CT image reveals large filling defects in both pulmonary arteries (*arrows*). **B.** Coronal maximum projection CT image reveals multiple thrombi (*arrows*).

What tests should be ordered?

Laboratory tests: Elevated serum BNP and troponin I and T may be elevated and indicate myocardial strain. D-dimer will be elevated, and, although is not usually helpful for diagnosis, it may help serially for resolution. CBC (anemia in malignancy, erythrocytosis in polycythemia), metabolic panel (creatinine, electrolytes), coagulation panel (INR, PTT, fibrinogen may be indicated if DIC is considered), and other serology (qualitative urine β-human chorionic gonadotropin [hCG] levels in women of childbearing age).

Imaging: CT pulmonary angiography is the imaging test of choice for suspected PE, based on the presence of an intraluminal "filling defect" in the contrast-enhanced pulmonary arterial vasculature (**Fig. 2.30**). Chest x-ray may reveal focal oligemia distal to the embolus (Westermark sign) or a shallow wedge-shaped opacity in the lung periphery (Hampton hump).

V/Q scan: Areas of ventilation without perfusion are concerning for an intrinsic vascular defect such as PE (**Fig. 2.31**). The utility of V/Q scans is lower in those with underlying pulmonary disease (e.g., COPD, asthma, pleural effusions, pneumonia) due to an increase in the number of false positives.

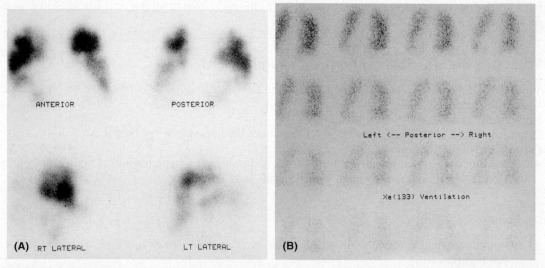

FIGURE 2.31. Ventilation–perfusion (V/Q) scan. **A.** Perfusion scan shows dark, photopenic areas throughout both lungs, which represent regions with diminished perfusion secondary to a PE. **B.** Ventilation scan reveals normal ventilation of the same regions.

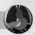 SOLITARY PULMONARY NODULE

Presentation

A 52-year-old male presents for follow-up of a solitary pulmonary nodule found incidentally on a chest CT scan obtained during work-up of his shortness of breath.

Definition

A solitary pulmonary nodule is a single, discrete pulmonary opacity ≤3 cm in diameter that is surrounded by normal lung tissue and is not associated with lymphadenopathy or atelectasis.

What are common causes?

The most common etiologies are summarized below.

Tumor	Bronchial adenoma, primary lung carcinoma, hamartoma, metastatic cancer
Infection	Granulomas due to mycobacteria (e.g., *Mycobacterium tuberculosis*, *Mycobacterium leprae*), bacteria (e.g., *Brucella*, *Actinomyces*, and *Listeria* species), or fungi (e.g., blastomycosis, histoplasmosis, coccidioidomycosis)
Simulated nodule	Nipple, bone lesion, skin tumor, foreign body, artifact

What is the differential diagnosis?

Lung nodule: The differential diagnosis includes arteriovenous malformation (AVM), atelectasis, rheumatoid arthritis, sarcoidosis, tumors, and infection.

What symptoms might be observed?

Asymptomatic unless the underlying etiology, such as malignancy, has progressed, in which case it may present with cough, hemoptysis, fever, night sweats, and unintentional weight loss.

What are the possible findings on examination?

Vital signs: Typically normal, depending on the location of the nodule, postobstructive pneumonia with associated fever may be present.
Inspection: Persistent cough, wheezing, or dyspnea.
Percussion: Dullness over affected lung fields.
Auscultation: Wheezes, rales, or diminished breath sounds.

What tests should be ordered?

Laboratory tests: Minimal role in evaluation of an asymptomatic solitary pulmonary nodule. However, if malignancy or infection is suspected, then obtain CBC (leukocytosis, anemia), basic metabolic panel (hyponatremia, hypercalcemia), and other serology (elevated erythrocyte sedimentation rate [ESR]).
Imaging: CT scans are the gold standard because of their higher resolution, allowing detection of nodules as small as 2 mm and characterization of their morphologic features (**Figs. 2.32 and 2.33**). However, solitary pulmonary nodules are often first detected on chest x-ray. Lateral films, as well as bone subtraction, can enable distinction between pulmonary and extrapulmonary nodules. Chest x-rays can also provide information on size, shape, cavitation, growth rate, and presence of calcifications. Serial imaging is helpful to assess the rate of change in nodule size, based on Fleischner Society guidelines.

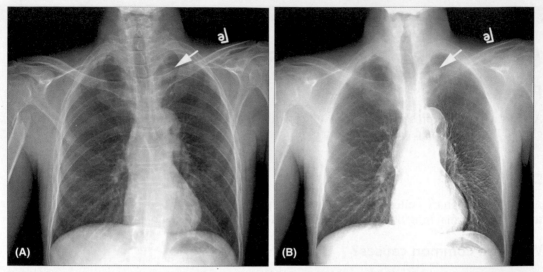

FIGURE 2.32. Chest x-ray of lung nodule. **A.** Normal frontal view with *arrow* denoting left upper lung nodule. **B.** Frontal lung window with bones subtracted.

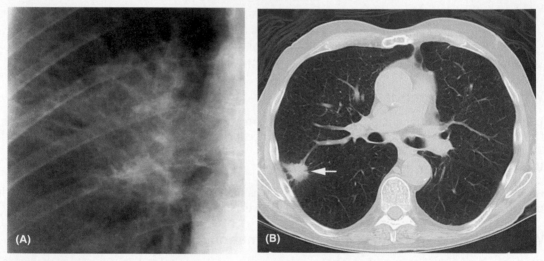

FIGURE 2.33. Spiculation in lung mass as seen on **(A)** chest x-ray and **(B)** CT image. A spiculated margin in a mass (*arrow*) indicates it is invading the surrounding tissue and is a sign of malignancy.

 # LUNG CANCER

Presentation

A 61-year-old male presents with a 3-month history of cough and wheezing. He has a long history of smoking, but quit last year after he required intubation for pneumonia.

Definition

Lung cancer is uncontrolled growth of abnormal cells, usually those lining the airways. The two main types are small-cell and non–small-cell lung cancer, which are diagnosed based on histopathology.

What are common causes?

The most common causes are summarized below.

Tobacco	The vast majority (90%) of lung cancers are related to tobacco use. The risk of lung cancer increases with the number of pack-years of smoking history and with exposure to secondhand smoke.
Asbestos	Fibers can persist in lung tissue for a lifetime following exposure, resulting in a five-fold increase in risk of lung cancer.
Radon	Natural radioactive gas, which is a natural decay product of uranium, can travel through soil and enter homes through gaps in the foundation, pipes, drains, or other openings.

What is the differential diagnosis?

Lung mass: The differential diagnosis includes bronchogenic carcinoid tumor, adenoma, hamartoma, lymphoma, and granuloma.

What symptoms might be observed?

Symptoms include persistent cough, wheezing, dyspnea, and hemoptysis.

What are the possible findings on examination?

Vital signs: Tachypnea and labored breathing and may present with fever, if postobstructive pneumonia.
Inspection: May have persistent cough, wheezing, or appear short of breath.
Percussion: Dullness due to consolidation or accumulation of pleural effusion.
Auscultation: Wheezes, rales, and diminished breath sounds over affected lung fields.

What tests should be ordered?

Laboratory tests: Blood tests are not diagnostic, and nonspecific serum markers include oncofetal carcinoembryonic antigen (β2 microglobulin, bombesin, and neuron-specific enolase).
Imaging: CT imaging is the gold standard to detect nodules as small as 1–2 mm and to characterize their morphologic features (**Fig. 2.34**). It can reveal bone destruction and is useful in the evaluation of mediastinal adenopathy, presence of other pulmonary masses, and liver involvement. Chest x-rays can also provide information on nodule size, shape, cavitation, growth rate, and presence of calcifications (**Fig. 2.35**).

Special Tests

Lung biopsy: Tissue samples confirm the diagnosis and help determine treatment and prognosis.

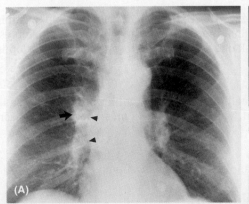
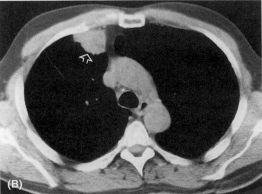

FIGURE 2.34. Lung carcinoma. **A.** Frontal x-ray reveals a mass (*arrow*) just above the hilum of the right lung. The mass does not obscure the ascending aorta (*arrowheads*), so it must be either anterior or posterior to it. **B.** CT image reveals the location of the mass adjacent to the pleura in the anterior segment of the right upper lobe (*arrow*).

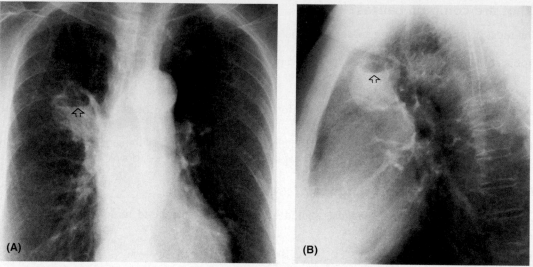

FIGURE 2.35. Cavitating lung lesion. Frontal **(A)** and lateral **(B)** views reveal an air–fluid level (*arrows*) indicative of cavitation in a right upper lobe carcinoma.

MESOTHELIOMA

Presentation

A 72-year-old male presents with dyspnea and a 1-week history of constant left-sided chest pain. He had worked in construction 30 years prior and was responsible for installing insulation material.

Definition

Mesothelioma is a malignancy that most frequently arises from cells of the pleura, peritoneum, or pericardium. Histologically, the tumors can be epithelial, sarcomatous, or mixed, with the latter two having a worse prognosis.

What are common causes?

The most common cause is exposure to asbestos, usually exposed through industries including mining, shipbuilding, ceramics, paper milling, auto parts, railroad repair, and insulation. Family members of workers exposed to asbestos can also be placed at risk due to transfer of fibers embedded in clothing.

What is the differential diagnosis?

Pleural lesions: Non–small-cell carcinoma, small-cell lung carcinoma, other primary lung malignancies, pulmonary fibrosis, infection (bacterial, viral, fungal), and mesothelial hyperplasia.

What symptoms might be observed?

Symptoms include dyspnea, fatigue, night sweats, and nonpleuritic chest pain.

What are the possible findings on examination?

Vital signs: Typically normal. Occasionally, fever, tachycardia, and tachypnea may be present.
Inspection: May appear generally unwell, cachectic, and short of breath.

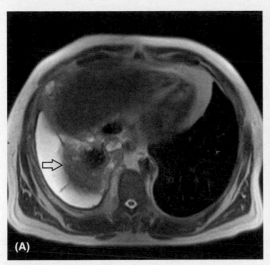
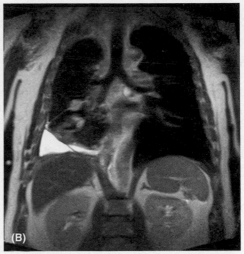

FIGURE 2.36. MRI image of mesothelioma. **A.** Axial image shows bright pleural effusion and adjacent pleural mass (*arrow*). **B.** Coronal image shows disease confined to the right chest without extension below the diaphragm. MRI is valuable for staging mesothelioma with its superior contrast resolution.

Percussion: Dullness over affected lung fields.
Auscultation: Diminished breath sounds over affected lung fields due to underlying pleural effusion.

What tests should be ordered?

Laboratory tests: Typically nondiagnostic, although serum biomarkers such as soluble mesothelin and megakaryocyte potentiating factor can be tested.
Imaging: Chest x-rays can reveal nodular or sheet-like thickening of the pleura. Pleural effusions are common and may obscure underlying pleural abnormalities. CT scans can delineate involvement of the mediastinum and concentric pleural thickening, which are highly suggestive of malignant pleural disease. MRI scans are superior in demonstrating solitary foci of chest wall invasion and diaphragmatic invasion (**Fig. 2.36**). PET/CT scans are expensive, but are used for baseline staging and assessment of treatment response.

Special Tests

Thoracentesis: Most patients present with a pleural effusion, which typically is nondiagnostic, with < 1,000 leukocytes/μL, elevated protein, and normal LDH levels. Cytology is diagnostic in 32% and suggestive in 56% of cases.
Biopsy: A biopsy should be performed and is diagnostic in 98% of cases.

 ## ATELECTASIS

Presentation

A 60-year-old female with a history of asbestosis exposure presents with a 1-week history of dyspnea after a long hospitalization for pneumonia.

Definition

Atelectasis occurs when lung tissue collapses and can be classified as obstructive or nonobstructive. Obstructive atelectasis is the blockage of an airway with resultant collapse of distal alveoli, whereas nonobstructive atelectasis is the collapse of lung tissue due to scarring, infiltrates, parenchymal compression, or surfactant dysfunction.

What are common causes?

The most common etiologies are summarized below.

Obstructive	Mucus plug, foreign body, aspiration, tumor within airway, and narrowing of airway from chronic infection or scarring
Nonobstructive	Chest wall trauma, tumor (nonobstructive to airway), chronic parenchymal infection or scarring, pneumonia, pleural effusion, and pneumothorax

What is the differential diagnosis?

Dyspnea and chest pain: The differential diagnosis includes pulmonary malignancy, loculated pleural effusion, pneumonia, atypical infection, asbestosis, and paraspinal masses.

What symptoms might be observed?

Symptoms include dyspnea, nonpleuritic chest pain, and cough.

What are the possible findings on examination?

Vital signs: Tachypnea and fever may be present.
Inspection: May appear cachectic.
Percussion: Dullness over affected lung fields.
Auscultation: Rales, wheezes, rhonchi, egophony, and decreased breath sounds over affected lung fields.

What tests should be ordered?

Laboratory tests: CBC (isolated leukocytosis).
Imaging: Chest x-rays can reveal collapse of lung tissue (**Fig. 2.37**), and similar changes may also be seen on CT scans.

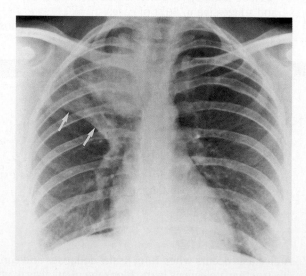

FIGURE 2.37. Right upper lobe consolidation and atelectasis. Frontal x-ray shows the superior mediastinal silhouette has been obscured on the right. Volume loss is evidenced by the elevation of the minor fissure (*arrows*).

SARCOIDOSIS

Presentation

A 32-year-old female presents with cough, dyspnea, and chest pain for 3 weeks and is found to have hilar adenopathy.

Definition

Sarcoidosis is an inflammatory disease with noncaseating granulomas that results in bilateral hilar adenopathy, pulmonary reticular opacities, and skin, joint, or eye lesions.

What are common causes?

The etiology of sarcoidosis is unknown and is thought to be related to environmental exposures, pathogens, and possible genetic contributions through T-cell abnormalities.

What is the differential diagnosis?

Hilar adenopathy: The differential diagnosis includes infection (bacterial or fungal), hypersensitivity pneumonitis, drug-induced hypersensitivity, and diseases associated with vasculitis (e.g., granulomatosis with polyangiitis, and eosinophilic granulomatosis with polyangiitis).

What symptoms might be observed?

Symptoms include cough, dyspnea, chest pain, weight loss, fever, and malaise.

What are the possible findings on examination?

Vital signs: Fever.
Inspection: Extrapulmonary manifestations of sarcoidosis include erythema nodosum, or appearance of plaques or nodules on the skin.
Auscultation: Wheezes, rales, and decreased breath sounds.

What tests should be ordered?

Laboratory tests: CBC (rule out infection), metabolic panel (creatinine, electrolytes), and other serology (elevated angiotensin-converting enzyme [ACE] levels in ~75% of cases).
Imaging: Chest x-ray shows bilateral hilar or right paratracheal lymphadenopathy, reticular opacities predominantly in the upper zones (**Fig. 2.38**). Chest CT scan shows hilar or mediastinal lymphadenopathy, peribronchovascular nodules, subpleural nodules, noncaseating granulomas, calcification, cavitation, bronchiectasis, ground-glass opacities, cysts, and fibrosis.

Special Tests

PFTs: Restrictive pattern with reduced diffusion capacity.
Bronchoalveolar lavage: Elevated CD4:CD8; ratio >4:1 with >16% lymphocytes and biopsy showing noncaseating granulomas has a 100% positive predictive value for sarcoidosis. CD4:CD8 ratio <1 has a 100% negative predictive value for sarcoidosis.
Biopsy: Noncaseating granulomas, commonly located in the alveolar septa, bronchial walls, and pulmonary vessels.

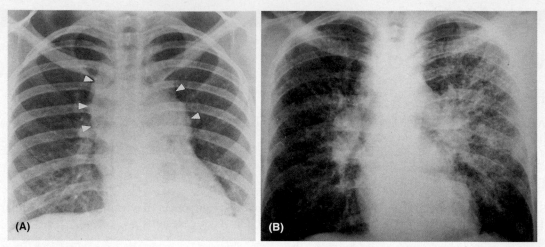

FIGURE 2.38. Sarcoidosis. **A.** Nodal pattern with "bumps" (*arrowheads*). **B.** Mixed parenchymal and nodal pattern. Note enlargement of mediastinal and hilar lymph nodes as well as diffuse interstitial disease, particularly on the left.

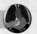 # CARDIAC VALVULAR DISEASE

Presentation

An 80-year-old male presents with progressive dyspnea on exertion and decreased exercise tolerance over the past month.

Definition

Valvular disease occurs when any of the four cardiac valves (tricuspid, pulmonic, mitral, and aortic) function suboptimally due to stenosis or insufficiency (**Fig. 2.39**).

What are common causes?

The common etiologies are summarized below.

Age-related changes	Males >65 years old and females >75 years old are prone to calcium deposition on heart valves, which can lead to valvular stiffening and stenosis.
Infection	Endocarditis, in which bacteria (e.g., group D *Streptococci*, *S. aureus*) or, less frequently, fungi (e.g., *Aspergillus*) enter the bloodstream and form vegetations on valve leaflets, can cause valvular insufficiency. Rheumatic fever caused by untreated streptococcal infection classically affects the mitral valve, leading to scarring and stenosis.
Connective tissue disease	Mitral valve prolapse (MVP) is a common condition affecting 1%–2% of the population, in which redundancy of the leaflets causes them to balloon into the left atrium during systole.
Congenital disease	Most often affects the aortic or pulmonic valves, causing leaflets to be malformed, fused, or incorrectly attached to the valve annulus

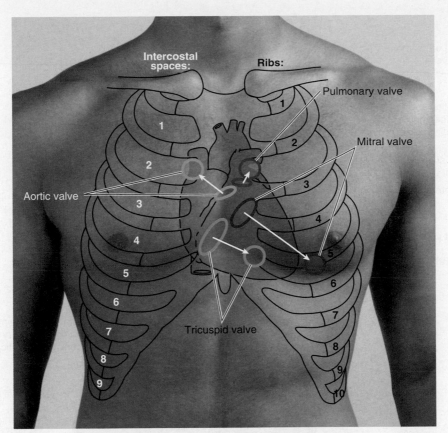

FIGURE 2.39. Surface marking of the heart valves and their auscultation areas. The aortic and pulmonary auscultation areas are in the 2nd intercostal space to the right and left of the sternal border. The tricuspid area is in the 5th or 6th intercostal space near the L sternal border. The mitral valve is best auscultated at the apex of the heart, in the 5th intercostal space in the midclavicular line.

What is the differential diagnosis?

Dyspnea: The differential diagnosis includes CHF, unstable angina, asthma, COPD, PE, anemia, and hypothyroidism.

What symptoms might be observed?

Symptoms include shortness of breath, orthopnea, palpitations, lower extremity edema, weight gain, and decreased exercise tolerance.

What are the possible findings on examination?

Vital signs: Hypoxemia.
Inspection: Signs of IV drug use (track marks on the skin) in a febrile patient may raise suspicion for endocarditis.
Auscultation: Characteristic murmurs reveal the underlying valvular pathology (**Figs. 2.40 and 2.41**).

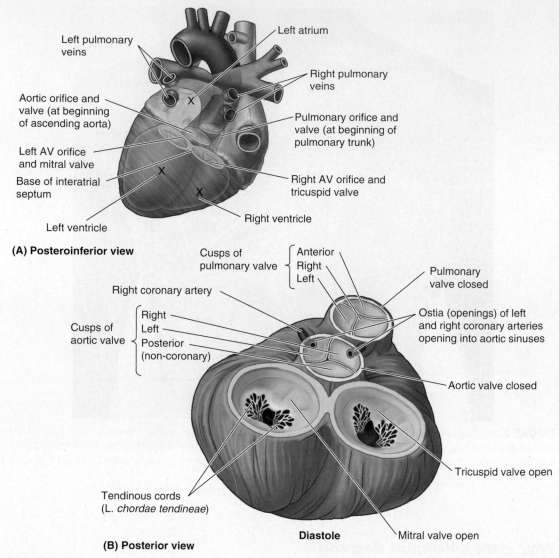

FIGURE 2.40. Valves of the heart and great vessels. **A.** Coronary valves are depicted in situ. *AV,* atrioventricular. **B.** Aortic and pulmonary valves close at the beginning of diastole, after which the tricuspid and mitral valves open.

What tests should be ordered?

Laboratory tests: If suspicious for infection, then obtain CBC (leukocytosis, if infection; anemia) and blood cultures and consider serology (ESR, C-reactive protein [CRP]) to assess for inflammatory conditions related to valvular disease.

Imaging: TTE is the test of choice to evaluate valvular pathology. It allows for assessment of valve anatomy as well as of chamber size and ventricular function. Doppler studies permit estimation of pressure gradients and valve area, particularly useful in characterizing the severity of aortic stenosis. Chest x-rays and CT scans can reveal valve calcification or ascending aortic dilation suggestive of long-standing aortic stenosis (**Fig. 2.42**).

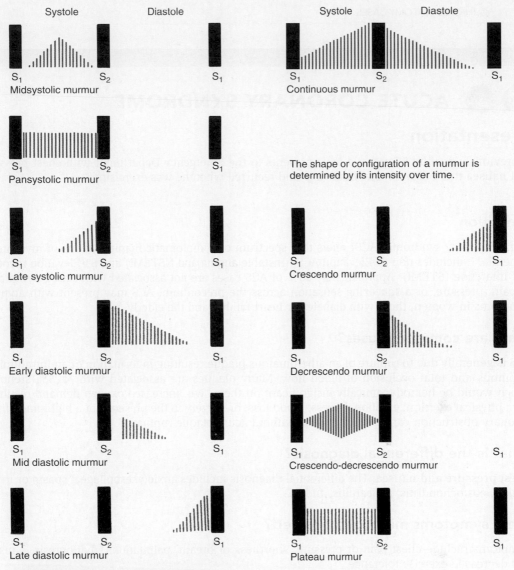

FIGURE 2.41. Characteristics of systolic and diastolic cardiac murmurs.

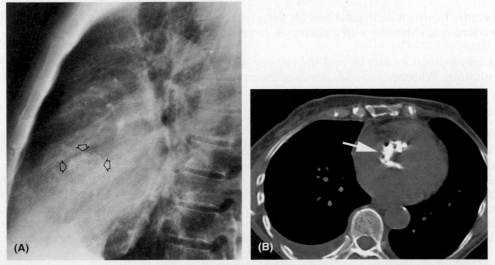

FIGURE 2.42. Aortic valve calcification. **A.** Lateral chest view shows aortic valve calcifications (*arrows*). Once these calcifications appear on chest x-ray, the stenosis is generally severe. **B.** Axial CT image with same finding (*arrow*).

ACUTE CORONARY SYNDROME

Presentation

A previously healthy 55-year-old male presents to the Emergency Department with chest pressure and nausea that began several hours ago and recurred when he was exercising.

Definition

Acute coronary syndrome (ACS) refers to a spectrum of symptomatic manifestations of myocardial ischemia. It includes non-ST-Elevation ACS (unstable angina and NSTEMI) and ST-Elevation myocardial infarction (STEMI). Approximately 50% of ACS cases are not associated with classic symptoms of pain, pressure, or a squeezing sensation across the precordium. ACS may present with atypical symptoms in women, those with diabetes or heart failure, and the elderly.

What are common causes?

ACS is generally due to rupture of an atheromatous plaque resulting in formation of an intraluminal thrombus and total occlusion of blood flow. Many plaques are associated with <75% stenosis, which would be hemodynamically insignificant on their own. Increased oxygen demand resulting from physical exertion, emotional stress, blood loss, or surgery in the presence of a high-grade fixed coronary obstruction can produce an ACS without acute plaque rupture.

What is the differential diagnosis?

Chest pressure and nausea: The differential diagnosis includes anxiety, esophageal spasm or irritation, costochondritis, pericarditis, and PE.

What symptoms might be observed?

Symptoms include chest pain or pressure, shortness of breath, palpitations, diaphoresis, nausea, and decreased exercise tolerance.

What are the possible findings on examination?

Vital signs: Tachycardia, hypotension (or hypertension), or hypoxemia.
Inspection: Acute distress with diaphoresis, increased work of breathing, and jugular venous distension.
Palpation: Extremities may be cool and clammy with cardiogenic shock.
Auscultation: Wheezes and rales due to pulmonary edema. Cardiac S_3 and S_4 may be present.

What tests should be ordered?

Laboratory tests: CBC (leukocytosis), metabolic panel (creatinine, electrolytes), coagulation panel, and serology (cardiac troponin, elevated ESR and CRP); up to 80% of cases with acute MI will have elevated troponin within 2–3 hours of onset of symptoms.
Imaging: Cardiac catheterization is the gold standard for defining coronary anatomy. Chest x-rays are helpful in assessing cardiomegaly and pulmonary edema and may also provide clues to alternative causes of symptoms, such as aortic dissection or pneumonia. TTE can identify regional wall motion abnormalities and assess overall function of the ventricles. In addition, TTE can identify complications such as acute mitral regurgitation, left ventricular rupture, and pericardial effusion. Coronary CT scans can distinguish between calcified and soft plaques, which cannot be done during cardiac catheterization, and allow for reconstruction of three-dimensional images.

Special Tests

Electrocardiogram (EKG): An EKG recorded during an episode of the presenting symptoms is helpful. ST-segment elevations or depressions and dynamic T-wave inversions and normalization that develop during a symptomatic period and then resolve with the symptoms are strongly suggestive of underlying coronary artery disease (CAD).

Diagnostic Scores

TIMI risk score: In those presenting with unstable angina or NSTEMI, the thrombolysis in MI (TIMI) risk score helps to predict the 14-day risk of death, MI, or recurrent ischemia that will require urgent revascularization. In addition, the TIMI risk score can be used to determine the urgency with which coronary revascularization should be performed.

 ACUTE AORTIC DISSECTION

Presentation

A 61-year-old male with a history of hypertension, hyperlipidemia, and smoking presents with sudden sharp chest pain that radiates to the back.

Definition

An acute aortic dissection occurs when a tear develops in the intima of the aortic wall, and blood then enters the tear and separates the intima from the media creating a false lumen. The Stanford classification categorizes dissections involving the ascending aorta (proximal to the left subclavian artery) as "Type A" and those not involving the ascending aorta as "Type B."

What are common causes?

Acute aortic dissection results from the degeneration and weakening of the medial layers of the aortic wall, thereby increasing aortic wall stress and predisposing the patient to aortic dilatation and eventual dissection.

What is the differential diagnosis?

Chest pain: The differential diagnosis includes anxiety, esophageal spasm or irritation, costochondritis, pericarditis, and PE. Also see **Table 2.1.**

What symptoms might be observed?

Symptoms include sudden-onset chest pain, "tearing" or "ripping" chest pain, syncope, or abdominal pain.

What are the possible findings on examination?

Vital signs: Tachycardia and hypotension raise concern for cardiac tamponade. Pulsus paradoxus should be performed (see Pericarditis and Cardiac Tamponade, Clinical Cases). BP in the upper extremities should be assessed, and a difference in systolic BP of > 20 mm Hg is considered significant.

Inspection: Cold, discolored skin and sluggish capillary refill may be seen in limb hypoperfusion.

Palpation: Pulse deficit in carotid, radial, femoral, dorsalis pedis, and posterior tibial arteries increases the likelihood of dissection.

Auscultation: New diastolic murmur in the aortic region increases concern for a dissection causing aortic valvular insufficiency (low specificity and low sensitivity).

Neurologic: Presence of focal deficits increases the likelihood of dissection.

● CLINICAL PEARL

Complications of aortic dissection include cardiac tamponade, acute aortic valve insufficiency, and obstruction of arterial branches by propagation of the false lumen.

What tests should be ordered?

Laboratory tests: CBC (anemia, if blood loss), metabolic panel (elevated BUN and creatinine, electrolytes), cardiac enzymes (elevated troponin, NT-BNP), and coagulation panel. If there is low clinical suspicion for aortic dissection, serum D-dimer levels of < 500 ng/mL (Sn 0.97) can help rule out aortic dissection if performed within 24 hours of symptom onset.

Imaging: Chest CT angiography with iodinated contrast is the most widely used test for the rapid diagnosis of aortic dissection (Sn 0.90–1.00, Sp 0.87–1.00) (**Fig. 2.43**). Chest x-rays are recommended in all cases of chest pain. Notably, nearly 20% of cases with aortic dissection have a normal x-ray; however, a widened mediastinum may be seen. Chest x-rays are most useful in ruling out other thoracic pathologies that may be causing the symptoms. TTE is useful in rapid assessment of the proximal aorta, as dissections in this area often cause acute aortic regurgitation, cardiac tamponade, and/or ischemia (Sn 0.59–0.85, Sp 0.93–0.96).

● CLINICAL PEARL

Almost all Type A dissections are managed surgically given that the mortality rate increases by 1%–2% every hour after onset of symptoms.

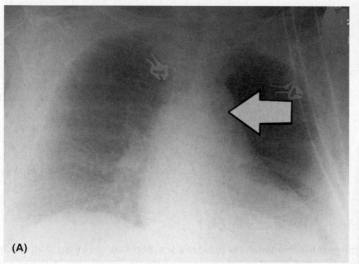
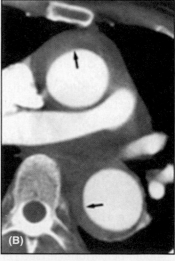

FIGURE 2.43. Aortic dissection. **A.** Portable frontal chest x-ray shows thickening of the aortic knob and medial displacement of the calcified intima suspicious for an aortic dissection (*arrow*). **B.** Axial CT image shows an intramural hematoma in the aortic wall (*arrows*).

CONGESTIVE HEART FAILURE

Presentation

A 51-year-old male with diabetes and a history of smoking presents with progressive weight gain, dyspnea on exertion, and lower extremity swelling.

Definition

CHF is failure of the heart to pump blood to meet the metabolic demands of the peripheral tissues or the ability to do so only at elevated cardiac filling pressures. The American College of Cardiology/American Heart Association has developed a system to describe stages in the development of heart failure. The New York Heart Association functional classification system conveys the severity of physical impairment due to heart failure.

What are common causes?

The most common etiologies are summarized below.

Ischemic	Risk factors for CAD: diabetes mellitus, hypertension, hypercholesterolemia, active smoking, and family history of CAD
Structural	Valvular heart disease (e.g., aortic stenosis or mitral regurgitation), congenital anomalies, and cardiomyopathy (e.g., peripartum, hypertrophic, familial, and idiopathic)
Infection and inflammation	Viral myocarditis and lupus pericarditis
Drug induced	Recreational (e.g., alcohol and cocaine) or therapeutic (e.g., anthracyclines such as doxorubicin)

What is the differential diagnosis?

Dyspnea: The differential diagnosis includes acute kidney injury, hepatic cirrhosis, COPD, pneumonia, PE, and pulmonary fibrosis.

What symptoms might be observed?

Symptoms of CHF include rest and exertional dyspnea, orthopnea, paroxysmal nocturnal dyspnea, fatigue, weakness, anorexia, and nausea.

What are the possible findings on examination?

Vital signs: Tachycardia, tachypnea, and decreased oxygen saturation.
Inspection: Altered mental status, lethargy, and confusion may be present. Cough, audible wheezes, or may appear short of breath with labored breathing; may have elevated JVP and abnormal hepatojugular reflux (Sn 0.73, Sp 0.87 for right atrial pressure > 8 mm Hg).

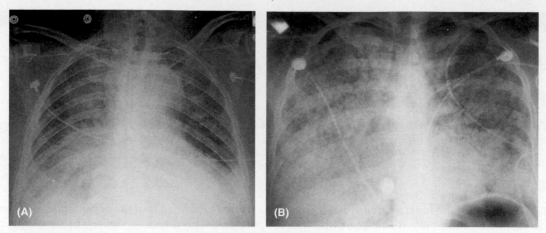

FIGURE 2.44. Pulmonary edema. **A.** Alveolar pulmonary edema is primarily central. Note the bilateral pleural effusions creating haziness in the lower lungs. **B.** Interstitial and alveolar pulmonary edema. Note the fluffiness of the densities and the indistinct cardiac borders.

Palpation: PMI may be displaced laterally and downward if cardiomegaly is present (Sn 0.66, Sp 0.96) and may have hepatomegaly (Chapter 3).

Percussion: Dullness at the bases may reflect the presence of pleural effusions.

Auscultation: Rales and decreased breath sounds may be present at the lung bases if pleural effusions are present. A left-sided S_3 is best heard in the left lateral decubitus position at the cardiac apex. An S_4 is best heard with the bell of the stethoscope over the cardiac apex.

What tests should be ordered?

Laboratory tests: CBC (anemia) and metabolic panel (hyponatremia, elevated BUN, creatinine, liver enzymes); BNP is a sensitive test in patients with dyspnea (BNP < 100 pg/mL).

Imaging: Echocardiography is the main imaging modality to distinguish systolic from diastolic dysfunction and to identify potential etiologies (e.g., MI from hypertrophic cardiomyopathy). Chest x-rays may reveal evidence of pulmonary edema (**Fig. 2.44**) such as cephalization and Kerley B lines (**Fig. 2.45**), pleural effusions, and cardiomegaly.

FIGURE 2.45. Kerley lines. Magnified view of the right lower lung showing Kerley B lines.

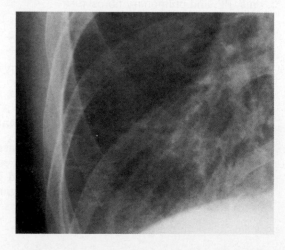

PERICARDITIS AND CARDIAC TAMPONADE

Presentation

A 53-year-old female with diabetes and hypertension presents to the Emergency Department with sharp nonexertional chest pain and progressive dyspnea for 3 days. Two weeks prior, she had a cold with fever, runny nose, and sore throat.

Definition

Pericarditis is an inflammation of the pericardium and can range from acute to chronic pericarditis, in which dense fibrosis, calcification, and adhesions occur between the visceral and parietal pericardial layers (**Fig. 2.46**). When pericarditis is associated with increased secretion of fluid into the pericardial space, it can result in cardiac tamponade. Cardiac tamponade is a state of hemodynamic compromise caused by fluid in the pericardial cavity, resulting in decreased ventricular filling; pulmonary edema; cardiogenic shock; and, possibly, death.

What are common causes?

The common etiologies are summarized below.

Malignancy	More than 50% of cases of cardiac tamponade are associated with an underlying neoplasm, with lung cancer being the most common, followed by breast and renal carcinoma, lymphoma, and leukemia.
Drug related	Medications include hydralazine, procainamide, isoniazid, and minoxidil.
Infection	Viral (e.g., coxsackievirus, echovirus, human immunodeficiency virus [HIV]), bacterial (*M. tuberculosis*, *S. pneumoniae*), and fungal infections (e.g., histoplasmosis, blastomycosis) can also result in accumulation of pericardial fluid.
Connective tissue disease	Systemic lupus erythematosus, rheumatoid arthritis, and dermatomyositis are associated with serositis.
Myocardial infarction	MI can lead to ventricular free wall rupture or Dressler syndrome.
Others	Uremia

FIGURE 2.46. Layers of the pericardium.

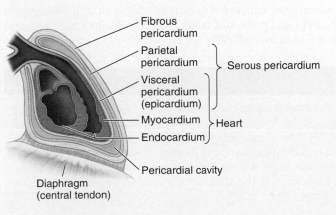

Fibrous pericardium
Parietal pericardium
Visceral pericardium (epicardium)
Serous pericardium
Myocardium
Endocardium
Heart
Pericardial cavity
Diaphragm (central tendon)

What is the differential diagnosis?

Dyspnea and chest pain: The differential diagnosis includes sepsis, MI, decompensated heart failure, and PE. Cardiac tamponade physiology has been reported with large pleural effusions and with tension pneumothorax.

What symptoms might be observed?

Symptoms include dyspnea and nonexertional chest pain.

What are the possible findings on examination?

Vital signs: Those with cardiac tamponade may have tachycardia and hypotension with a narrow pulse pressure (e.g., < 35 mm Hg). However, BP may remain normal or be slightly elevated until hemodynamic collapse occurs.

Inspection: Altered mental status and cold mottled extremities due to circulatory collapse may be present. JVP is often elevated, and breathing may be labored as a result of pulmonary edema.

Auscultation: Cardiac sounds may be muffled, and pericardial friction rub is rarely present.

Kussmaul sign: Paradoxical increase in JVP and systolic BP on inspiration. This is typically seen in constrictive pericarditis and rarely with cardiac tamponade.

Beck triad: Triad of elevated JVP, hypotension, and muffled heart sounds is present in 10%–40% of cases of cardiac tamponade.

Ewart sign: Dullness with bronchial breath sounds and increased tactile fremitus below the left scapular angle due to lung atelectasis caused by a large pericardial effusion.

What tests should be ordered?

Laboratory tests: CBC (leukocytosis), metabolic panel (creatinine, electrolytes, liver enzymes, thyroid-stimulating hormone), and cardiac enzymes (CK and troponin may be elevated).

Imaging: TTE is the first-line modality to diagnose pericardial disease. It is widely available and cost-effective, can be performed at the bedside, does not require radiation or IV contrast to outline the pericardial space, and provides critical physiologic data. Inversion of the right atrium in ventricular systole is usually an early sign of tamponade, followed by compression of the right ventricular outflow tract during diastole. With a large effusion, the heart can swing to and fro within the pericardial fluid with each beat, a finding that correlates with electrical alternans on EKG (**Fig. 2.47**). Chest x-rays can reveal enlargement of the cardiac silhouette (**Fig. 2.48**). Cardiac CT scans can reveal pericardial thickening and irregular contours (**Fig. 2.49**). If an effusion is present, attenuation measurement will enable its initial characterization. Cardiac MRI scans can provide more detailed quantification and localization of the effusion and along with CT scan can be used to guide pericardiocentesis (**Fig. 2.50**).

Special Tests

EKG: Findings in pericarditis include widespread concave ST-segment elevation and PR-segment depression in most limb (I, II, III, aVL, aVF) and precordial leads (V2–V6). Reciprocal ST-segment depression and PR-segment elevation are seen in lead aVR (± V1).

● CLINICAL PEARL

In patients with pericardial effusion, the presence of pulsus paradoxus (Sn 0.82) significantly increases the likelihood of cardiac tamponade. To assess for pulsus paradoxus, a manual BP cuff is inflated until just above the systolic BP, then slowly released until Korotkoff sounds become audible. At first, they will be audible only during expiration (BP reading is noted), but upon further deflation, Korotkoff sounds will become audible throughout the respiratory cycle (BP at the first instance of this is noted). Pulsus paradoxus is the difference between these two pressure readings and is a positive finding if >12 mm Hg.

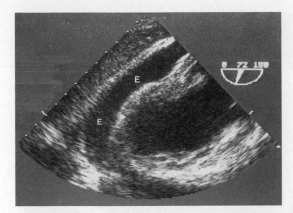

FIGURE 2.47. Pericardial effusion demonstrated on a parasternal long-axis echocardiogram image. *E*, pericardial effusion.

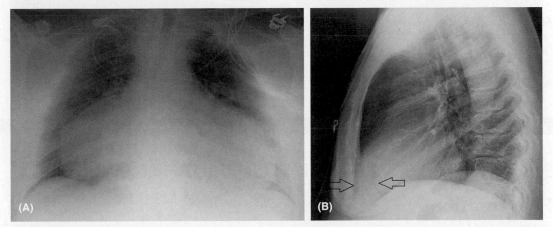

FIGURE 2.48. Pericardial effusion on chest films. **A.** Portable chest film shows massive enlargement of the cardiac silhouette or the "water bottle" heart. **B.** Lateral view shows the "Oreo cookie" sign with outer black stripes and a central white stripe that represents the pericardial effusion (*arrows*). The sign is very specific, but not sensitive.

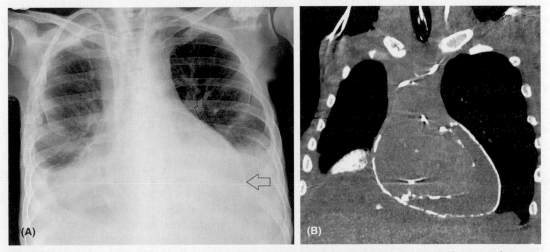

FIGURE 2.49. Uremic constrictive pericarditis. **A.** Frontal view shows thickening and calcification of the pericardium (*arrow*) due to fibrinous deposition. **B.** Coronal CT scan reveals calcification of the visceral and parietal pericardium, which can eventually result in constrictive physiology.

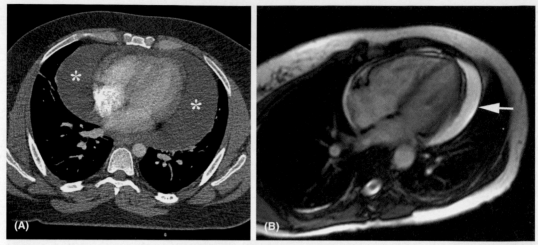

FIGURE 2.50. Pericardial effusion. **A.** Axial CT image shows a serous fluid collection (*asterisk*) in the pericardial sac enshrouding the heart. **B.** Axial MRI scan shows a bright serous fluid collection (*arrow*) surrounding the heart.

 # ACHALASIA AND DIFFUSE ESOPHAGEAL SPASM

Presentation

A 65-year-old male presents with nonradiating substernal chest pain and significant difficulty swallowing solids and liquids for the past 5 days.

Definition

Diffuse esophageal spasm is the uncoordinated simultaneous contraction of esophageal muscles resulting in aberrant propulsion of solids and liquids. Achalasia is the loss of normal esophageal peristalsis and abnormal relaxation of the lower esophageal sphincter. Both conditions cause significant dysphagia to solids and liquids and often present with chest discomfort.

What are common causes?

Diffuse esophageal spasm is poorly understood with no clear consensus on etiologies. Achalasia is an autoimmune destruction or neurodegeneration of the ganglion cells in the esophageal myenteric plexus.

What is the differential diagnosis?

Chest pain and dysphagia: The differential diagnosis includes motility disorders (achalasia, diffuse esophageal spasm, Chagas disease, scleroderma, esophagitis, gastroesophageal reflux disease [GERD], lymphocytic infiltration, and eosinophilic esophagitis), structural disorders (foreign body, tumors, strictures, esophageal webs/rings, and Zenker diverticulum), and neurologic disorders (brainstem stroke, Parkinson disease, dementia, multiple sclerosis, amyotrophic lateral sclerosis, and Guillain-Barré syndrome).

What symptoms might be observed?

Symptoms include dysphagia, chest pain, heartburn, regurgitation, belching, nausea, vomiting, and odynophagia.

What are the possible findings on examination?

The physical examination is largely unrevealing, except if occurring in the context of other disorders or systemic conditions (e.g., systemic sclerosis).

What tests should be ordered?

Laboratory tests: No specific laboratory tests. If suspicious for systemic sclerosis, then check serum antinuclear antibody (may be elevated), Scl-70, and anticentromere antibodies (elevated in sclerosis).

Imaging: Barium swallow is the gold standard test (**Fig. 2.51**). In diffuse esophageal spasm, areas of severe nonperistaltic contractions may be visualized giving the appearance of a "rosary bead" or "corkscrew" esophagus. Findings suggestive of achalasia include dilation of the esophagus with narrowing at the level of the lower esophageal sphincter, giving it a "bird-beak" appearance.

Special Tests

Esophageal manometry: This test is performed by inserting a probe along the length of the esophagus and past the lower esophageal sphincter. This probe contains numerous pressure-sensing sites at known distances from one another. As the esophagus contracts and relaxes at the level of the lower esophageal sphincter, the pressures are recorded. Findings suggestive of achalasia include lack of peristalsis and insufficient relaxation of the lower esophageal sphincter.

Esophagogastroduodenoscopy (EGD): The role of EGD in the diagnosis of motility disorders is primarily to rule out other causes of dysphagia, primarily esophageal malignancy and esophagitis.

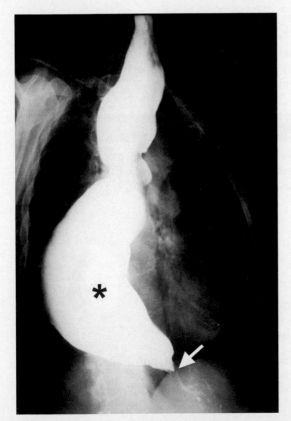

FIGURE 2.51. Achalasia. Single-contrast esophagram demonstrates bird's beak narrowing at the gastroesophageal junction (*arrow*) and upstream dilation of the esophagus (*asterisk*).

ESOPHAGEAL PERFORATION

Presentation

A 60-year-old healthy male presents with substernal chest pressure, fever, and dyspnea 2 hours after multiple episodes of nonbloody emesis.

Definition

Esophageal perforation, or Boerhaave syndrome, is transmural rupture of the esophageal wall. Intraluminal content and air leak into the surrounding space resulting in the presence of subcutaneous emphysema, pneumomediastinum, and pleural effusion. The extravasation of luminal contents into the surrounding tissue causes an intense systemic inflammatory response.

What are common causes?

The common etiologies are summarized below.

Iatrogenic	The most common cause is during endoscopic procedures when the lumen has narrowed and/or pathology is present. Common comorbid conditions associated with esophageal perforation include malignancy, GERD, achalasia, stricture, scleroderma, and hiatal hernia.
Spontaneous rupture (Boerhaave syndrome)	Occurs after vomiting or retching where increased esophageal luminal pressure causes transmural rupture of the esophageal wall at sites of weakness
Trauma	Blunt trauma to the chest rarely causes esophageal perforation. Penetrating trauma can cause injury anywhere along the esophagus.
Miscellaneous	Ingestion of foreign bodies, particularly those with sharp contours. Ingestion of alkaline substances produces more severe esophageal damage than does that of acidic substances.

● CLINICAL PEARL

Violent retching or vomiting can cause nontransmural damage to the distal esophagus resulting in mucosal lacerations. This is termed *Mallory-Weiss syndrome* and often presents with significant hematemesis due to rupture of submucosal arteries.

What is the differential diagnosis?

Chest pain: See **Table 2.1**.

What symptoms might be observed?

Symptoms include pain, dyspnea, nausea, vomiting, and hematemesis.

What are the possible findings on examination?

Vital signs: Fever and tachycardia depending on the severity of inflammation and sepsis.
Inspection: Evidence of blunt and/or penetrating trauma.
Palpation: Subcutaneous emphysema may be palpated (see Subcutaneous Emphysema, Clinical Cases).

Percussion: Dullness at the lung base indicates the presence of a pleural effusion.

Auscultation: "Crunching" noise (Hamman crunch) over the cardiac apex that is synchronous with systole and is indicative of pneumomediastinum.

> ● **CLINICAL PEARL**
>
> Neck pain and stiffness are often seen with perforation of the cervical esophagus and are less common with distal esophageal perforations.

What tests should be ordered?

Laboratory tests: CBC (anemia, leukocytosis), metabolic panel (elevated creatinine, electrolytes), and coagulation panel (INR and PTT) as may require blood products to reduce potential bleeding.

Imaging: Contrast-enhanced esophagography is the gold standard test with a false-negative rate of 10%. Barium is more sensitive than water-soluble contrast (Gastrografin), but is caustic to extraluminal surfaces and can cause fibrosing mediastinitis if a perforation is present. Chest x-ray may reveal subcutaneous emphysema, pleural effusions, pneumothorax, and/or pneumomediastinum. Chest CT findings include mediastinal or extraluminal air, esophageal wall thickening, extravasation of contrast material, and pleural effusion.

Special Tests

Thoracentesis: Pleural fluid (low pH, elevated amylase if effusion secondary to esophageal perforation).

> ● **CLINICAL PEARL**
>
> The triad of subcutaneous emphysema, chest pain, and vomiting is referred to as *Mackler triad*, which is pathognomonic of spontaneous esophageal rupture.

ESOPHAGEAL CANCER

Presentation

A 55-year-old male with a history of chronic alcohol abuse and smoking presents with 2 months of progressive dysphagia and unintentional 20-lb weight loss.

Definition

Esophageal cancer is uncontrolled growth of malignant cells originating from the lining and glandular epithelium of the esophagus (**Fig. 2.52**). Esophageal squamous cell carcinoma and adenocarcinoma are the two most common types of esophageal cancer. Squamous cell carcinoma tends to occur in the upper to middle regions of the esophagus, whereas esophageal adenocarcinoma occurs in the distal esophagus.

What are common causes?

The most common etiologies are summarized below.

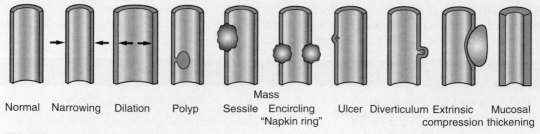

| Normal | Narrowing | Dilation | Polyp | Sessile | Mass Encircling "Napkin ring" | Ulcer | Diverticulum | Extrinsic compression | Mucosal thickening |

FIGURE 2.52. Patterns of disease and the radiographic appearances that can affect tubular structures.

Squamous cell carcinoma	Smoking, alcohol consumption, low consumption of fruits and vegetables
Adenocarcinoma	GERD/Barrett esophagus, smoking, increased body mass index, low consumption of fruits and vegetables

What is the differential diagnosis?

Dysphagia: The differential diagnosis includes achalasia, esophageal spasm, GERD, and pharyngeal infection. Also see Achalasia and Diffuse Esophageal Spasm, Clinical Cases.

What symptoms might be observed?

Symptoms include dysphagia to solids (described as a "sticking" sensation), retrosternal burning discomfort, hematemesis, and melena.

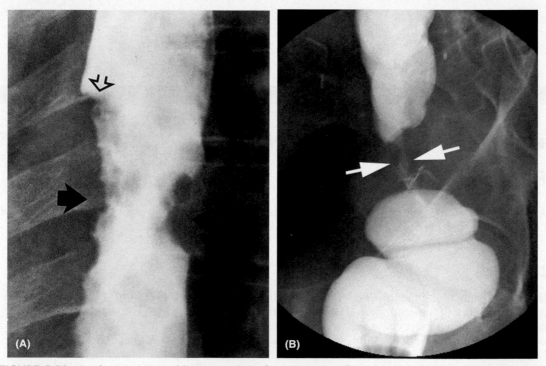

FIGURE 2.53. Apple-core mucosal lesion resulting from the circumferential growth of the tumor within the lumen of the tube. **A.** Esophageal carcinoma demonstrating the abrupt mucosal margins of the constricting lesion (*solid arrows*), termed a "tumor shoulder" (*open arrow*). **B.** Note the resemblance of the lesion (*arrow*) to an apple core lesion.

What are the possible findings on examination?

Vital signs: Typically unremarkable, although an accurate weight is required to document changes.
Inspection: May appear cachectic with sunken temporal fossae and prominent clavicles and ribs. The abdomen may also be scaphoid.

What tests should be ordered?

Laboratory tests: CBC (anemia), metabolic panel (hypoalbuminemia), and other serology (elevated ESR and CRP).
Imaging: Barium esophagography can help visualize the lumen (single contrast) and mucosa (double contrast) of the esophagus to visualize irregularities within the esophagus. Cancers of the GI tract may cause a circumferential narrowing of the lumen creating an "apple-core" appearance (**Fig. 2.53**). Endoscopy with biopsy is the primary method for the diagnosis of esophageal cancer with or without preceding barium esophagography (**Fig. 2.54**).

● **CLINICAL PEARL**

Barrett esophagus is a condition in which the normal squamous epithelium lining the distal esophagus is replaced by metaplastic columnar epithelial cells. This is most often due to chronic GERD and is a significant risk factor for the development of esophageal adenocarcinoma.

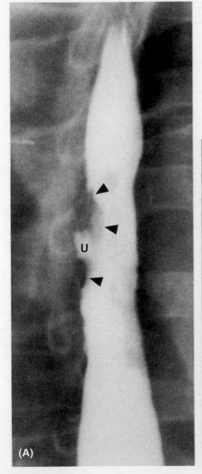
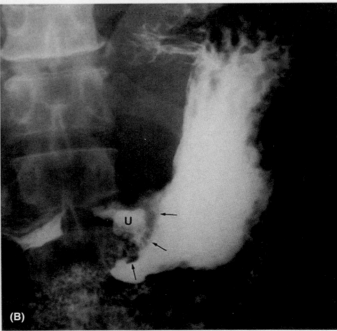

FIGURE 2.54. Ulcerating malignancy. Ulcerating esophageal carcinoma. An ulcer crater is present within the mucosal mass (*arrowheads* and *arrows*). *U,* ulcer crater.

Abdomen

JONATHAN S. ZIPURSKY • ERNEST CHIU • JEFFREY E. ALFONSI
• TANYA CHAWLA • PIERO TARTARO • SAMUEL A. SILVER

3

The abdomen is continuous with the pelvis (Chapter 4) and contains organs of the digestive, upper urinary, and circulatory systems. It is divided into intraperitoneal and retroperitoneal spaces by the peritoneum (**Figs. 3.1 and 3.2**). The intraperitoneal organs in the abdomen include the stomach, first part of the duodenum, jejunum, ileum, transverse colon, sigmoid colon, upper third of the rectum, liver, and spleen. The retroperitoneal space, which is situated external and posterior to the peritoneum, contains the adrenal glands, kidneys, aorta, inferior vena cava, pancreas, second to fourth parts of the duodenum, ascending and descending colon, and part of the rectum.

■ INITIAL EVALUATION AND ASSESSMENT

Abdominal pathology may manifest with a wide range of symptoms, and a differential diagnosis can be developed based on organ(s) most likely to be involved (**Table 3.1**) or the location of abdominal pain (**Table 3.2**; **Fig. 3.3**).

General Abdominal Examination

To further evaluate abdominal pathology, a physical examination is performed with the patient positioned supine with arms at the sides to relax the abdominal muscles. The anterior abdominal

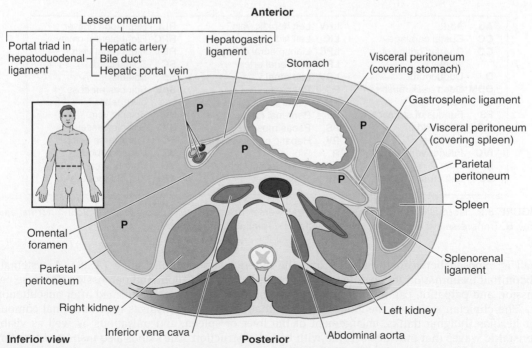

FIGURE 3.1. Transverse section of abdomen at the level of omental bursa. The orientation figure indicates the level of the transverse section. The peritoneum (*blue*) is marked *P*, and the stomach, portal triad, and spleen are seen. The retroperitoneum organs at this section include the kidneys, aorta, and inferior vena cava.

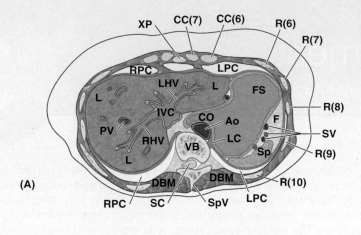

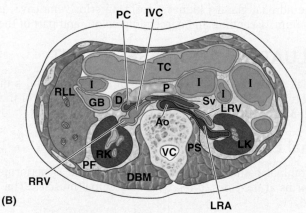

Ao	Aorta	LHV	Left hepatic vein	RLL	Right lobe of liver
CC	Costal cartilage	LK	Left kidney	RPC	Right pleural cavity
CO	Cardiac orifice of stomach	LPC	Light pleural cavity	RRV	Right renal vein
D	Duodenum	LRA	Left renal artery	SC	Spinal cord
DBM	Deep back muscles	LRV	Left renal vein	Sp	Spleen
F	Fat	P	Pancreas	SpV	Spinous process of vertebra
FS	Fundus of stomach	PC	Portal confluence	Sv	Splenic vein
GB	Gallbladder	PF	Perirenal fat	SV	Splenic vessels
I	Intestine	PS	Psoas muscle	TC	Transverse colon
IVC	Inferior vena cava	PV	Hepatic portal vein (triad)	VB	Vertebral body
L	Liver	R	Rib	VC	Vertebral canal
LC	Left crus	RHV	Right hepatic vein	XP	Xiphoid process
		RK	Right kidney		

FIGURE 3.2. Normal abdominal anatomy. **A.** Transverse cut at the T10 vertebra level depicting normal anatomy. **B.** Transverse cut at the L1–L2 vertebrae level depicting normal anatomy.

wall is exposed between the nipples and the anterior superior iliac spine (ASIS). A systematic abdominal examination involves inspection, auscultation, palpation, and percussion. Because percussion and palpation can affect bowel sounds, these maneuvers are performed after auscultation.

The clinician stands at the foot of the examination table and inspects the abdominal contours for hernias, bulging flanks, enlargement of the liver or spleen, and pulsations as well as visible peristaltic waves that may be observed with bowel obstruction. The skin is also inspected for scars, visible veins, rashes, or striae.

Following inspection, all quadrants of the abdomen are auscultated for bowel sounds and vascular bruits. Bowel sounds represent intestinal peristalsis and are typically heard every 2–20 seconds

TABLE 3.1. Causes of abdominal symptoms categorized by anatomical region

Anatomical Region/System	Symptoms
Upper GI tract (from esophagus to second part of duodenum)	Dysphagia and odynophagia (Chapter 2), early satiety, nausea, vomiting, bloating, eructation, dyspepsia, and gastric reflux symptoms (water brash, cough, retrosternal discomfort)
Hepatobiliary (liver and gallbladder)	Jaundice, pruritus, dark-colored urine, acholic stool, increased abdominal girth, and confusion
Bowel (small and large intestines)	Constipation, diarrhea, nausea, abdominal pain, change in stool caliber, hematochezia, melena, mucus in stool, bowel urgency, and tenesmus
Perianal	Pain with defecation, anal mass, and hematochezia
Blood vessels (aorta, mesenteric arteries, and veins)	Postprandial abdominal pain, hematochezia, vomiting, and sharp pain that radiates to the back
Renal (kidneys, ureters, and bladder)	Flank pain, hematuria, dysuria, urinary frequency, edema, and hypertension

TABLE 3.2. Causes of abdominal pain categorized by abdominal region

Epigastric Region

- Pancreatitis
- Peptic ulcer disease, esophagitis
- Hepatitis and liver abscess/mass
- Abdominal aorta aneurysm rupture, superior mesenteric artery syndrome, myocardial infarction (MI)

Right Upper Quadrant (RUQ) Region	Left Upper Quadrant (LUQ) Region
<ul><li>Cholecystitis, cholangitis, choledocholithiasis, biliary colic (cholelithiasis)</li><li>Hepatitis, liver abscess/mass, Budd-Chiari syndrome</li><li>Pancreatitis</li><li>Right lower lobe pneumonia/empyema</li><li>Appendicitis in pregnancy</li><li>Renal colic, pyelonephritis, infected renal cyst</li></ul>	<ul><li>Splenic infarct or rupture</li><li>Colitis</li><li>Renal colic, pyelonephritis, infected renal cyst</li></ul>

Right Lower Quadrant (RLQ) Region	Left Lower Quadrant (LLQ) Region
<ul><li>Ectopic pregnancy, tubo-ovarian abscess, ovarian torsion, pelvic inflammatory disease (PID), mittelschmerz (Chapter 4)</li><li>Appendicitis, Crohn disease (ileitis), inferior mesenteric artery ischemia, inguinal hernia</li><li>Testicular torsion (Chapter 4)</li></ul>	<ul><li>Ectopic pregnancy, tubo-ovarian abscess, ovarian torsion, PID, mittelschmerz (Chapter 4)</li><li>Diverticulitis, inferior mesenteric artery ischemia, inguinal hernia</li><li>Testicular torsion (Chapter 4)</li></ul>

Generalized Abdominal Pain

Metabolic: diabetic ketoacidosis, Addison disease, hypercalcemia, porphyria, angioedema (hereditary or acquired), celiac disease

Mechanical: small and large bowel obstruction, ileus, intussusception/volvulus

Inflammatory: inflammatory bowel disease (IBD) (Crohn disease and ulcerative colitis [UC]) and complications including toxic megacolon, fistulae, strictures, and intra-abdominal abscesses

Infectious: familial Mediterranean fever, small intestinal bacterial overgrowth

Multifactorial: peritonitis, colitis (infectious, ischemic, or inflammatory)

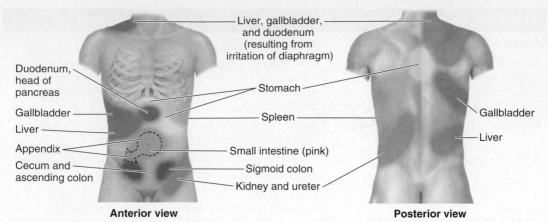

FIGURE 3.3. Location of pain based on pathology. Pain related to abdominal viscera can also be referred to the back and shoulders.

but may be heard up to 2 minutes apart. Bowel sounds may be dampened by excessive abdominal fat or peritoneal fluid. Next, auscultate for vascular bruits, which are generated by turbulent blood flows around an obstruction such as atherosclerosis, stenosis, or aneurysm. Major abdominal arteries are summarized in **Figure 3.4**.

Blood supply to the viscera of the abdomen is based on embryological derivatives. Abdominal foregut derivatives (esophagus, stomach, first and second parts of duodenum, liver, pancreas, and spleen) receive blood from branches of the celiac artery (**Fig. 3.5**). Midgut derivatives (second and third parts of duodenum, small intestine, ascending and transverse colon, and appendix) receive blood from branches of the superior mesenteric artery. Hindgut derivatives (descending and sigmoid colon and rectum) receive blood from branches of the inferior mesenteric artery. Portal venous and lymphatic drainage and sympathetic innervation parallel this pattern, coursing with the corresponding arteries as they drain to the portal vein, celiac lymph nodes, and superior and inferior mesenteric lymph nodes, and synapse in celiac and superior and inferior mesenteric ganglia, respectively.

After auscultation, the abdomen is percussed. Normally, percussion elicits a tympanic sound. Areas that sound dull may have an underlying mass, fluid collection, or organomegaly. Areas that sound hyperresonant may have free air in the abdominal cavity or excess air in the stomach or intestines. Following percussion, the abdomen is palpated. Light palpation can help identify tenderness, rigidity, and guarding, and deep palpation can help identify peritonitis. Peritonitis is inflammation of the peritoneum and may be caused by infection, visceral perforation, or trauma and constitutes a surgical emergency. Deep palpation can also detect masses in the subcutaneous fat and tissue, deep fascia, muscle (rectus abdominis or external oblique, internal oblique, and transversus abdominis muscles), peritoneum, and, in some circumstances, abdominal viscera.

Laboratory Tests

Common laboratory investigations to help diagnose abdominal pathology include a complete blood count (CBC) to diagnose infection, liver disease, or splenic sequestration of blood cells; CBC may also help diagnose a hematological malignancy. Serum liver enzymes (aspartate aminotransferase [AST], alanine transaminase [ALT], alkaline phosphatase [ALP]) and bilirubin levels may be elevated in liver or gallbladder pathology. Elevations in bilirubin have a range of etiologies beyond gallbladder pathology (Box 3.1). Gallbladder pathology can be further assessed by checking serum γ-glutamyl transpeptidase (GGT) levels. If AST and ALT are elevated more than ALP and GGT, this is referred to as a *hepatocellular* pattern and is more common in liver pathology. Note that muscle pathology can also result in an elevated AST and ALT. Alternatively, if the increase in GGT and ALP is greater than that of AST and ALT, this is referred to as a *cholestatic* pattern of liver enzyme disturbance. The kidneys are assessed by measuring the creatinine, blood urea nitrogen (BUN), and electrolytes, and performing a urinalysis. A coagulation profile is performed in the case of bleeding, if procedures and

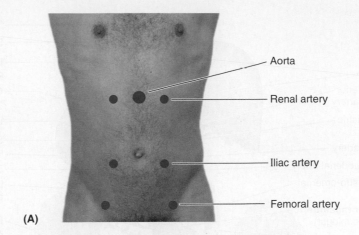

(A)

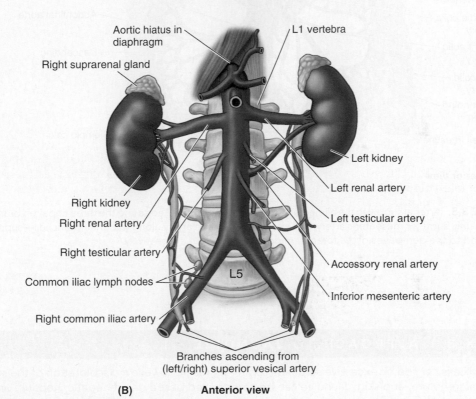

(B)   **Anterior view**

FIGURE 3.4. Arteries of the abdomen. **A.** Anatomical locations to auscultate the abdomen for bruits. **B.** Abdominal aorta and major branches. The abdominal aorta lies anterior to the L1–L4 vertebral bodies. The renal arteries usually arise at L1 vertebral body. An accessory left renal artery is present. The aorta bifurcates usually around the L4 vertebral body.

surgeries are intended, or with liver failure. Other laboratory tests and cultures of body fluids may be necessary based on the presenting symptoms.

Abdominal Imaging

Common imaging modalities for the abdomen include conventional x-rays, ultrasound, magnetic resonance imaging (MRI), and computed tomography (CT). In certain situations, endoscopic retrograde cholangiopancreatography (ERCP), percutaneous transhepatic cholangiography (PTC), and

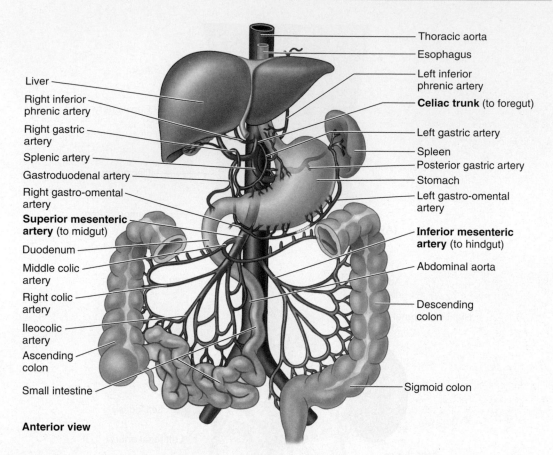

Liver

Right inferior phrenic artery

Right gastric artery

Splenic artery

Gastroduodenal artery

Right gastro-omental artery

Superior mesenteric artery (to midgut)

Duodenum

Middle colic artery

Right colic artery

Ileocolic artery

Ascending colon

Small intestine

Thoracic aorta

Esophagus

Left inferior phrenic artery

Celiac trunk (to foregut)

Left gastric artery

Spleen

Posterior gastric artery

Stomach

Left gastro-omental artery

Inferior mesenteric artery (to hindgut)

Abdominal aorta

Descending colon

Sigmoid colon

Anterior view

FIGURE 3.5. Arterial supply to the alimentary system. The abdominal aorta and the three unpaired branches—celiac trunk, superior mesenteric artery, and inferior mesenteric artery along with their branches—supply arterial blood to the derivatives of the foregut, midgut, and hindgut, respectively.

BOX 3.1 APPROACH TO JAUNDICE

Jaundice is caused by excessive serum bilirubin that results in yellow discoloration of the sclera, lingual frenulum, and skin. Jaundice can be categorized based on prehepatic, hepatic, or posthepatic etiologies. By comparing the ratio of conjugated (direct) bilirubin to unconjugated (indirect) bilirubin, along with serum assays for liver enzymes, CBC, and a peripheral blood smear, the etiology of jaundice can be determined.

Prehepatic etiologies result from an increased destruction of RBCs and metabolism of intracellular iron (heme), and the excess serum bilirubin is primarily unconjugated. Examples of prehepatic causes include hemolysis and large hematomas. Hepatic etiologies result from liver pathology or obstruction of intrahepatic ducts, and the excess serum bilirubin is a mixture of conjugated and unconjugated forms. Examples of hepatic causes include Gilbert syndrome, portal hypertension, cirrhosis, acquired immunodeficiency syndrome (AIDS) cholangiopathy, medications (e.g., tamoxifen, oral contraceptives, amoxicillin–clavulanate, cyclosporine, and azathioprine), and toxins such as ethanol. Posthepatic etiologies result from obstruction of the biliary system, and the excess serum bilirubin is primarily conjugated. Examples of posthepatic causes include gallstones, cholangitis, and malignancy (e.g., pancreatic carcinoma, cholangiocarcinoma, and ampullary or periampullary carcinoma).

nuclear imaging (e.g., cholescintigraphy or hepatobiliary iminodiacetic acid [HIDA] scan) may be performed.

Abdominal x-rays (**Fig. 3.6**) are a common initial investigation to assess abdominal pathology. One approach to reading x-rays is as follows:

1. Identify x-ray orientation (e.g., anterior–posterior, supine, or upright/erect).
2. Assess bony structures for fractures or joint space disease (Chapter 6).
3. Assess the gas pattern in the stomach and intestines. Normally, gas present in the stomach and intestines serves as a natural contrast agent to identify the location and diameter of the intestines. The small intestine is typically located at the center of the x-ray with characteristic circular rings called *plicae circulares* (or *valvulae conniventes*). The large intestine is typically located at the periphery of the x-ray and can be differentiated from the small intestine by the presence of haustra (**Figs. 3.7 and 3.8**). The normal size of the intestine varies depending on the anatomical location (**Table 3.3**).
4. Assess for free air under the diaphragm. In upright x-rays, the presence of radiolucency below the diaphragm can represent free air in the abdominal cavity and suggests that abdominal viscera may be perforated.

Abdominal ultrasound can determine the size of organs such as the liver, spleen, and kidneys and detect pathology such as free fluid, stones in the biliary system, abdominal aorta aneurysms (AAA), and hydronephrosis. Bedside ultrasound can be performed to confirm the presence of ascites. The ultrasound probe is placed at the right lower intercostal space in the midaxillary line and moved cranially and caudally to examine for fluid in the hepatorenal recess (Morison pouch), a potential space separating the right kidney from the liver.

CT scans provide excellent visualization of the abdominal organs and can diagnose conditions such as hernias, masses, abscesses, renal calculi, and gallstones. The use of oral and/or intravenous contrast can enhance a CT scan and characterize vascular abnormalities, such as aneurysms, bowel obstructions, and abdominal masses. MRI scans can also evaluate abdominal organs, particularly the liver and biliary system.

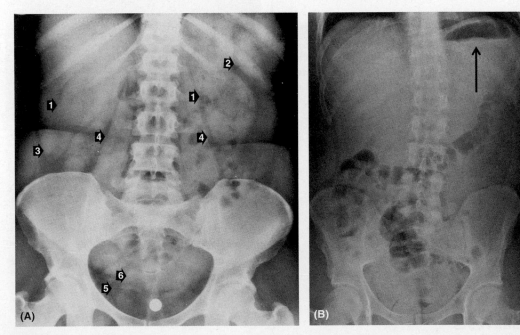

FIGURE 3.6. Abdominal x-rays. **A.** Normal supine abdomen demonstrating a normal bowel gas pattern. Although not ideal for soft tissue, the numbered arrows represent the kidneys (1), spleen (2), liver margin (3), psoas muscles (4), bladder (5), and uterus (6) are visible. **B.** Normal upright view demonstrating an air–fluid level in the stomach (*black arrow*). This is not free air under the diaphragm.

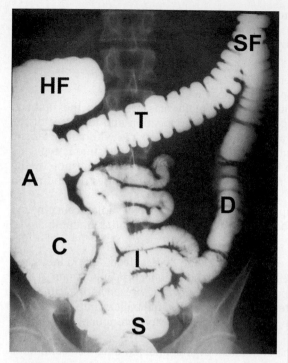

FIGURE 3.7. Barium enema showing the small and large bowel. Note how the large bowel is peripheral to the small bowel. *A,* ascending colon; *C,* cecum; *D,* descending colon; *HF,* hepatic flexure; *I,* ileum; *S,* sigmoid colon; *SF,* splenic flexure; *T,* transverse colon.

TABLE 3.3. Normal bowel size on abdominal x-rays by anatomical location	
Location	**Normal Bowel Diameter**
Small bowel	<3 cm
Cecum	<12 cm
Proximal large bowel	<9 cm
Distal large bowel	<6 cm

Adapted from Daffner, *Clinical Radiology: The Essentials,* Chapter 7.

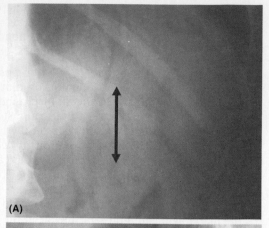

(A)

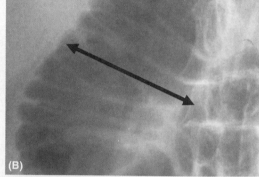

(B)

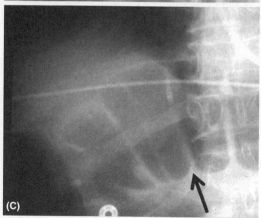

(C)

FIGURE 3.8. Radiology of the alimentary canal. **A.** X-ray of the stomach demonstrating gastric folds running parallel to the long axis of the stomach (*arrow*). **B.** X-ray of the small intestine demonstrating circumferential folds (valvulae conniventes) (*arrow*). **C.** X-ray of the large intestine demonstrating folds that go part way from side to side (haustra) (*arrow*).

Special Tests

Special investigations of the abdomen include biopsies, for example, of the liver or colon. Endoscopy may be performed of the upper and lower gastrointestinal (GI) tract to look for causes of bleeding or for malignancy. Other investigations may be specific to the presenting symptoms.

SYSTEMS OVERVIEW

◼ LIVER

Overview

The liver is divided superficially into two anatomic lobes (right and left lobes) and two accessory lobes (quadrate and caudate lobes). Typically, most of the liver lies inferior to the right hemidiaphragm and deep to the 7th to 11th ribs (**Fig. 3.9**). Nutrients and drugs absorbed in the GI tract are carried to the liver by the hepatic portal venous system.

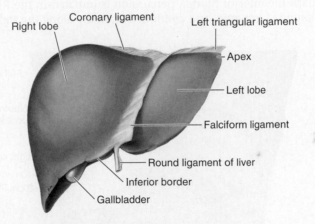

(A) Anterior view, diaphragmatic surface

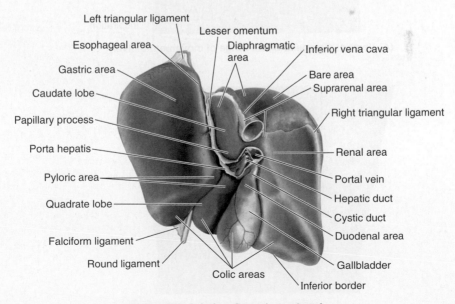

(B) Postero–inferior view, visceral surface

FIGURE 3.9. Peritoneal and visceral relationships of liver. **A.** The liver is divided into right and left lobes by the falciform and coronary ligaments. **B.** The posterior–inferior aspect of the liver.

The liver is also responsible for producing bile to emulsify dietary fats. Within the liver, bile produced by hepatocytes is secreted into the bile canaliculi and carried to the interlobular biliary ducts, the collecting bile ducts, the left or right hepatic duct, and, eventually, the common hepatic duct. The tributaries of the common hepatic duct along with the branches of the hepatic artery and hepatic portal vein form portal triads.

Physical Examination

Examination of the liver begins by inspecting for causes and consequences (stigmata) of liver disease (see Hepatitis). Following inspection, the RUQ is auscultated for vascular bruits or a friction rub; the latter may be due to local inflammation. The liver is a dense organ that sounds dull on percussion. By percussing above and below the liver borders for variations in percussion sounds, the liver span can be estimated. Percussion is initiated at the junction of the midclavicular line and right third intercostal space, where the underlying lung normally sounds resonant, and continued caudally until resonance is replaced by dullness (**Fig. 3.10**). This marks the superior border of the liver. To mark the inferior border, percussion is initiated in the RLQ, where the underlying bowel normally sounds tympanic, and continued cranially along the right midclavicular line until

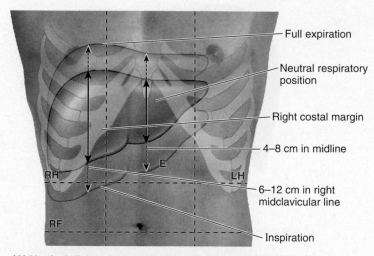

Full expiration

Neutral respiratory position

Right costal margin

4–8 cm in midline

6–12 cm in right midclavicular line

Inspiration

(A) Vertical dimensions and range of movement of liver

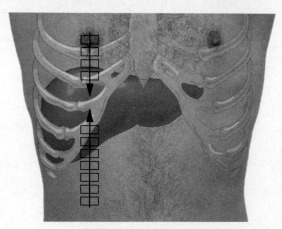

(B) Percussing liver span

FIGURE 3.10. Examination of the liver. A. Surface anatomy of the liver and its change with inspiration and expiration. *E*, epigastric region; *RF*, right flank; *LH*, left hypochondrium; *RH*, right hypochondrium. B. Percussion of the liver superiorly and inferiorly.

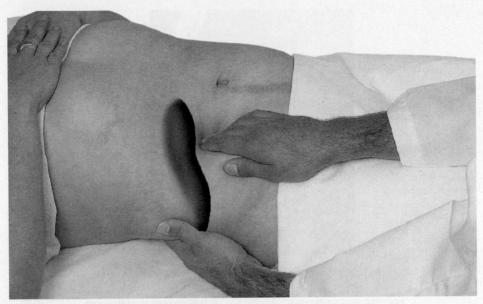

FIGURE 3.11. Technique for palpating the liver edge.

dullness is appreciated. This marks the inferior border of the liver. The distance between the superior and inferior borders represents the liver span and typically ranges from 8 to 12 cm. After percussion, the liver is palpated starting in the RLQ at the level of the umbilicus and continued cranially as the patient inspires until the liver edge is palpated (**Fig. 3.11**). If palpable, the presence of masses or nodules should be documented.

Imaging

Radiographic images can enhance the assessment of the liver. MRI and ultrasound imaging are demonstrated in **Figure 3.12**.

◼ BILIARY SYSTEM

Overview

The biliary system includes the bile ducts and gallbladder. The gallbladder is typically 7–10 cm in length and is divided into the fundus, body, and a neck that tapers and joins the cystic duct. Bile produced in the liver is stored in the gallbladder. In response to dietary fat, bile is secreted and travels along the cystic duct into the common bile duct. The pancreas and gallbladder share a common entry into the second part of the duodenum (**Fig. 3.13**).

Physical Examination

To examine the gallbladder, the clinician's fingers are wrapped under the right costal margin lateral to the rectus abdominis muscles, and the patient is instructed to take a deep breath. If this maneuver elicits pain or abrupt cessation in inspiration, the test is positive (Murphy sign) and raises concern for cholecystitis. Note that abdominal tenderness on palpation and jaundice may also be present during the general abdominal examination.

Imaging

Radiographic images can enhance the assessment of the biliary system. MRI (magnetic resonance cholangiopancreatography [MRCP]) and ERCP are demonstrated in **Figure 3.14**.

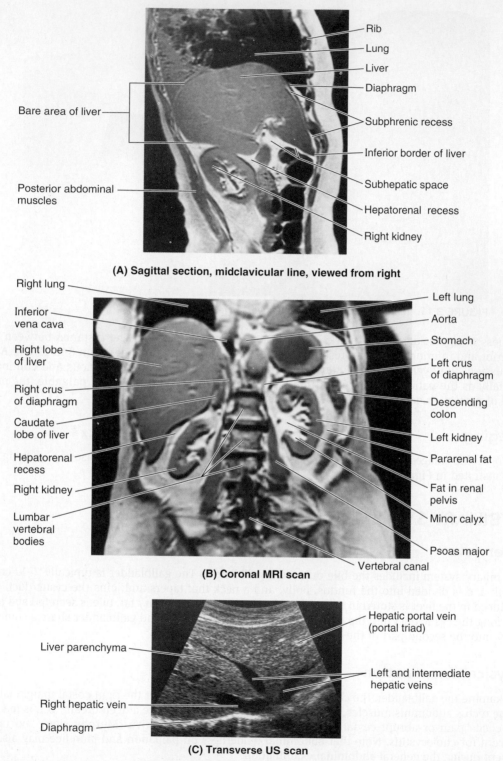

Rib
Lung
Liver
Diaphragm
Subphrenic recess
Inferior border of liver
Subhepatic space
Hepatorenal recess
Right kidney

Bare area of liver

Posterior abdominal muscles

(A) Sagittal section, midclavicular line, viewed from right

Right lung
Inferior vena cava
Right lobe of liver
Right crus of diaphragm
Caudate lobe of liver
Hepatorenal recess
Right kidney
Lumbar vertebral bodies

Left lung
Aorta
Stomach
Left crus of diaphragm
Descending colon
Left kidney
Pararenal fat
Fat in renal pelvis
Minor calyx
Psoas major
Vertebral canal

(B) Coronal MRI scan

Liver parenchyma
Right hepatic vein
Diaphragm

Hepatic portal vein (portal triad)
Left and intermediate hepatic veins

(C) Transverse US scan

FIGURE 3.12. Liver imaging. **A.** Sagittal magnetic resonance imaging section demonstrating the liver, diaphragm, lung, and kidney. **B.** A coronal magnetic resonance imaging image demonstrating the liver's anatomical location. **C.** Ultrasonography of the liver showing the hepatic veins.

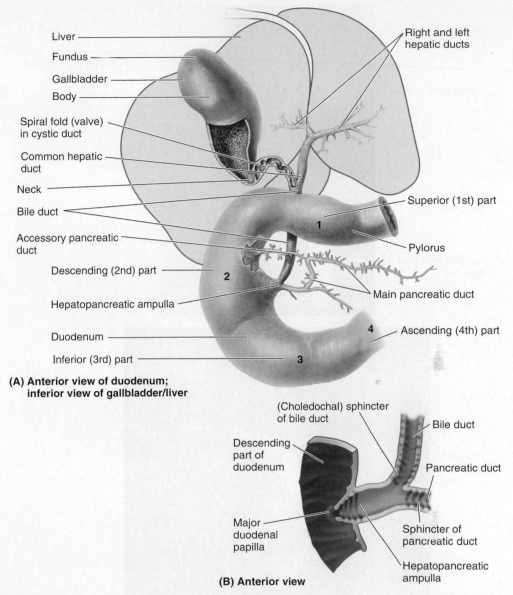

Liver

Fundus

Gallbladder

Body

Spiral fold (valve) in cystic duct

Common hepatic duct

Neck

Bile duct

Accessory pancreatic duct

Descending (2nd) part

Hepatopancreatic ampulla

Duodenum

Inferior (3rd) part

Right and left hepatic ducts

Superior (1st) part

Pylorus

Main pancreatic duct

Ascending (4th) part

(A) Anterior view of duodenum; inferior view of gallbladder/liver

(Choledochal) sphincter of bile duct

Bile duct

Descending part of duodenum

Pancreatic duct

Major duodenal papilla

Sphincter of pancreatic duct

Hepatopancreatic ampulla

(B) Anterior view

FIGURE 3.13. Biliary system. A. The gallbladder and the biliary tree in relation to the liver and second part of the duodenum. B. The bile duct and the pancreatic ducts joining the duodenum.

■ SPLEEN

Overview

The spleen is an ovoid structure inferior to the left hemidiaphragm and deep to the 9th to 11th ribs. The spleen is typically 12 cm long and 7 cm wide and is covered by a delicate fibroelastic capsule that allows for expansion. Functionally, the spleen is involved in removing platelets and old red blood cells (RBCs); for recycling their intracellular globin, heme, and iron; and for initiating an immune response to some bloodborne antigens.

Physical Examination

Examination of the spleen begins with inspection of the left upper quadrant (LUQ) for asymmetry in the abdominal contour that may represent a mass or enlarged spleen, followed by auscultation

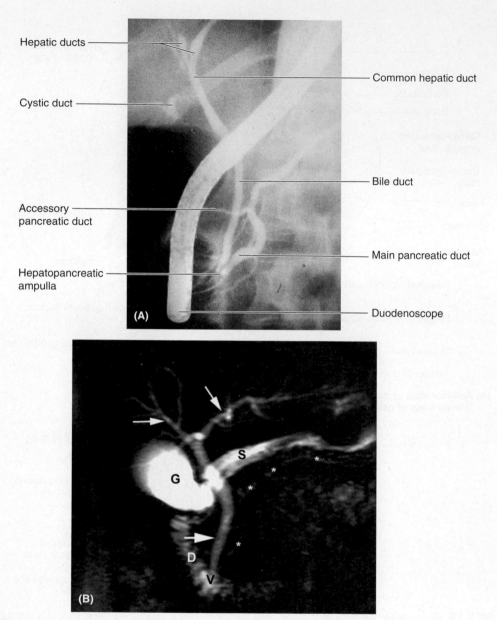

Hepatic ducts

Cystic duct

Accessory pancreatic duct

Hepatopancreatic ampulla

Common hepatic duct

Bile duct

Main pancreatic duct

Duodenoscope

(A)

(B)

G

S

D

V

FIGURE 3.14. Biliary system imaging. **A.** Endoscopic retrograde cholangiopancreatogram (ERCP). **B.** Normal magnetic resonance cholangiopancreatogram (MRCP) showing the biliary system. The gallbladder is normal. The intrahepatic ducts (*small arrows*) and the common bile duct (*large arrow*) are of normal caliber. The pancreatic duct (*asterisks*) is thin. It joins the common bile duct at the ampulla of Vater and empties into the duodenum. *G*, gallbladder; *V*, ampulla of Vater; *D*, duodenum; *S*, stomach.

for rubs or vascular bruits. Three common techniques for percussing the spleen are presented in **Table 3.4** and **Figure 3.15**.

The spleen is typically only palpable when it is enlarged. Palpation is initiated in the RLQ and continued across the abdomen toward the LUQ. Simultaneously applying gentle pressure to the left flank moves the spleen superficially and may aid in palpation (**Fig. 3.16**).

Imaging

Radiographic images can enhance the assessment of the spleen. CT scan and angiography are demonstrated in **Figure 3.17**.

TABLE 3.4. Techniques to percuss the spleen and assess for splenomegaly		
Technique	**Description**	**Performance**
Nixon method	With the patient in right lateral decubitus position, percussion is initiated midway along the left costal margin and advancing cranially along a line perpendicular to the costal margin. Dullness that persists for 8 cm or more is suggestive of splenomegaly.	Sn 0.59 Sp 0.94
Castell method	With the patient supine, the junction of the lowest intercostal space and left anterior axillary line is percussed while the patient fully inspires and expires. A change from resonance (during expiration) to dullness (during inspiration) is suggestive of splenomegaly (**Fig. 3.14**).	Sn 0.82 Sp 0.83
Percussion of Traube space	With the patient supine, the triangular space created by the 6th rib, midaxillary line, and left costal margin is percussed. Dullness to percussion is suggestive of splenomegaly.	Sn 0.62 Sp 0.72

Sn, sensitivity; Sp, specificity (see Introduction for definitions and formulae).

INGUINAL HERNIA

Overview

Inguinal hernias occur when bowel protrudes in the inguinal region. Herniated bowel that passes through the internal (deep) inguinal ring lateral to the inferior epigastric artery and veins is referred to as an *indirect inguinal hernia*. Indirect hernias are typically congenital and more frequently found in males; in contrast, a *direct inguinal hernia* lies medial to the inferior epigastric artery and veins through a weakened area in the anterior abdominal wall but also protrudes through the external (superficial) inguinal ring. Direct inguinal hernias are more likely to occur in adulthood (**Fig. 3.18**). Femoral hernias are found more commonly in women than are inguinal hernias.

Physical Examination

To examine for an inguinal hernia, the patient stands upright with feet together and hands by the side. The inguinal area is inspected for presence of a mass, which can be accentuated when the patient coughs or bears down. Palpate along the inguinal ligament for possible masses (**Fig. 3.19**).

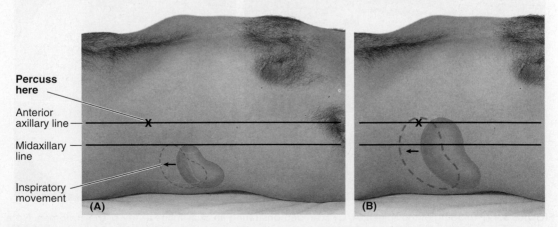

FIGURE 3.15. Percussion of the spleen using Castell method. **A.** Negative splenic percussion sign. **B.** Positive splenic percussion sign.

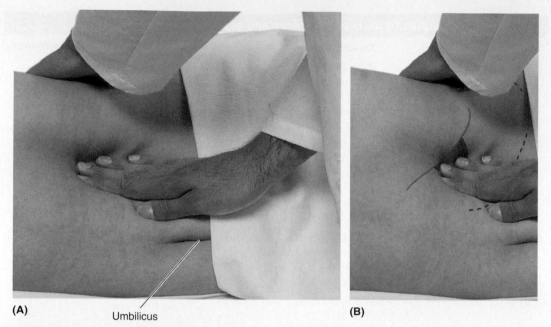

(A) Umbilicus   **(B)**

FIGURE 3.16. **A.** Technique for palpation of the spleen. **B.** The enlarged spleen is palpable about 2 cm below the left costal margin on deep inspiration.

In males, the inferior margin of the scrotal sac, spermatic cord, and superficial inguinal ring are also palpated for masses.

Hernias are described based on size, location, temperature, and reducibility. A reducible hernia can easily be returned to the peritoneal cavity by applying manual pressure, whereas an irreducible hernia cannot be returned to the peritoneal cavity. An obstructed hernia occurs when the herniated bowel is compressed causing bowel obstruction, although the blood supply remains intact. A strangulated hernia occurs when blood supply to the herniated bowel is compromised resulting in ischemia. Strangulated hernias are a surgical emergency.

Imaging

Radiographic images can enhance the assessment of a hernia (**Fig. 3.20**).

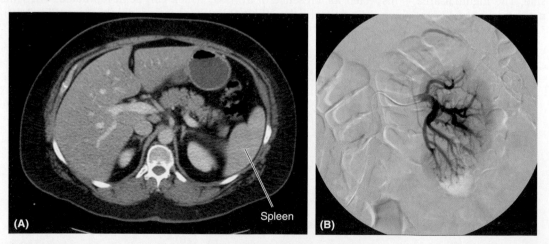

(A)   Spleen   **(B)**

FIGURE 3.17. Imaging of the spleen. **A.** CT scan demonstrating an axial image at T12 of the abdomen. Note the spleen in the left upper quadrant. **B.** Splenic angiogram demonstrating the arteries of the spleen.

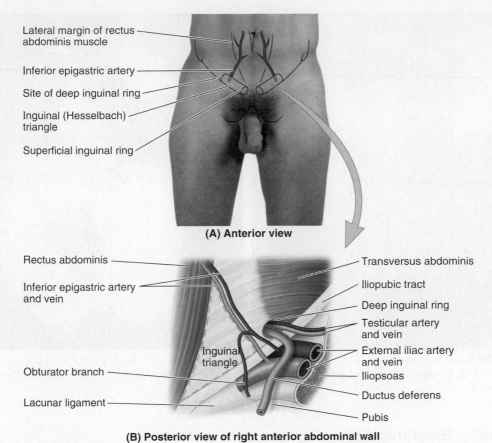

Lateral margin of rectus abdominis muscle

Inferior epigastric artery

Site of deep inguinal ring

Inguinal (Hesselbach) triangle

Superficial inguinal ring

(A) Anterior view

Rectus abdominis

Inferior epigastric artery and vein

Inguinal triangle

Obturator branch

Lacunar ligament

Transversus abdominis

Iliopubic tract

Deep inguinal ring

Testicular artery and vein

External iliac artery and vein

Iliopsoas

Ductus deferens

Pubis

(B) Posterior view of right anterior abdominal wall

FIGURE 3.18. (A) Surface anatomy and (B) anatomical structures, relevant to inguinal hernias.

■ RECTUM AND ANUS

Overview

The rectum is a 12-cm section of the colon that begins after the sigmoid colon (rectosigmoid junction). The rectum is connected to the anal canal, the final part of the large intestine.

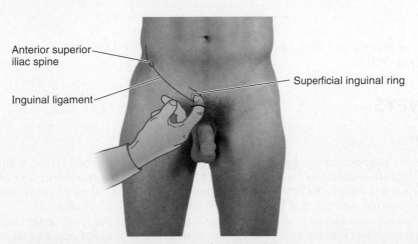

Anterior superior iliac spine

Inguinal ligament

Superficial inguinal ring

FIGURE 3.19. Examination technique for inguinal hernia.

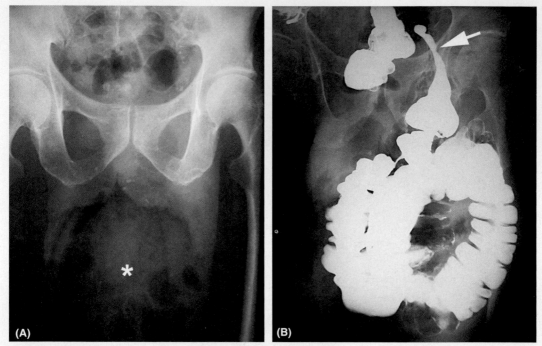

FIGURE 3.20. Scrotal hernias. **A.** X-ray demonstrating soft tissue with air in the scrotum consistent with bowel (*asterisk*). **B.** Barium enema demonstrating bowel in the colon. The neck of the hernia is narrowed (*arrow*) in the inguinal region.

Physical Examination

The anus and rectum are evaluated via a digital rectal examination (DRE). With the patient in the lateral decubitus position with knees and hips flexed, the buttocks are separated, and the anus is inspected for hemorrhoids, fistulas, or skin tags. Lubrication gel is applied to the gloved index finger, and, after informing the patient, the index finger is inserted into the anus. The wrist is rotated clockwise and counterclockwise to sweep the circumference of the rectum and palpate for masses, ulcers, or stool; an assessment of bowel tone can also be made by asking the patient to bear down. The clinician withdraws the index finger and cleans the lubrication gel on the skin. Lastly, the stool remaining on the glove is studied for blood, mucus, or fecal occult blood (FOB) using an FOB test kit. The examination of the prostate is discussed in Chapter 4.

Imaging

Imaging of the rectum and anus can be performed using CT or MRI. Barium studies can also be performed (**Fig. 3.21**).

◼ KIDNEYS

Overview

The kidneys are retroperitoneal organs that span from T12 to L3 vertebral levels, with the left kidney located slightly superior to the right kidney. The nephron is the functional unit of the kidney. The kidneys are responsible for filtering toxins from the blood, regulating blood volume and blood pressure, electrolytes, and pH, and producing erythropoietin for RBC production.

Macroscopically, the kidney is divided into renal pyramids and the renal cortex. Urine is filtered from the renal pyramids into the minor calyces via renal papilla, the major calyces, and eventually the renal pelvis before emptying into the ureter (**Fig. 3.22**).

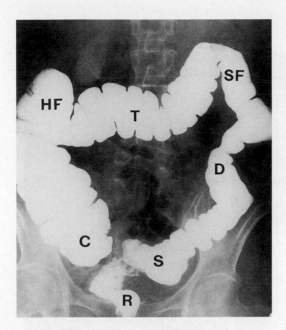

FIGURE 3.21. Normal barium edema showing single contrast. Note the rectum (*R*) at the distal aspect of the large intestine. *C*, cecum; *D*, descending colon; *HF*, hepatic flexure; *S*, sigmoid; *SF*, splenic flexure; *T*, transverse colon.

Physical Examination

Examination of the kidney begins with inspection of the abdomen and flanks for asymmetry or masses. Following inspection, the epigastric region is auscultated for vascular bruits, which may indicate renal artery stenosis. Next, the kidneys are palpated by placing one hand on the ipsilateral lumbar back to push the kidney anteriorly while palpating with the other hand for masses or

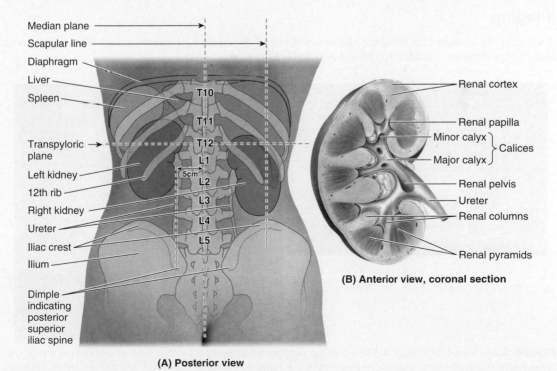

FIGURE 3.22. The kidney anatomy. A. Surface anatomy of the kidneys. B. A coronal section of the kidney showing the organ's internal structure. The renal pyramids contain the collecting tubules and form the medulla of the kidney. The renal cortex contains the renal corpuscles.

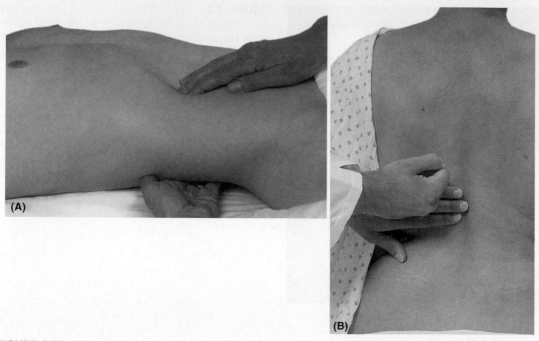

FIGURE 3.23. Physical examination of the kidney. **A.** Palpation of the right kidney. **B.** Assessing costovertebral tenderness.

irregularities (**Fig. 3.23**). The patient is then instructed to sit upright, and the costovertebral angles are percussed for signs of tenderness.

Imaging

Radiographic images can enhance the assessment of the kidney as summarized below. Common imaging modalities include ultrasound and MRI (**Fig. 3.24**).

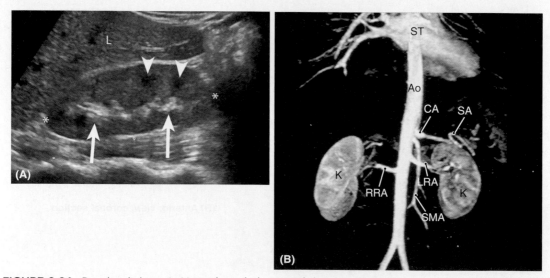

FIGURE 3.24. Renal radiology. **A.** Normal renal ultrasound showing a sagittal view of the kidney. Fat in the renal hilum is bright or echogenic (*arrows*), while the renal pyramids (*arrowheads*) are darker or hypoechoic. *Asterisks* mark the superior and inferior poles of the kidney. *L*, liver. **B.** MR angiogram of the abdominal aorta and its branches, and the kidneys. *Ao*, Aorta; *CA*, celiac artery; *K*, kidney; *LRA*, left renal artery; *RRA*, right renal artery; *SA*, splenic artery; *SMA*, superior mesenteric artery; *ST*, stomach.

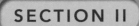

SECTION II

CLINICAL CASES

 ACUTE PANCREATITIS

Presentation

A 65-year-old male presents with sudden-onset epigastric pain that radiates to the back. He has had three episodes of nonbloody emesis.

Definition

Pancreatitis is an acute inflammatory process from direct or indirect toxicity to the pancreas (**Fig. 3.25**) resulting in excess secretion and premature activation of pancreatic enzymes that damage the pancreas. Pancreatitis causes interstitial edema and, in 5%–10% of cases, results in necrotizing pancreatitis that can become infected. Pancreatitis is classified as mild when there is no organ failure or systemic symptoms; moderate when there is organ failure that resolves within 48 hours; and, severe when there is persistent or multiorgan failure. Chronic pancreatitis is caused by recurrent bouts of inflammation leading to fibrosis and subsequent exocrine and endocrine dysfunction.

What are common causes?

Etiologies of acute pancreatitis are summarized below. Chronic pancreatitis is related to alcohol use in 70%–80% of cases.

Gallstones	Most common cause of pancreatitis; females are at higher risk than males
Alcohol	Second most common cause of pancreatitis; males are at higher risk than females
Obstruction	Physical obstruction of the pancreatic duct secondary to malignancy (e.g., malignancies of the pancreas or ampulla of Vater) and anatomic variants (e.g., papillary stenosis, pancreas divisum, and annular pancreas)
Infection	Coxsackievirus, Epstein–Barr virus (EBV), cytomegalovirus (CMV), human immunodeficiency virus (HIV), herpes simplex virus (HSV), hepatitis A, hepatitis B, mycobacteria (e.g., tuberculosis), *Mycoplasma*, *Candida*, *Cryptococcus*, *Toxoplasma*, and ascariasis
Autoimmune	Increased levels of immunoglobulin (Ig)G4 are associated with autoimmune pancreatitis and may reflect systemic IgG4-related disease
Drugs	Common drugs include didanosine, pentamidine, metronidazole, stibogluconate, tetracycline, furosemide, thiazides, sulfasalazine, 5-ASA[a], L-asparaginase, azathioprine, valproic acid, sulindac, calcium, and estrogen
Trauma	Blunt trauma or ERCP
Metabolic	Hypertriglyceridemia and hypercalcemia
Ischemia	Vasculitis (e.g., polyarteritis nodosa, systemic lupus erythematosus), cholesterol emboli, and shock
Toxins	Scorpion stings cause hyperstimulation of the pancreas leading to inflammation

[a]5-ASA: Mesalazine is a medication to reduce inflammation of the GI tract in IBD.

What is the differential diagnosis?

RUQ pain: The differential diagnosis includes hepatitis, gallbladder pathology, and diaphragmatic irritation (e.g., RLL pneumonia) (**Table 3.1**).

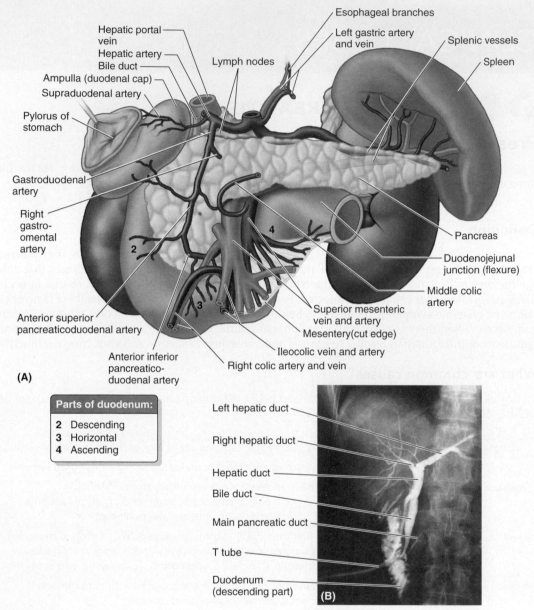

FIGURE 3.25. The pancreas. **A.** The pancreas and anatomical structures. **B.** ERCP showing the bile and pancreatic ducts.

Epigastric pain: The differential diagnosis includes peptic ulcer disease (PUD), hiatal hernia, dyspepsia, pancreatitis, and myocardial infarction (MI) (**Table 3.1**).

What symptoms might be observed?

Symptoms of pancreatitis include acute-onset (10–20 minutes) epigastric or RUQ pain that radiates to the back (**Fig. 3.26**) and is relieved by leaning forward (Ingelfinger sign), nausea, and vomiting. Dyspnea may be present in advanced disease secondary to diaphragmatic irritation, pleural effusion, or acute respiratory distress syndrome (ARDS).

What are the possible findings on examination?

Vital signs: Tachycardia, tachypnea, hypoxia, and hypotension may be present in severe pancreatitis with distributive shock.

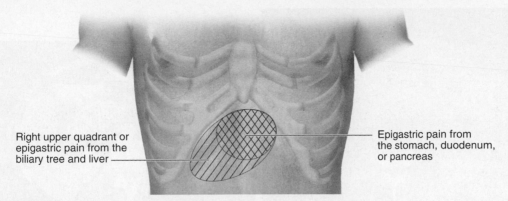

Right upper quadrant or epigastric pain from the biliary tree and liver

Epigastric pain from the stomach, duodenum, or pancreas

FIGURE 3.26. Common location of pain associated with acute pancreatitis.

Inspection: Scleral, subfrenular icterus and jaundice may be present with biliary obstruction. Signs of hemorrhagic pancreatitis caused by pancreatic necrosis and retroperitoneal hemorrhage include periumbilical ecchymosis (Cullen sign) and flank ecchymosis (Grey Turner sign).

Auscultation: Decreased bowel sounds (adynamic ileus).

Percussion: Typically normal, but dullness may indicate a fluid-filled pancreatic pseudocyst.

Palpation: Tenderness in the epigastric area and guarding; an abdominal mass may indicate pancreatic cancer or a pancreatic pseudocyst.

What tests should be ordered?

Laboratory tests: CBC (hemoconcentration may cause all three cell lines to be elevated, isolated leukocytosis); metabolic panel (amylase and lipase, the latter being more specific; elevated more than three times the upper limit of normal is highly suggestive of pancreatitis. Elevated AST, ALT, ALP, and bilirubin are seen in gallstones or physical obstruction. Elevated GGT and macrocytic anemia may indicate alcohol pancreatitis. Elevated creatinine and BUN, elevated glucose, elevated lactate, and elevated lactase dehydrogenase may indicate severity of disease; lipid panel may reveal hypertriglyceridemia); other serology (IgG4 if autoimmune pancreatitis is suspected); and urine profile (qualitative β-human chorionic gonadotropin [HCG] to rule out ruptured ectopic pregnancy).

Imaging: An abdominal CT scan is not required; however, it is the gold standard to diagnose pancreatitis. On CT scan, pancreatitis with interstitial edema will demonstrate homogenous enhancement of the pancreas parenchyma with fat stranding. A CT scan can also assess the severity of pancreatitis and possible complications, such as necrosis, infection (extraluminal gas in the pancreatic tissue), pseudocyst, or pseudoaneurysms (**Fig. 3.27**). The full effects of necrosis may take several days to manifest on a CT scan. In chronic disease, calcification of the pancreas may be seen on CT scan. Abdominal ultrasound is optimal to visualize the biliary system and determine the presence of gallstones. MRCP may be used to diagnose cholelithiasis or choledocholithiasis as visualization of bile ducts on ultrasound may be suboptimal.

Diagnostic Scores

BISAP: The bedside index of severity in acute pancreatitis (BISAP) is a widely accepted risk stratification tool for acute pancreatitis[3]. It is calculated based on BUN >25 mg/dL, Glasgow Coma Scale (GCS) score of <15, presence of systemic inflammatory response syndrome (SIRS), age over 60 years, and the presence of a pleural effusion.

● **CLINICAL PEARL**

SIRS is a systemic inflammatory state defined by two or more of the following: temperature <36°C (96.8°F) or >38°C (100.4°F), heart rate >90 beats per minute, respiratory rate >20 or PCO_2 <32 breaths per minute, and a leukocyte count <4 or >12 × 10^9 cells/L.

The sequential organ failure assessment (SOFA) is a new definition of sepsis that may replace SIRS. Other risk calculators include Acute Physiology and Chronic Health Evaluation (APACHE) II[4], Ranson criteria (evaluation at diagnosis and at 48 hours)[5], and CT severity index ([CTSI] or Balthazar score)[6].

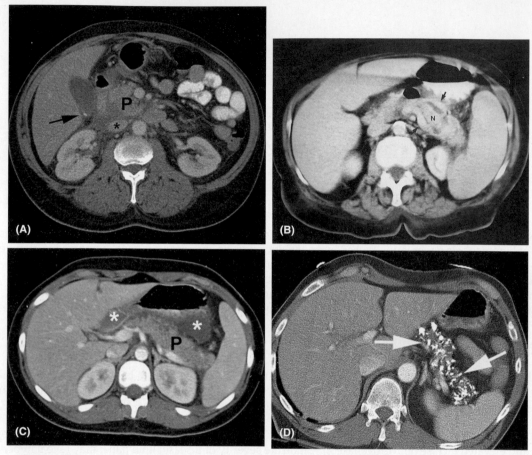

FIGURE 3.27. CT scans demonstrating pancreatitis. **A.** Axial CT image with inflammation and fluid surrounding the pancreatic head and second part of the duodenum. Also note retroperitoneum fluid (*asterisk*) and a gallstone (*arrow*) in the gallbladder. *P*, pancreatic head. **B.** Axial CT image demonstrating an enlarged pancreas (*arrows*) with necrotic tissue. *N*, necrotic tissue. **C.** Axial CT image demonstrating an enlarged pancreas with fluid (*asterisks*) anteriorly. *P*, pancreas. **D.** Axial CT image with multiple calcifications (*arrows*) of the pancreas consistent with chronic pancreatitis.

 # BILIARY TRACT DISEASE

Presentation

A 57-year-old female presents with acute-onset RUQ pain with associated nausea, vomiting, and temperature of 38.5°C (101.3°F). She has experienced similar painful attacks over the last few months, usually after consuming a large, fatty meal.

Definition

Biliary tract disease comprises pathology of the biliary system and gallbladder and includes cholelithiasis (gallstones in the gallbladder), biliary colic (gallstones that transiently obstruct the cystic duct causing pain but no inflammation), cholecystitis (inflammation and/or infection of the

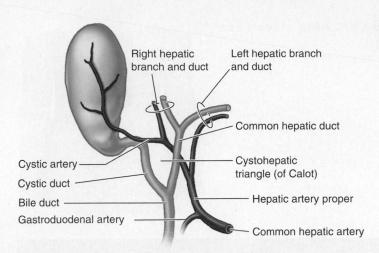

FIGURE 3.28. A simplified diagram of the biliary tree and arterial supply.

gallbladder due to obstruction of the cystic duct), choledocholithiasis (gallstones in the bile duct), and cholangitis (ascending suppurative infection of the biliary tree due to obstruction of the common bile duct) (**Figs. 3.13 and 3.28**).

What are common causes?

The most common causes are summarized below.

Cholelithiasis	Gallstones are either cholesterol based (90%) or pigmented (10%). Cholesterol stones form when bile contains more cholesterol than can be solubilized by bile salts and phospholipids. Pigmented stones are either black or brown. Black stones are formed from unconjugated bilirubin (e.g., in hemolysis, ileal resection, or cirrhosis). Brown stones are associated with intraductal biliary infections and stasis.
Cholecystitis	Acute cholecystitis is calculous in more than 90% of cases. Calculous cholecystitis is caused by an impacted stone in the cystic duct, resulting in gallbladder inflammation and swelling. Acalculous cholecystitis occurs in the absence of stones and is often caused by gallbladder stasis and ischemia in critically ill patients.
Choledocholithiasis	The presence of one or more gallstones in the bile duct.
Cholangitis	Infection as a result of bile duct obstruction. Gallstones are the most common cause of biliary obstruction. Other causes include strictures, malignancy, and parasitic infection, such as *Clonorchis sinensis*, *Fasciola hepatica*, and *Opisthorchis viverrini*. Cholangitis is a medical emergency and requires urgent ERCP.

What is the differential diagnosis?

RUQ pain: The differential diagnosis includes hepatitis, gallbladder pathology, and diaphragmatic irritation (e.g., RLL pneumonia) (**Table 3.1**).

Epigastric pain: The differential diagnosis include PUD, hiatal hernia, dyspepsia, pancreatitis, and MI (**Table 3.1**).

What symptoms might be observed?

Symptoms of cholelithiasis can range from asymptomatic to RUQ or epigastric pain (**Fig. 3.29**) radiating to the scapula or shoulder, and nausea. Symptoms of choledocholithiasis are similar to those of cholelithiasis but may also include pruritus and nausea. Symptoms of cholangitis are similar to those of choledocholithiasis, but patients are generally unwell and may be confused or obtunded.

FIGURE 3.29. Location of pain in the RUQ typical of biliary tract disease.

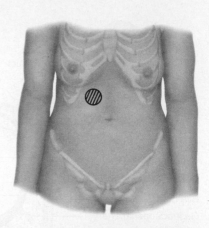

● **CLINICAL PEARL**

Cholangitis classically presents with fever, RUQ pain, and jaundice (Charcot triad). Charcot triad in association with shock and mental status changes is referred to as *Reynolds pentad*.

What are the possible findings on examination?

General: With cholangitis, the patient may appear unwell and confused.
Vital signs: Typically normal in cholelithiasis and choledocholithiasis; fever, tachycardia, and hypotension are often present in cholecystitis and cholangitis.
Inspection: Scleral icterus and jaundice may be present.
Auscultation: Typically normal; however, decreased bowel sounds may be present.
Percussion: Tenderness in RUQ.
Palpation: Tenderness in RUQ, especially in cholecystitis (Sn 0.21, Sp 0.80).

Special Tests

Murphy sign: A positive sign (see Systems Overview) is suggestive of cholecystitis (Sn 0.65, Sp 0.87).

What tests should be ordered?

Laboratory tests: Summarized in **Table 3.5**. In cholangitis, AST and ALT rise rapidly, whereas ALP and bilirubin often show a delayed rise after 1–3 days.
Imaging: RUQ ultrasound is the preferred test to evaluate for gallstones (Sn >0.95, Sp >0.95). For suspected cholecystitis, RUQ ultrasound can identify gallbladder wall thickening, pericholecystic fluid, gallbladder distention, and the presence of a sonographic Murphy sign. CT scan can also demonstrate gallbladder edema and stones (**Fig. 3.30**).

Cholescintigraphy (HIDA scan) is indicated if ultrasound is unrevealing and clinical suspicion of cholecystitis remains high. For suspected choledocholithiasis or cholangitis (**Fig. 3.31**), ERCP is used for both diagnosis and treatment. If ERCP is unsuccessful or unavailable, PTC is performed to insert a percutaneous biliary drain (PBD).

TABLE 3.5. Laboratory test results in biliary tract diseases

	Cholelithiasis	Cholecystitis	Choledocholithiasis	Cholangitis
Leukocyte count	Normal	↑	Normal	↑
Bilirubin	Normal	↑	↑	↑
ALP	Normal	↑	↑	↑
AST/ALT		↑ (<500)	↑ (>500)	↑ (>500)
Amylase		↑	↑ Mild	↑ Mild
Blood culture		Rarely positive		Positive

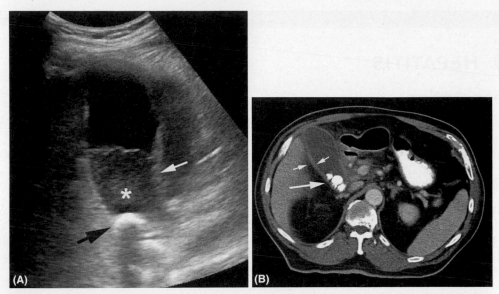

FIGURE 3.30. Cholecystitis. **A.** An abdominal ultrasound demonstrating thickening of the gallbladder wall (*white arrow*) and internal echoes representing "sludge" formed by crystals and salt (*asterisk*) along with a gallstone (*black arrow*). **B.** CT image demonstrating thickening of the gallbladder wall (*small arrows*) and multiple gallstones (*large arrow*).

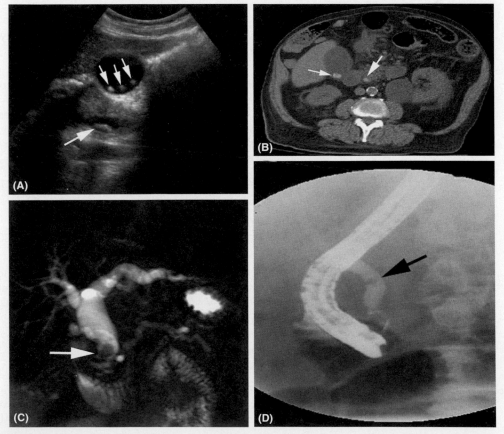

FIGURE 3.31. Choledocholithiasis. **A.** An abdominal ultrasound demonstrating cholelithiasis (*small arrows*) and choledocholithiasis (*large arrow*). **B.** Axial image of an abdominal CT scan demonstrating cholelithiasis (*small arrow*) and choledocholithiasis due to a gallstone within the distal common bile duct (*large arrow*). **C.** MRCP demonstrating a filling defect secondary to a gallstone (*arrow*) in the common bile duct. **D.** ERCP demonstrating a gallstone in the common bile duct (*arrow*). The radiolucent tube represents the endoscope.

HEPATITIS

Presentation

A 25-year-old male presents with malaise, decreased appetite, nausea, vomiting, and RUQ pain. He returned from vacation in Mexico 4 weeks ago.

Definition

Hepatitis is an inflammation of the liver. Hepatitis is a histologic diagnosis; however, it is often characterized biochemically by elevation in serum AST and ALT levels. Hepatitis is considered acute if it lasts <6 months and chronic if it lasts longer. Fulminant hepatitis is a rapidly progressing and life-threatening form of hepatitis (defined by the presence of coagulopathy [international normalized ratio (INR) >1.5] and encephalopathy) in a previously healthy patient.

What are common causes?

Common causes are summarized below.

Viral	**Hepatitis A (HAV):** Single-stranded RNA virus that accounts for 30%–45% of hepatitis cases. It is transmitted by the fecal–oral route via contaminated food, water, and shellfish. The incubation period is 2–6 wk, and the illness is usually acute and self-limited and typically does not result in fulminant hepatic failure, chronic hepatitis, or cirrhosis.
	Hepatitis B (HBV): Double-stranded DNA virus that accounts for 45% of hepatitis cases. It is transmitted via blood transfusions, via sexual intercourse, and perinatally. The incubation period is 6–24 wk, and the illness is characterized by acute and chronic phases; 95%–99% of adults with acute HBV will spontaneously clear the virus. Of those patients chronically infected, 25%–40% will develop hepatocellular carcinoma (HCC).
	Hepatitis C (HCV): Single-stranded RNA virus that accounts for 10%–30% of hepatitis cases. It is transmitted via blood (e.g., blood transfusion prior to 1992 or intravenous [IV] drug use) and less commonly through sexual intercourse. The incubation period is 4–20 wk. Of those infected, 70% will develop chronic infection, and 30% will develop cirrhosis.
	Hepatitis D (HDV): Single-stranded RNA virus that requires the presence of HBV to cause a simultaneous or superimposed infection. It is transmitted via blood transfusions, via IV drug use, or through sexual intercourse.
	Hepatitis E (HEV): Single-stranded RNA virus that causes acute hepatitis with 10%–20% mortality in pregnancy. It is transmitted by the fecal–oral route via contaminated food, water, and shellfish.
	Other: EBV, HSV, varicella–zoster virus (VZV), CMV, and HIV.
Alcohol	May be acute or chronic (mean 100 g of alcohol per day). Patients present with jaundice and liver failure. Serum aminotransferases are elevated, but <300 IU/mL; and AST is often elevated to twice the level of ALT.
Drugs	The most common cause of liver injury is acetaminophen and typically requires an ingestion of 7.5 or more grams in a 24-h period.
Autoimmune	Results in injury of hepatocytes; occurs predominantly in females.

| Vascular | Decreased perfusion of the liver secondary to congestive heart failure, sepsis, hypotension, or shock. Aminotransferases may rise to levels above 1,000 IU/mL with a rapid fall in hepatocellular enzymes after initial peak and resolution of the inciting condition. A thrombus of the hepatic veins or inferior vena cava may also cause venous congestion and cause hepatitis. |
| Nonalcoholic fatty liver disease (NAFLD) | Fatty infiltration of the liver in the absence of alcoholic liver disease; major risk factors include type 2 diabetes mellitus and metabolic syndrome. |

What is the differential diagnosis?

RUQ pain: The differential diagnosis includes hepatitis, gallbladder pathology, and diaphragmatic irritation (e.g., RLL pneumonia) (**Table 3.1**).

Jaundice: The differential diagnosis includes hemolysis, hepatitis, and gallbladder or pancreatic disease causing obstruction (Box 3.1).

What symptoms might be observed?

Hepatitis can result in a range of symptoms including RUQ pain, dark urine, acholic stool, pruritus, weakness, anorexia, nausea, and vomiting.

What are the possible findings on examination?

Vital signs: Fever, tachycardia, and hypotension may be present in fulminant hepatic failure; mental status may be altered in hepatic encephalopathy.

Inspection: Scleral icterus and jaundice.

Auscultation: Typically normal.

Percussion: Increased liver span.

Palpation: RUQ tenderness, hepatomegaly.

What tests should be ordered?

Laboratory tests: CBC (elevated WBC secondary to infection, or low platelets secondary to infection or liver failure); metabolic panel (elevated AST, ALT, ALP, and bilirubin. The pattern of liver enzyme elevation may help determine the etiology. If ALT is greater than AST, viral hepatitis or NAFLD/nonalcoholic steatohepatitis [NASH] should be suspected; if AST is elevated twice as much as ALT, alcoholic hepatitis is more likely; lactate may be elevated in ischemic causes of hepatitis; albumin may be low); coagulation profile (elevated INR); other serology (elevated brain natriuretic peptide [BNP] if right-sided heart failure is responsible for hepatitis, antinuclear antibody [ANA], immunoglobulin quantification, total protein, anti–smooth muscle antibody [ASMA], anti-liver kidney microsomal antibodies, and antiliver antibodies may be positive in autoimmune hepatitis; serum and urine toxicology screen); and viral serology (**Table 3.6**).

Imaging: Abdominal ultrasound is performed to visualize vascular abnormalities or venous thrombosis (**Fig. 3.32**). On ultrasound, increased echogenicity of the portal triads relative to the hypoechoic liver ("starry sky" appearance) and thickening of the gallbladder wall may be present. Liver CT and MRI scans are useful to detect and quantify infiltrates such as fat (**Fig. 3.33**).

Diagnostic Scores

Rumack-Matthew nomogram: Predicts the risk of hepatotoxicity when the time of ingestion and serum acetaminophen level are known. It helps to guide therapy with N-acetylcysteine.

Maddrey discriminant function: Predicts if a patient with alcoholic hepatitis will benefit from corticosteroids. The discriminant function is calculated with the formula:

$$[4.6 \times \text{PT-control} + \text{total serum bilirubin (mg/dL)}]$$

If the value is >32, the patient should be started on corticosteroids. After 7 days of corticosteroids, the Lille model[6] is used to determine if the patient will respond to ongoing treatment. The Lille model is based on age, serum bilirubin (at day 0 and 7 of treatment), creatinine, albumin, and prothrombin time (PT). A Lille score above 0.45 implies a poor prognosis and favors discontinuing corticosteroids.

TABLE 3.6. Viral serology studies for hepatitis

Hepatitis A virus (HAV)	Presence of HAV IgM antibodies (anti-HAV) indicates active infection, and presence of HAV IgG antibodies indicates prior infection or vaccination.
Hepatitis B virus (HBV)	Presence of HBV surface antigen (HBsAg) indicates active or chronic infection; HBV surface antibody (anti-HBs) indicates prior infection or vaccination. HBV core antibody (IgM anti-HBc) indicates active infection and is the earliest antibody detectable. If either anti-HBc or HBsAg is positive, then HBe antigen (HBeAg) and antibody (anti-HBe) and HBV DNA should be measured to determine infectivity.
Hepatitis C virus (HCV)	Presence of HCV antibodies (anti-HCV) indicates active infection. If positive, HCV viral load (RNA level) and HCV genotype should be measured for prognosis and to plan treatment.
Hepatitis D virus (HDV)	Presence of HDV antibodies (anti-HDV) antibody indicates active infection.
Hepatitis E virus (HEV)	Presence of HEV antibodies (IgM anti-HEV) indicates active infection.
Other	Serology for HSV, VZV, EBV, CMV, and HIV

IgM, immunoglobulin M; *HSV*, herpes simplex virus; *VZV*, varicella-zoster virus; *EBV*, Epstein-Barr virus; *CMV*, cytomegalovirus; *HIV*, human immunodeficiency virus.

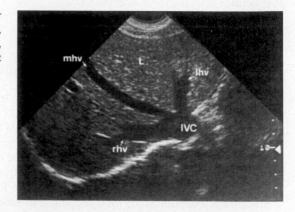

FIGURE 3.32. Abdominal ultrasound of the liver demonstrating the hepatic veins, liver parenchyma, and diaphragm. *L*, liver; *IVC*, inferior vena cava; *rhv*, right hepatic vein; *mhv*, middle hepatic vein; *lhv*, left hepatic vein.

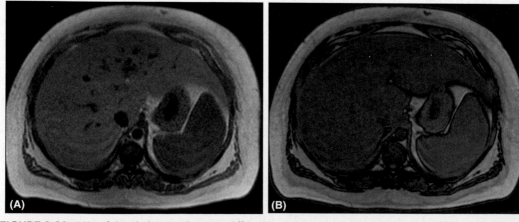

FIGURE 3.33. MRI of the abdomen showing diffuse hepatic steatosis. T1-weighted images are performed in **(A)** and out **(B)** of phase to highlight microscopic fat (steatosis).

CIRRHOSIS

Presentation

A 52-year-old male presents with fatigue, weakness, and abdominal distention. He has a history of hepatitis C.

Definition

Cirrhosis is the histologic development of regenerative nodules surrounded by fibrous bands, in response to chronic liver injury, that leads to portal hypertension and end-stage liver disease (**Fig. 3.34**).

What are common causes?

Common causes are summarized below.

Alcohol (60%–70%)	Alcohol is the most common cause of cirrhosis and typically results in tiny regenerative nodules (micronodular cirrhosis).
Viral hepatitis (10%)	Chronic hepatitis B, C, and D infection.
Autoimmune hepatitis[2]	Autoimmune process leading to cirrhosis, with liver biopsy revealing plasma cell infiltrates. This is more common in females.
Metabolic diseases (5%)	Hereditary hemochromatosis: a recessive disorder of iron sensing and transport leading to tissue iron overload. Most patients (85%) have mutations in the HFE gene (C282Y or H63D alleles).
	Wilson disease: a recessive disorder leading to impaired copper transport and copper overload. Patients often have a mutation in the ATP7B gene.
	α_1-antitrypsin deficiency: an autosomal disorder resulting in abnormal α_1-antitrypsin protein that polymerizes in the liver causing cirrhosis; also affects lung tissue leading to emphysema.
Vascular diseases	Right-sided heart failure, constrictive pericarditis, and Budd-Chiari syndrome lead to chronic venous congestion and cirrhosis.
NAFLD (10%–15%)	The most common cause of cryptogenic cirrhosis, often seen in patients who are obese or meet criteria for the metabolic syndrome.
Biliary tract diseases	Primary biliary cirrhosis, primary sclerosing cholangitis, and secondary biliary cirrhosis (e.g., strictures, cholelithiasis, neoplasm, and biliary atresia).
Drugs	Toxins (e.g., acetaminophen, nonsteroidal anti-inflammatory drugs [NSAIDs], methotrexate, and isoniazid).

What is the differential diagnosis?

Ascites: Ascites is a common finding in cirrhosis. Analyzing the ascitic fluid with paracentesis can help narrow the differential diagnosis. Ascitic fluid is checked for infection based on cell count, Gram stain, and culture and sensitivity; malignancy based on cytology; and etiology based on biochemistry (specifically albumin). The serum ascites albumin gradient (SAAG) is calculated by subtracting the serum albumin level by the ascites albumin level.

FIGURE 3.34. Nodular appearance of the surface of the liver secondary to cirrhosis.

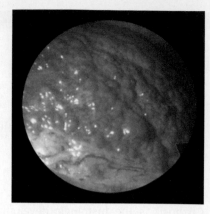

SAAG = (serum albumin) − (albumin level of ascitic fluid)

When the SAAG is >1.1 g/dL (>11 mmol/L) (transudative), portal hypertension forces fluid into the perineum. Causes include acute hepatitis, heart failure, Budd-Chiari syndrome, portal or splenic vein thrombosis, and cirrhosis.

When the SAAG is <1.1 g/dL (<11 mmol/L) (exudative), nonportal hypertension related or causes of ascites include peritonitis (e.g., tuberculosis or a ruptured viscous), peritoneal carcinomatosis, reduced albumin states (e.g., nephrotic syndrome, protein-losing enteropathy, or malnutrition), Meigs syndrome (a benign ovarian tumor with ascites and pleural effusion), lymphatic leak, and bowel obstruction or infarction.

What symptoms might be observed?

Symptoms of cirrhosis include anorexia, pruritus, fatigue, easy bleeding and bruising, abdominal and leg swelling, and shortness of breath.

What are the possible findings on examination?

Vital signs: Tachycardia, hypotension, and fever may be present especially with a GI bleed or infection.

Inspection: Scleral icterus or jaundice (Sn 0.28, Sp 0.93); inspect for signs of excess estradiol that include palmar erythema (Sn 0.46, Sp 0.91), spider angioma (Sn 0.46, Sp 0.89) (**Fig. 3.35**A), frontal balding, gynecomastia (Sn 0.18–0.58, Sp 0.98), and testicular atrophy (Sn 0.18, Sp 0.97); inspect the hands for clubbing, hypertrophic osteoarthropathy, and Dupuytren contractures; inspect the nails for Muehrcke lines and Terry nails (Sn 0.44, Sp 0.98) (**Fig. 3.35**B); inspect the abdomen for caput medusa (**Fig. 3.35**C) and bulging flanks (Sn 0.81, Sp 0.59)[7] or distention; and inspect the lower extremity for edema (Sn 0.37, Sp 0.90).

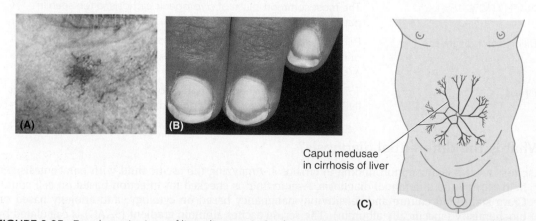

Caput medusae
in cirrhosis of liver

FIGURE 3.35. Extrahepatic signs of liver disease. A. Spider angioma. B. Terry nails. C. Caput medusae.

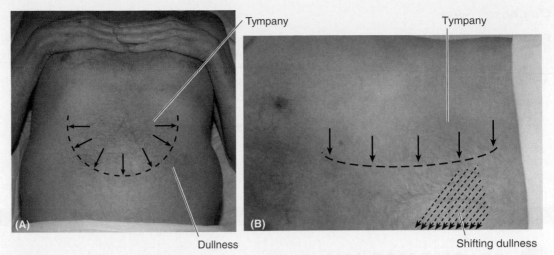

FIGURE 3.36. Physical examination of the abdomen for ascites. **A.** Ascites causing bulging flanks on inspection. On percussion, dullness will be heard over the flanks secondary to ascitic fluid. **B.** When the patient rolls to one side, ascitic fluid will shift based on gravity, which will change the location at which percussion changes from tympanic to dull. This is referred to as *shifting dullness*.

Auscultation: Bowel sounds may appear distant in the presence of ascites.

Percussion: RUQ dullness may be present with hepatomegaly (Sn 0.74, Sp 0.69), LUQ dullness may be present with splenomegaly, and flank dullness may be present with ascites (**Fig. 3.36**).

Palpation: Liver nodules along the edge of the liver (Sn 0.73, Sp 0.81), hepatomegaly, and/or splenomegaly.

Special Tests

Digital rectal examination: Hemorrhoids and hematochezia may be present in an acute GI bleed.

What tests should be ordered?

Laboratory tests: CBC (neutropenia, anemia, thrombocytopenia), metabolic panel (elevated bilirubin, AST, ALT; serum sodium may be low and creatinine may be elevated secondary to decreased renal perfusion; low glucose may occur in advanced disease), coagulation profile (elevated INR), and other serology (tests for viral hepatitis [see Hepatitis] and metabolic diseases such as HFE gene mutation for hemochromatosis, reduced serum ceruloplasmin for Wilson disease, and α_1-antitrypsin gene testing).

Imaging: Abdominal ultrasound is performed to confirm the presence of cirrhosis, portal hypertension, alterations in portal blood flow, or evidence of a portal vein thrombosis. Ultrasound is also used to screen for HCC. CT or MRI scans are ordered to monitor sequelae of cirrhosis and definitively diagnose HCC. Fibroscan or transient elastography is a small ultrasound probe used to noninvasively assess liver stiffness. Scores above 6 kPa indicate fibrosis and scores above 14 kPa indicate cirrhosis.

Special Tests

Paracentesis: Is used to diagnose the cause of ascites and spontaneous bacterial peritonitis based on an ascites neutrophil count above 250 cell/mm³ or a positive bacterial culture. Paracentesis should be performed on all patients with new ascites or a change in clinical status.

Endoscopy: Is performed in all patients diagnosed with cirrhosis to screen for esophageal and gastric varices.

Biopsy: Percutaneous or transjugular liver biopsy is the gold standard for diagnosing cirrhosis.

Diagnostic Score

FibroTest: Predicts the degree of hepatic fibrosis using α-2-macroglobulin, GGT, ALT, haptoglobin, apolipoprotein A1, and total bilirubin. The score has been validated in patients with cirrhosis secondary to chronic HBV/HCV, alcohol, and NAFLD/NASH.

AST to platelet ratio index (APRI): Predicts the likelihood of cirrhosis in hospitalized patients with hepatitis C, HIV, or chronic alcoholic ingestion. It is calculated using the formula:

$$[(AST/ULN \text{ of } AST)/\text{platelet count}] \times 100$$

A score >1.0 implies cirrhosis (Sn 0.76, Sp 0.72).

SPLENOMEGALY

Presentation

A 20-year-old female presents to her health care provider with fatigue, swollen cervical lymph nodes, and a sore throat. During the abdominal examination, an enlarged spleen was suspected.

Definition

Splenomegaly is a spleen that is heavier than 250 g or larger than 12 × 7 cm on diagnostic imaging.

What are common causes?

Common causes are summarized below.

Increased splenic function	Removal of defective RBCs secondary to spherocytosis, hemoglobinopathies such as α and β thalassemias and sickle cell anemia, and nutritional anemia (e.g., vitamin B$_{12}$, folate, and iron deficiency)
	Infection: bacterial (e.g., typhoid, brucellosis, leptospirosis, tuberculosis, and ehrlichiosis), viral (e.g., mononucleosis, HIV, and hepatitis), fungal (histoplasmosis), and parasitic (e.g., malaria, leishmaniasis, trypanosomiasis, schistosomiasis, and echinococcosis)
	Disordered immunoregulation may occur in connective tissue disease (e.g., rheumatoid arthritis and lupus), serum sickness, autoimmune hemolytic anemia, sarcoidosis, and adverse drug reactions
	Extramedullary hematopoiesis secondary to decreased bone marrow function related to myelofibrosis, bone marrow infiltration, or bone marrow damage from medications or radiation
Abnormal splenic blood flow	Venous congestion secondary to thrombosis of the hepatic vein, portal vein, or splenic vein; cirrhosis
Infiltration of the spleen	Metabolic diseases (e.g., Gaucher disease, Niemann-Pick disease, and amyloidosis)
	Malignant infiltration secondary to leukemia, lymphoma, myeloproliferative disease, and metastases (e.g., from malignant melanoma)
	Benign infiltration secondary to hemangioma, lymphangioma, splenic cysts, and hamartoma

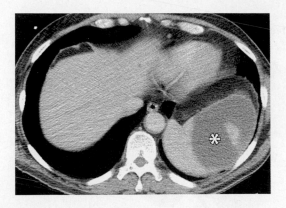

FIGURE 3.37. An axial image from a contrast-enhanced CT scan of the upper abdomen demonstrating splenomegaly on the left side of the slice (*asterisk*).

What is the differential diagnosis?

Splenomegaly: See common causes.

What symptoms might be observed?

Symptoms of splenomegaly may include LUQ or shoulder (referred) pain, early satiety, fatigue, easy bruising, and bleeding.

What are the possible findings on examination?

Vital signs: Typically normal; however, fever may be present.
Inspection: LUQ mass may be present.
Auscultation: Typically normal; however, vascular bruits or a rub in the LUQ.
Percussion: Dullness in the LUQ (Chapter 1).
Palpation: Spleen edge may be palpated in the RLQ or LUQ.

What tests should be ordered?

Laboratory tests: CBC (leukocytosis or leukopenia, anemia, thrombocytopenia; peripheral blood smear may reveal fragmented RBCs and/or schistocytes), metabolic panel (low haptoglobin, elevated bilirubin, and lactate dehydrogenase [LDH] in hemolysis. An elevated LDH may also be seen in lymphoma. Elevated liver enzymes may indicate hepatic congestion), and microbiology (blood cultures for infectious etiologies).
Imaging: Abdominal ultrasound is the gold standard for assessing the size of the spleen. Ultrasound can also look for venous thrombosis. CT (**Fig. 3.37**), MRI, or PET scans can confirm splenomegaly and identify other intra-abdominal pathology.

 # PEPTIC ULCER DISEASE

Presentation

A 42-year-old male presents to the Emergency Department with intermittent epigastric pain that resolves with eating. He has noticed intermittent black tarry stools over the past 2 weeks.

Definition

PUD is a break in the mucosa with perceptible depth that develops in the stomach or duodenum. Ulcers are four times more common in the duodenum than in the stomach and can cause significant upper GI bleeding, perforation, or obstruction (**Fig. 3.38**).

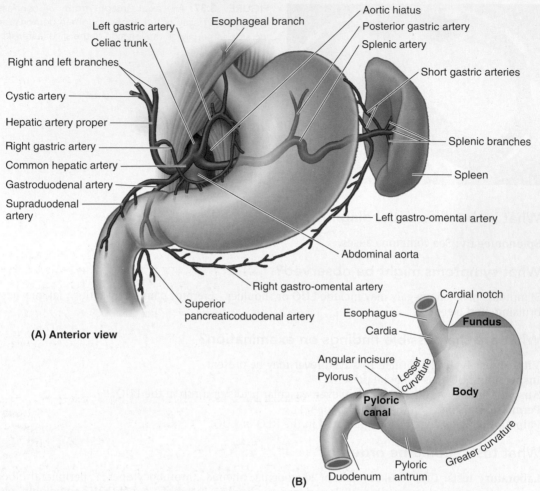

FIGURE 3.38. The stomach. **A.** Arterial supply to the stomach, duodenum, and spleen, which arise from the celiac artery. **B.** Anatomical parts of the stomach.

What are common causes?

Common causes are summarized below.

Helicobacter pylori	H. pylori causes 80% of duodenal and 60% of gastric ulcers. Approximately 50% of the population worldwide is colonized with H. pylori; however, only 5%–10% will develop PUD.
NSAIDs	NSAIDs inhibit cyclooxygenase, a set of enzymes that regulate prostaglandin production; prostaglandins are involved in gastric protection, and inhibiting their production can lead to erosion and ulcers.
Malignancy	Adenocarcinoma, GI stromal tumors ([GISTs] or masses that arise from the interstitial cells of Cajal), and lymphoma account for 5%–10% of gastric ulcers.
Hypersecretory states	Zollinger-Ellison syndrome [ZES] (gastrin-secreting tumor that stimulates parietal cells in the stomach to secrete acid) and carcinoid tumor (neuroendocrine tumor that releases substances such as serotonin into the bloodstream) are less common causes of ulcers related to increased acid production.
Other	Other etiologies include critical illness, smoking, viral infections (e.g., CMV and HSV), radiation-induced ulcers, Crohn disease, nasogastric tubes, hiatal hernias (Cameron lesion), and drugs (e.g., steroids, chemotherapy, spironolactone, and high-dose acetaminophen).

What is the differential diagnosis?

Dyspepsia: The differential diagnosis includes functional dyspepsia, malignancy (e.g., gastric carcinoma and mucosa-associated lymphoid tissue [MALT]), inflammatory disease (e.g., celiac or Crohn disease), drug-induced dyspepsia (commonly associated with NSAIDs, theophylline, caffeine, and alcohol), esophagitis, granulomatosis with polyangiitis (formerly Wegener granulomatosis), Ménétrier disease (causes hyponatremic hypertrophic gastritis), and mycobacterial infection of the stomach and/or duodenum.

Upper GI bleed: The differential diagnosis includes esophageal or gastric varices, esophagitis, gastritis, PUD, Mallory-Weiss tear, Dieulafoy lesion, gastric antral vascular ectasia ([GAVE] or watermelon stomach), GI angiodysplasia, GI malignancy, and an aortoenteric fistula.

What symptoms might be observed?

Symptoms of PUD include pain that may be alleviated (duodenal ulcer) or exacerbated (gastric ulcer) by food, dyspepsia, early satiety, nausea, and vomiting.

What are the possible findings on examination?

Vital signs: Tachycardia, hypotension, or orthostatic changes may be present with GI bleeding.
Inspection: Abdominal distention may be present with gastric or intestinal perforation.
Auscultation: Typically normal or reduced bowel sounds.
Percussion: Tenderness or hyperresonance may be present with gastric or intestinal perforation.
Palpation: Epigastric tenderness.

What tests should be ordered?

Laboratory tests: CBC (anemia), metabolic panel (elevated BUN, elevated creatinine), coagulation profile (elevated INR or partial thromboplastin time [PTT] may require reversal of anticoagulation), microbiology (*H. pylori* serology [Sn >0.80, Sp >0.90] to diagnose first-time infection but not repeat infections as serology will often remain positive; rapid urease breath test for active infection if patient is not on a proton pump inhibitor [PPI]; *H. pylori* stool antigen is not indicated for diagnosis but can help to confirm eradication).
Imaging: Upright abdominal x-ray may reveal free air under the diaphragm if the ulcer has caused a perforation. Ulcers can be visualized on an upper GI series with barium contrast (**Fig. 3.39**). Rarely, a CT scan is ordered to identify complications related to ulcers, such as hemorrhage, perforation, fistulas, and gastric outlet obstruction (**Fig. 3.40**).

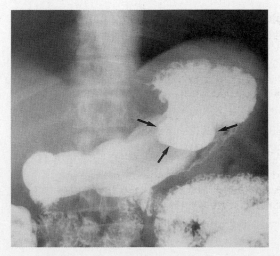

FIGURE 3.39. Upper gastrointestinal series, which consists of x-rays or fluoroscopy, enhanced with oral barium contrast. A large gastric ulcer is visible (*arrows*).

FIGURE 3.40. An axial image from an abdominal CT scan of a perforated duodenal ulcer. The image is enhanced with oral contrast that is visible in the duodenal bulb. Contrast is seen spilling out around the liver (*small arrows*). There is also a small amount of free air or pneumoperitoneum visible (*large arrow*). D, duodenal bulb.

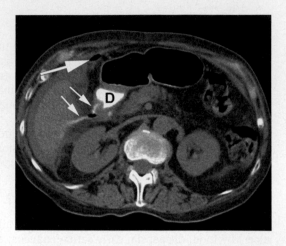

Special Tests

Endoscopy: Upper endoscopy (esophagogastroduodenoscopy) is required to make a definitive diagnosis of PUD and perform biopsies for *H. pylori* or malignancy. The morphology and location of the ulcer can help to discriminate benign from malignant ulcers. Benign ulcers are typically located on the lesser curve of the stomach, posterior wall, or antrum and have a well-defined mucosal defect with smooth, radiating folds.

BOWEL OBSTRUCTION

Presentation

A 78-year-old female presents to the Emergency Department with 1 day of abdominal pain and distention, along with numerous episodes of vomiting. She has had several abdominal surgeries including a cholecystectomy, hernia repair, and hysterectomy.

Definition

A bowel obstruction occurs when the flow of intraluminal contents is interrupted by a mechanical obstruction. Obstruction leads to dilation of the intestine proximal to the blockage and decompression and collapse distal to the blockage.

What are common causes?

Common causes are summarized below.

Small bowel obstruction	Adhesions are the most common cause (70%); prior surgery and IBD are major risk factors. Other causes include malignancy of the small and large bowel, lymphoma, ovarian cancer, sarcoma, and peritoneal carcinomatosis, hernias, and volvulus (**Fig. 3.41**). Less common causes may be related to endometriosis, congenital malformations, radiation-induced strictures, intussusception, gallstones, bezoar, foreign bodies, and parasites (e.g., *Ascaris lumbricoides* and *Strongyloides stercoralis*).
Large bowel obstruction	Tumors are the most common cause; other causes include adhesions and volvulus.

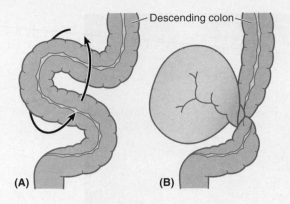

FIGURE 3.41. Diagrammatic representation of a volvulus. **(A)** Formation of volvulus. **(B)** Volvulus.

What is the differential diagnosis?

Bowel obstruction: The differential diagnosis includes constipation, adynamic ileus, toxic megacolon, and acute colonic pseudo-obstruction (Ogilvie syndrome).

What symptoms might be observed?

Symptoms of small bowel obstruction include cramping, colicky periumbilical abdominal pain, abdominal distention, nausea and vomiting (may be feculent), obstipation, and anorexia. Symptoms of large bowel obstruction include lower abdominal pain (between the umbilicus and pubic tubercle) and obstipation.

What are the possible findings on examination?

Vital signs: Tachycardia, hypotension, and fever may be present in bowel ischemia, necrosis, or perforation.
Inspection: Prior surgical scars or hernias may explain the cause of the obstruction.
Auscultation: Acute obstruction is characterized by high-pitched "tinkling" bowel sounds on auscultation; with progression, the lumen distends and bowel sounds may become hypoactive.
Percussion: Bowel distention causes hyperresonance; dullness if fluid-filled bowel is present.
Palpation: Pain, masses may be present with an abscess, tumor, volvulus, or hernia.

Special Tests

Digital rectal examination: Stool impaction or palpable rectal mass.

What tests should be ordered?

Laboratory tests: CBC (leukocytosis, anemia), metabolic panel (hyponatremia, hypokalemia, elevated creatinine, elevated lactate may represent ischemic bowel or sepsis; arterial blood gas may reveal metabolic acidosis), and microbiology (blood cultures).
Imaging: Abdominal x-rays (Sn 0.64–0.79, Sp 0.82–0.83) should be performed to diagnose a bowel obstruction (Chapter 1) (**Fig. 3.42**). A CT scan is ordered if x-rays (**Fig. 3.43**) are inconclusive as they are more sensitive in identifying transition site, severity, and etiology of the obstruction (Sn 0.93, Sp 1.00) (**Fig. 3.44A**). Both x-rays (**Fig. 3.44B**) and CT scans can be used to detect free air in the abdomen secondary to intestinal perforation.

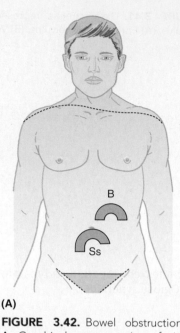

(A)

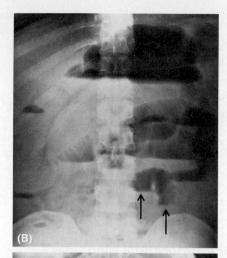

(B)

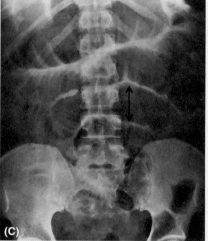

(C)

FIGURE 3.42. Bowel obstruction. **A.** Graphical representation of air–fluid levels, which can be a finding of bowel obstruction. *B*, balanced air–fluid levels; *Ss*, stair-step appearance air–fluid levels. **B.** Upright x-ray demonstrating multiple air–fluid levels related to a small bowel obstruction (*arrows*). **C.** Supine x-ray demonstrating dilated loops (*arrow*) of small bowel proximal to a bowel obstruction.

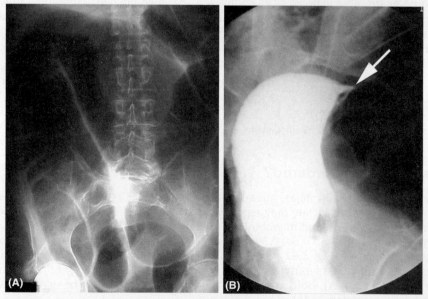

(A)

(B)

FIGURE 3.43. Radiological signs of a volvulus. **A.** Two adjacent loops of dilated bowel forming the "coffee bean" sign. **B.** Barium enema demonstrating a narrowing at the level where the bowel twists forming a "bird's beak" (*arrow*).

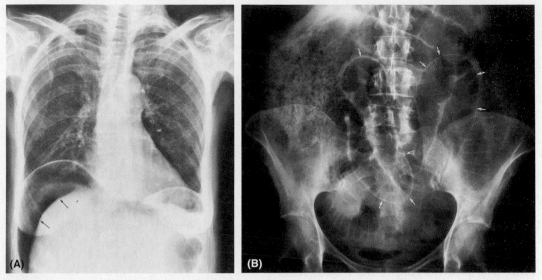

FIGURE 3.44. Pneumoperitoneum on imaging. **A.** Chest x-ray with air under the diaphragm and above the liver (*arrows*). **B.** Supine x-ray with air on both sides of the bowel wall. Note the definition of the serosal surfaces (*arrows*).

 # APPENDICITIS

Presentation

A 27-year-old male presents to the Emergency Department with RLQ pain, low-grade fever, nausea, and vomiting; 10 hours earlier, he had developed mild periumbilical pain.

Definition

Appendicitis is an acute inflammation of the appendix caused by obstruction of the appendiceal lumen resulting in a closed loop of bowel, inflammation, and, possibly, perforation, necrosis, and peritonitis. Typically, the appendix is located near the ileocecal junction (**Fig. 3.45**) resulting in RLQ pain; however, patients with a retrocecal or pelvic appendix may present differently, as discussed below.

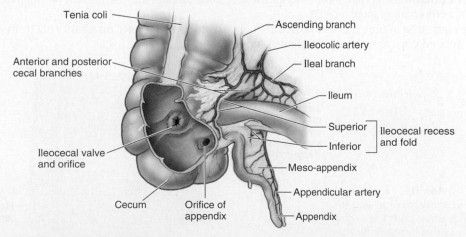

FIGURE 3.45. Blood supply to the appendix.

What are common causes?

The most common causes are summarized below.

Lumen obstruction	Obstruction can be caused by a fecalith or calculi, lymphoid hyperplasia (especially in children and adults with IBD and infections, such as gastroenteritis and mononucleosis), and tumors (benign, malignant, or carcinoid tumors).
Infection	Bacterial infections include *Yersinia pestis*, actinomycosis, mycobacteria species, and *Histoplasma* species.
	Viral infections include adenovirus and cytomegalovirus.
	Parasitic infections include schistosomiasis, pinworms, and *Strongyloides stercoralis*.

What is the differential diagnosis?

RLQ pain: The differential diagnosis includes renal stones and diverticulitis; additionally, in women, ectopic pregnancy, PID, and ovarian cysts (**Table 3.1**).

What symptoms might be observed?

Symptoms of appendicitis include RLQ pain (Sn 0.81, Sp 0.53), periumbilical pain that migrates to the McBurney point (Sn 0.64, Sp 0.82) (**Fig. 3.46**), nausea, diarrhea, and anorexia.

> ● **CLINICAL PEARL**
>
> Vomiting typically follows the onset of pain (Sn 1.00, Sp 0.64).

What are the possible findings on examination?

Vital signs: Low-grade fever, hypotension, and tachycardia may be present with peritonitis.
Inspection: Typically normal, but may appear in distress.
Auscultation: Increased bowel sounds.
Percussion: Tenderness.
Palpation: RLQ pain, specifically at the McBurney point (the point one third of the distance from the right ASIS to the umbilicus). Guarding, rebound tenderness, and abdominal rigidity may be present (Sn 0.27, Sp 0.83).

Special Tests

Digital rectal examination: Pain may be present with retrocecal appendicitis.
Pelvic examination: Cervical motion tenderness or adnexal pain may be present with pelvic appendicitis, ectopic pregnancy, or PID.
Rovsing sign: In a supine patient, pressure is applied to the left lower quadrant (LLQ). In patients with appendicitis, this maneuver elicits pain in the RLQ.

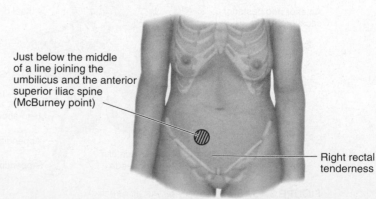

Just below the middle of a line joining the umbilicus and the anterior superior iliac spine (McBurney point)

Right rectal tenderness

FIGURE 3.46. The anatomical location of tenderness in appendicitis (McBurney point) is in the RLQ. Pain in this location may be absent early in the disease course.

Psoas sign (Sn 0.16, Sp 0.95): In a supine patient, the right hip is extended with the knee fully flexed. In patients with retrocecal appendicitis, this maneuver may elicit pain in the RLQ.

Obturator sign: In a supine patient, the hip is internally rotated with the hip and knee flexed. In patients with pelvic appendicitis, this maneuver may elicit pain in the RLQ.

Cough reflex: Tenderness at McBurney point.

What tests should be ordered?

Laboratory tests: CBC (leukocytosis), metabolic panel (elevated lactate and creatinine), and urine studies (qualitative β-HCG to rule out pregnancy).

Imaging: Abdominal ultrasound has excellent specificity and sensitivity and is the primary imaging modality in children, pregnant women, and young lean adults. A CT scan is the gold standard to diagnose appendicitis and is used in the setting of an inconclusive ultrasound or if complications such as perforation are suspected (**Fig. 3.47**). Abdominal x-ray can identify perforation and calcified fecaliths, which are seen in ~5% of cases.

Diagnostic Scores

Modified Alvarado score: Predicts the probability of appendicitis based on migratory right iliac fossa pain (one point), anorexia (one point), nausea or vomiting (one point), tenderness in the right iliac fossa (two points), rebound tenderness in the right iliac fossa (one point), temperature above 37.5°C (99.5°F) (one point), and leukocytosis (two points).

The diagnostic utility of the Alvarado score is to rule out appendicitis. A low score (<5) has more utility in ruling out appendicitis than a high score (>7) has in ruling appendicitis.

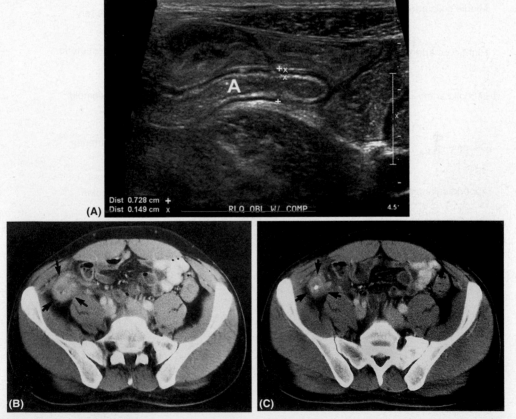

FIGURE 3.47. Imaging of the appendix. **A.** Abdominal ultrasound showing mild dilation and wall thickening of the appendix. *A*, appendix. **B.** Axial image of a CT scan of abdomen and pelvis showing a soft tissue inflammatory mass in the RLQ (*arrows*). **C.** Axial image of a CT scan of abdomen and pelvis showing a calcified fecalith (*arrows*) within a thickened appendix.

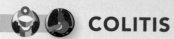 **COLITIS**

Presentation

A 24-year-old female presents with 3 weeks of colicky LLQ pain and diarrhea. She averages 12 loose bowel movements per day that contain both blood and mucus.

Definition

Colitis is inflammation of the colon and is categorized as inflammatory, ischemic, radiation induced, or infectious. The colon and its blood supply are summarized in **Figure 3.48.**

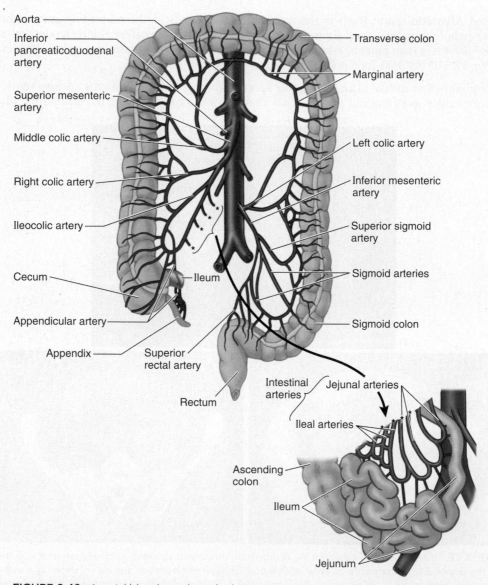

FIGURE 3.48. Arterial blood supply to the large intestine.

What are common causes?

Common causes are summarized below.

IBD	Crohn disease is a relapsing illness that causes transmural inflammation of the GI tract (from mouth to anus). In contrast to UC, there can be areas of normal mucosa interspersed within affected areas (skip lesions). GI biopsy shows transmural inflammation and noncaseating granulomas. Major complications include perianal disease, strictures, fistulas, abscesses, and malabsorption.
	UC is a relapsing nontransmural inflammation restricted to the colon. Typically, UC starts in the rectum and progresses proximally toward the cecum; some patients can develop backwash ileitis, which may falsely be interpreted as Crohn disease. Major complications of UC include toxic megacolon and colon cancer risk.
Ischemic	Nonocclusive vascular disease that occurs secondary to changes or anatomic variants in systemic circulation or local mesenteric vasculature. Ischemia is most common in the elderly population. It often occurs in watershed areas such as the splenic flexure and rectosigmoid colon.
Infectious	*Clostridium difficile* colitis is a cause of toxin-mediated diarrhea that can cause pseudomembranous colitis. Risk factors include antibiotic exposure, advanced age, IBD, and previous *C. difficile* infections.
	Bacterial infections caused by *Campylobacter* species, *Salmonella* species, *Shigella* species, *Escherichia coli* (enterohaemorrhagic E. coli), *Yersinia* species, *Mycobacterium tuberculosis*, and atypical mycobacteria (MAC).
	Parasitic infections caused by *Entamoeba histolytica*, *Cryptospora* species, *Isospora* species, *Trichuris trichiura*, and *Strongyloides* species.
	Viral infections caused by CMV, HSV, and HIV.

● CLINICAL PEARL

Smokers are at increased risk of Crohn disease and lower risk of UC.

What is the differential diagnosis?

Colitis: The differential diagnosis includes diverticulitis (see Diverticular Disease Clinical Case), microscopic colitis (collagenous and lymphocytic subtypes), eosinophilic gastroenteritis, graft-versus-host disease, radiation colitis, Behçet syndrome, sarcoidosis, malignancy, irritable bowel syndrome, celiac disease, and vasculitis.

What symptoms might be observed?

Symptoms of IBD include abdominal pain, tenesmus or bowel urgency, nausea and vomiting, diarrhea with or without blood and mucus, bloating or abdominal distention, and obstipation. Extra-abdominal symptoms can include rash, joint pain, and eye pain.

What are the possible findings upon examination?

Vital signs: Fever, tachycardia, and hypotension may be present.
Inspection: Observe for extraintestinal manifestations of IBD:

- Skin: dark red nodules on the shins (erythema nodosum) and deep necrotic ulcers that often occur on the legs or around stoma sites (pyoderma gangrenosum)
- Eyes: red eye and papillary changes (uveitis, particularly iritis)
- Oral mucosa: aphthous ulcers (**Fig. 3.49**)
- Musculoskeletal: arthritis (knee is most common) and sacroiliitis (Chapter 6)

Auscultation: Increased bowel sounds; in severe colitis, absent bowel sounds may indicate toxic megacolon.

FIGURE 3.49. Aphthous ulcer.

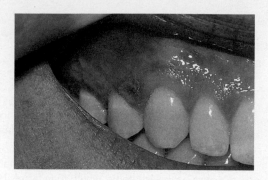

Percussion: Abdominal tenderness.

Palpation: Generalized abdominal tenderness; focal tenderness may indicate an abscess.

Special Tests

Digital rectal examination: Perianal disease such as fissures, fistulas, and perirectal abscess may be present in IBD; stool mixed with blood or mucus.

What tests should be ordered?

Laboratory tests: CBC (leukocytosis may be secondary to infection or corticosteroids, anemia, thrombocytosis as a marker of inflammation), metabolic panel (elevated lactic acid may indicate bowel ischemia; low albumin may indicate malnutrition), microbiology (blood cultures, stool ova and parasites, stool culture, *C. difficile* cytotoxin assay, and serology for *E. histolytica*), and other serology (elevated erythrocyte sedimentation rate [ESR] and C-reactive protein [CRP]; nutritional deficiencies may include low iron, vitamin B_{12}, and vitamin D; anti-*Saccharomyces cerevisiae* antibodies [ASCA] are sometimes positive in Crohn disease and perinuclear antineutrophil cytoplasmic antibodies [p-ANCA] in UC).

Imaging: Abdominal x-rays and CT scans may reveal thickening of the colon wall and complications of colitis such as fistulas, strictures, and abscesses (**Figs. 3.50 and 3.51**). CT or MR enterography may be helpful in imaging the small bowel, especially in the setting of Crohn disease in which the entire GI tract may be involved.

X-rays of the sacroiliac joints may also confirm extra-abdominal features of IBD (**Fig. 3.52**).

Pneumatosis intestinalis occurs when a gas cyst forms in the bowel wall. This may be seen in ischemic causes of colitis (**Fig. 3.53**).

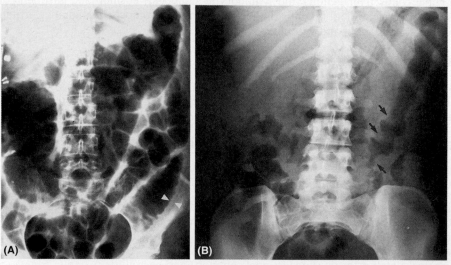

(A)

(B)

FIGURE 3.50. Mucosal thickening secondary to ulcerative colitis. **A.** Thickened bowel wall is seen on the right side of the x-ray (*arrowheads*). **B.** The thickened mucosa has a "thumbprint" appearance (*arrows*).

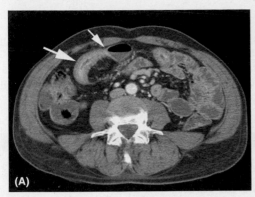
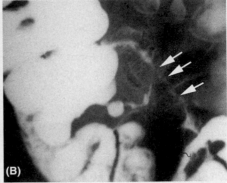

FIGURE 3.51. Radiology of inflammatory bowel disease. **A.** Thickening of the bowel wall along with hyper-enhancement of the mucosa (*large arrow*) and narrowing of the intestinal luminal (*small arrow*) secondary to Crohn disease. **B.** Small bowel follow-through study using barium as a contrast agent demonstrates narrowing of the terminal ileum (*arrows*).

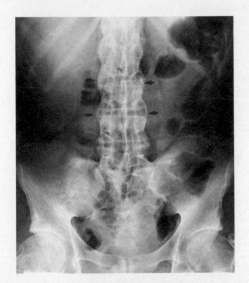

FIGURE 3.52. Spondyloarthropathy from inflammatory bowel disease. The abdominal x-ray demonstrates fusion (*ankyloses*) of the sacroiliac joints. There are also bony outgrowths from ligaments (*syndesmophytes*) that bridge the vertebral discs (*arrows*).

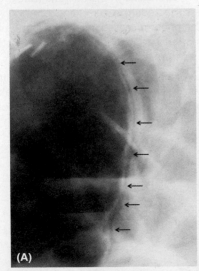
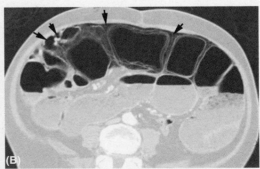

FIGURE 3.53. Pneumatosis intestinalis, or gas cysts within the bowel wall, related to ischemic colitis. **A.** X-ray of the left lower quadrant of the abdomen demonstrating a thin column of gas within the bowel wall (*arrows*). **B.** Axial CT images with an abnormal gas collection within the wall of the bowel (*arrows*).

Special Tests

Endoscopy: Colonoscopy and flexible sigmoidoscopy are important in the diagnosis of Crohn disease and UC. The characteristic endoscopic appearance of Crohn disease consists of nonfriable mucosa, cobblestoning, aphthous ulcers, and fissures; in UC, a granular friable mucosa with diffuse ulceration may be seen. In *C. difficile* colitis, pseudomembranes (caused by inflammatory exudate overlying sites of mucosal injury) may be present.

 # DIVERTICULAR DISEASE

Presentation

A 58-year-old male presents to the Emergency Department with severe LLQ abdominal pain and fever. He was diagnosed with sigmoid diverticula on a colonoscopy 2 years prior.

Definition

Diverticuloses are acquired herniations or "outpouchings" of the colonic mucosa and submucosa through the colonic wall (**Fig. 3.54**). Diverticulitis is inflammation of the diverticula commonly associated with gross or microperforation. Diverticular hemorrhage is a lower GI bleed as a consequence of diverticula.

What are common causes?

Common causes are summarized below.

Diverticulosis	May be caused by a low-fiber diet leading to increased stool transit time, increased intraluminal pressure, and herniation of the colonic mucosa/submucosa at sites of relative muscle weakness. The sigmoid colon is the segment with the smallest diameter and highest intraluminal pressure and is the most common site of diverticulosis.
Diverticulitis	Caused by stasis or obstruction in the diverticulum leads to local bacterial overgrowth and tissue ischemia that causes infection. Anaerobic bacteria (*Bacteroides*, *Peptostreptococcus*, *Clostridium*, and *Fusobacterium* species) are commonly implicated organisms. Diverticulitis can be uncomplicated (microperforation and localized infection) or complicated (macroperforation leading to abscess, fistula, phlegmon, peritonitis, obstruction, and strictures).
Diverticular hemorrhage	Accounts for 23%–30% of lower GI bleeds. As the vasa recta course over the outpouching of the diverticula, there is intimal thickening and medial thinning, which weaken the vascular wall and can cause arterial rupture. Even though diverticula are more common in the left colon, bleeding diverticula are more common in the right colon.

FIGURE 3.54. Diverticulosis of the colon.

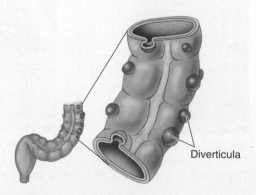

Diverticula

What is the differential diagnosis?

LLQ pain: The differential diagnosis include renal stones, diverticulitis, and, in women, ectopic pregnancy, PID, and ovarian cysts (**Table 3.1**).

Lower GI bleed: The differential diagnosis includes angiodysplasia, colorectal cancer (CRC), hemorrhoids, colitis (ischemic, infectious, inflammatory), anal fissure, postpolypectomy, radiation proctitis, and vasculitis.

What symptoms might be observed?

Diverticulosis is usually asymptomatic. Symptoms of diverticulitis include LLQ pain, nausea and vomiting, and constipation. Symptoms of a diverticular hemorrhage include abdominal cramping and syncope.

What are the possible findings on examination?

> ● **CLINICAL PEARL**
>
> Diverticulosis is asymptomatic and a normal examination is expected.

Vital signs: Tachycardia and hypotension may be present in both diverticulitis and diverticular hemorrhage. A fever may occur in diverticulitis.

Inspection: Rigid abdomen may be present with peritonitis associated with diverticulitis.

Auscultation: Decreased bowel sounds in diverticulitis and increased bowel sounds in diverticular hemorrhage.

Percussion: Pain or dullness in LLQ may represent an abscess related to diverticulitis.

Palpation: Tenderness in LLQ, guarding, rigidity, and rebound tenderness may be present with peritonitis associated with diverticulitis. Mild tenderness may be present in diverticular hemorrhage.

Special Tests

Digital rectal examination: Frank, bright red blood may be present in diverticular hemorrhage.

What tests should be ordered?

Diverticulitis

Laboratory tests: CBC (leukocytosis).

Imaging: A CT scan is the preferred imaging modality to diagnose and assess for complications such as perforation or abscess. Less commonly, x-rays with contrast can demonstrate diverticulosis (**Fig. 3.55**).

Diverticular hemorrhage

Laboratory tests: CBC (anemia), blood type and screen, and coagulation profile (check for an elevated PT/INR in case reversal of coagulopathy is needed).

Special tests: Colonoscopy is the preferred investigation for diagnosis. If the bleeding is brisk and an upper GI source has been ruled out, arteriography may be used for diagnosis and therapeutic embolization (**Fig. 3.56**).

FIGURE 3.55. Abdominal x-ray with contrast showing innumerable diverticula (outpouchings) in the descending colon.

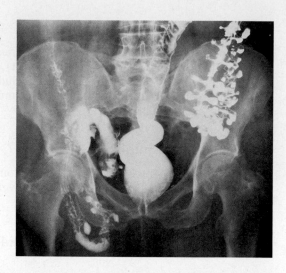

Colonoscopy is contraindicated in acute diverticulitis due to the risk of perforation and should be done 6 weeks after the acute episode to rule out IBD or malignancy.

Diagnostic Scores

The Hinchey classification scheme predicts the risk of death from diverticulitis: Stage 1 is defined by small confined pericolic or mesenteric abscess (5%); stage 2 is defined by a larger abscess confined to the pelvis (5%); stage 3 is defined by perforated diverticulitis causing purulent peritonitis (13%); stage 4 is defined by perforation with fecal contamination (43%).

FIGURE 3.56. Mesenteric arteriogram in a patient with a lower gastrointestinal bleed. The contrast enhancement (*arrow*) is at the site of a diverticular bleed in the descending colon.

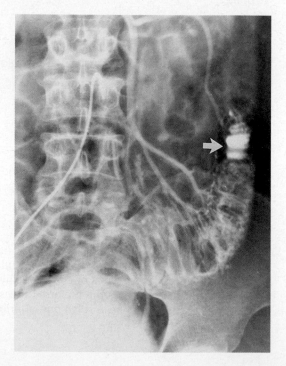

MESENTERIC ISCHEMIA

Presentation

A 75-year-old male with hypertension and hypercholesterolemia presents to the Emergency Department with postprandial abdominal pain. He has had a fear of eating for the past few months because it worsens his abdominal pain.

Definition

Mesenteric ischemia is an acute or chronic state of bowel ischemia due to occlusion of the mesenteric vasculature (**Fig. 3.57**).

What are common causes?

The most common cause of chronic mesenteric ischemia is atherosclerosis that often involves two or more major visceral arterial vessels. Risk factors for chronic mesenteric ischemia include hypertension, smoking, hyperlipidemia, and hypercholesterolemia.

The four major etiologies of acute mesenteric ischemia are:

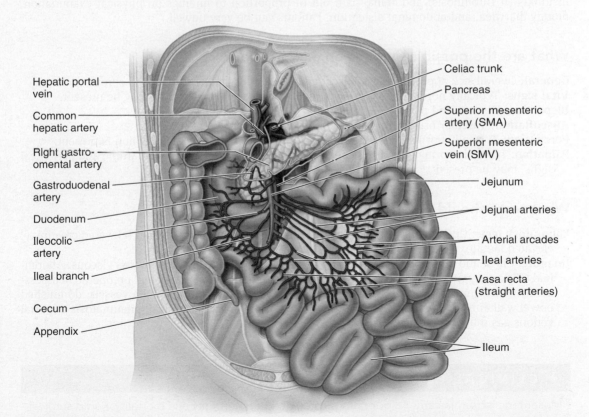

FIGURE 3.57. Arterial supply and mesenteries of the intestines. Except for the proximal duodenum, the small intestines are supplied by the SMA. The SMV drains blood from the same portions of the intestine into the hepatic portal vein.

Arterial embolism (40%–50%)	Arrhythmia, MI, rheumatic valve disease, endocarditis, cardiomyopathies, ventricular aneurysms, history of embolic events, and recent angiography
Arterial thrombosis (25%)	Atherosclerosis, prolonged hypotension, high estrogen state (oral contraceptive pill or hormone replacement therapy), and hypercoagulable states
Nonocclusive thrombosis (20%)	Hypovolemia, hypotension, low cardiac output state, digoxin, and β-agonists
Venous thrombosis (10%)	Right-sided heart failure, deep vein thrombosis, hepatosplenomegaly, hypercoagulable state, malignancy, hepatitis, pancreatitis, recent abdominal surgery or infection, high estrogen state, polycythemia, and sickle cell disease

What is the differential diagnosis?

Generalized abdominal pain: The differential diagnosis includes peritonitis, mesenteric ischemia, ruptured abdominal aortic aneurysm, and bowel obstruction (**Table 3.1**).

Severe abdominal pain: The differential diagnosis includes appendicitis, PUD, acute pancreatitis, ruptured viscera, nephrolithiasis, and acute cholecystitis.

What symptoms might be observed?

Symptoms of chronic mesenteric ischemia include postprandial pain that occurs 15–30 minutes after initiating a meal and that lasts for at least 1 hour, fear of eating, nausea and vomiting, and early satiety. Symptoms of acute mesenteric ischemia include sudden (if arterial embolism) or insidious (if thrombosis) abdominal pain out of proportion to findings on physical examination, bloody diarrhea, and abdominal distention. Patients can be very unwell.

What are the possible findings on examination?

General: Overall sick appearing if acute ischemia; weight loss may be present in chronic ischemia.
Vital signs: Typically normal; however, hypotension, fever, and tachycardia may be present.
Inspection: Distress and pain.
Auscultation: Vascular bruit in the upper abdominal region.
Percussion: Typically normal but resonance may be heard if abdominal distention is present.
Palpation: Typically normal, but diffuse abdominal pain, and in later stages, guarding and peritoneal signs, may be present.

What tests should be ordered?

Laboratory tests: CBC (hemoconcentration, leukocytosis) and metabolic panel (elevated creatinine, elevated lactate, metabolic acidosis with a large anion gap).

Imaging: Chest and abdominal x-rays should be performed to rule out a perforated viscous. Abdominal CT angiography (CTA) (**Fig. 3.58**) is the gold standard for diagnosis and preoperative assessment, which may reveal absent filling of major or minor mesenteric branch vessels, diminished bowel wall enhancement, and mural thickening. If ischemia is established, pneumatosis or portal venous gas may be detected.

● CLINICAL PEARL

Mesenteric ischemia carries a poor prognosis with high morbidity and mortality. Rapid surgical or interventional treatment is required to minimize infarction to the bowel.

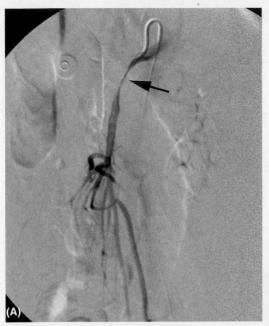
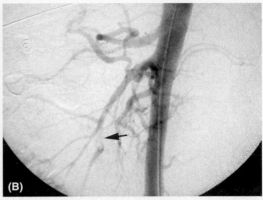

FIGURE 3.58. Mesenteric imaging. **A.** Inferior mesenteric arteriogram with major vessels labeled (*arrow*). **B.** Superior mesenteric artery (SMA) embolus causing a filling defect in the distal main trunk of the SMA (*arrow*).

 # ABDOMINAL AORTIC ANEURYSM

Presentation

A 68-year-old male presents to his health care provider after an incidental finding of a 4.2-cm infra-renal AAA on abdominal ultrasound.

Definition

AAA is a localized dilation of the abdominal aorta exceeding the normal diameter by >50% and is the most common form of aortic aneurysm (**Fig. 3.59**).

What are common causes?

The following risk factors are associated with the development of an AAA:

Age	Above 50 years old increases the risk of an AAA; on average, females tend to develop AAA 10 years later than do males
Gender	Males have five-fold increase in risk of AAA
Smoking	Fivefold increase in risk of AAA
Hypertension	Risk increases by 1.25×
Genetics	Family history and connective tissue disorders such as Marfan syndrome and Ehlers-Danlos syndrome
Atherosclerosis	Risk increases by 1.6×

FIGURE 3.59. Diagrammatic representation of an AAA.

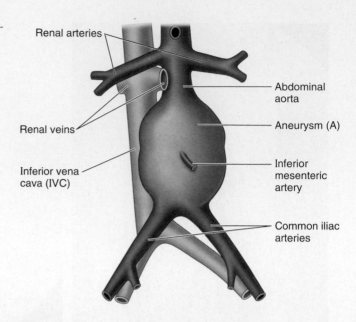

What is the differential diagnosis?

Epigastric pain: The differential diagnosis includes MI, aortic dissection, diverticular disease, pyelonephritis, biliary tree disease, pancreatitis, and PUD.

What symptoms might be observed?

Most AAAs are typically asymptomatic and diagnosed incidentally on abdominal imaging. Symptoms of a ruptured AAA include abdominal or back pain that can radiate to the flanks or groin, and patients often appear unwell.

What are the possible findings on examination?

General: Patients may appear sick, drowsy, or confused.
Vital signs: Typically normal; tachycardia and hypotension may be present in ruptured AAA.
Inspection: Typically normal, but patient may be in distress.
Auscultation: Vascular bruit over an AAA.
Percussion: Typically normal.
Palpation: With the patient supine and knees flexed, the area just cephalad to and left of the umbilicus is palpated for the aortic pulsation. The diameter of the aorta can be estimated by measuring the distance between the two points palpated (**Fig. 3.60**). Guarding or a palpable and pulsatile abdominal aorta may be felt (Sn 0.45–0.90). In asymptomatic patients, the likelihood of palpating the aorta is based on size:

- 3.0–3.9 cm (Sn 0.29, ≥3.0 cm [likelihood ratio] LR+ 15.6, LR− 0.51)
- 4.0–4.9 cm (Sn 0.50, ≥4.0 cm LR+ 15.6, LR− 0.51)
- ≥ 5.0 cm (Sn 0.76)

What tests should be ordered?

Laboratory tests: CBC (severe anemia in ruptured AAA), metabolic panel (creatinine and electrolytes to assess perfusion to the kidney, liver enzymes), and coagulation panel (INR, PTT in case reversal of bleeding is needed).
Imaging: Abdominal ultrasound may be used for the initial assessment and serial monitoring of an AAA (**Fig. 3.61**). CTA of the abdomen allows for assessment of the size and extent of an AAA and helps quantify the residual lumen. In addition, CTA depicts morphology and the relationship of the AAA to major arterial vessels and can help exclude complications, such as a leak or inflammatory changes.

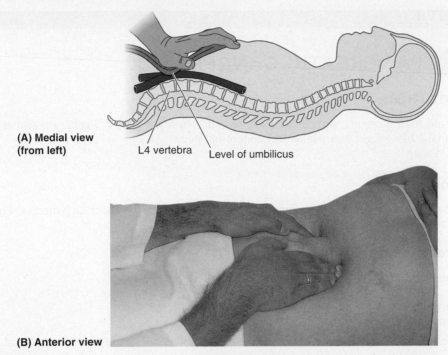

(A) Medial view (from left)

L4 vertebra   Level of umbilicus

(B) Anterior view

FIGURE 3.60. Physical examination for AAA. **A.** Diagrammatic representation of palpating an AAA. **B.** A clinician palpating the abdomen for a pulsatile mass.

● CLINICAL PEARL

AAA is monitored based on size and rate of growth. The average annual growth of an aneurysm is 0.2–0.5 cm. If the AAA is <4.0 cm, annual monitoring with abdominal ultrasound is indicated. If the AAA is 4–5 cm, the risk of rupture is 1%–3% per year; if the AAA is 5–7 cm, the risk of rupture is 6%–11% per year; if the AAA is more than 7 cm, the risk of rupture is 20%.

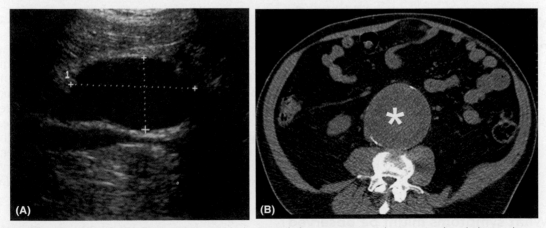

FIGURE 3.61. AAA radiology. **A.** Abdominal ultrasound demonstrating a large saccular abdominal aortic aneurysm. **B.** An axial image of a CT scan of abdomen demonstrating an aortic aneurysm (*asterisk*).

PANCREATIC CANCER

Presentation

A 79-year-old male presents with progressive jaundice over the past 2 weeks. He also reports an unintentional 30-lb weight loss. He denies abdominal pain.

Definition

Pancreatic cancer most commonly refers to a malignant tumor of the exocrine pancreas (**Fig. 3.25**). Approximately 60% of tumors are located in the pancreatic head.

What are common causes?

Common causes are summarized below.

Noncystic neoplasms of the pancreas[1,2]	
Pancreatic adenocarcinoma Other noncystic masses	Represents 85% of pancreatic neoplasms and often occurs in patients 60–80 years of age. Neuroendocrine tumor metastases (10%) and lymphoma are less common causes.
Cystic neoplasms of the pancreas[3]	
Intraductal papillary mucinous neoplasm (IPMN)	Neoplasms that arise in the main pancreatic duct or a branch and can be a precursor to adenocarcinoma (2%–3%).
Pancreatic mucinous cystic neoplasm (MCN)	MCNs are typically benign, multiloculated masses in the body or tail of the pancreas and have ovarian-type stroma. These lesions are precancerous and almost exclusively seen in females.
Serous cystadenoma	Typically benign lesions that are more common in females.
Solid pseudopapillary neoplasm (SPN)	SPNs are more commonly seen in young females and carry a moderate to high risk of malignant transformation.

What is the differential diagnosis?

Painless jaundice: Cholangiocarcinoma is a primary neoplasm of intrahepatic, perihilar, or extrahepatic biliary ducts. Patients may present with pruritus, dull RUQ pain, jaundice, and fever. Serum biomarkers such as carcinoembryonic antigen (CEA) and carbohydrate antigen 19-9 (CA19-9) may be elevated. Cholangiocarcinoma carries a poor prognosis, and patients typically present with advanced disease. Gallbladder carcinoma is a rare neoplasm of the gallbladder. Patients are often asymptomatic but may present with nausea, vomiting, anorexia, and painless jaundice. The diagnosis is often made incidentally on imaging or during a cholecystectomy. If the gallbladder polyps appear larger on serial imaging, they are at risk for transformation into cancer, and these patients should be referred for cholecystectomy. Ampullary carcinoma is a primary neoplasm that develops in the ampullary complex, distal to the confluence of the common bile duct and pancreatic duct (**Fig. 3.25**). For a differential diagnosis of jaundice, see Box 3.1.

What symptoms might be observed?

Symptoms of pancreatic cancer are often limited in early disease. Patients may experience painless jaundice; asthenia; abdominal, epigastric, or back pain; dark-colored urine; nausea and vomiting; diarrhea or steatorrhea; and lower extremity pain, swelling, or redness.

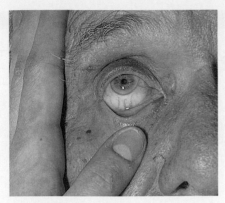

FIGURE 3.62. Jaundice is most easily and reliably seen in the sclera of the eyes or the mucous membranes.

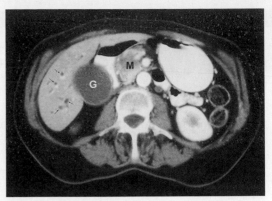

FIGURE 3.63. An axial image from a CT scan of abdomen showing a mass in the head of the pancreas consistent with pancreatic carcinoma. The gallbladder and intrahepatic bile ducts (*arrows*) are dilated. G, gallbladder; *M*, mass.

What are the possible findings on examination?

Vital signs: Typically normal.

Inspection: General cachexia and jaundice (**Fig. 3.62**); a distended abdomen may be present with ascites or peritoneal carcinomatosis.

Auscultation: Typically normal.

Percussion: Dullness in the RUQ may be present in hepatomegaly; flank dullness may be present with ascites.

Palpation: RUQ mass and a large, nontender gallbladder in the presence of jaundice (Courvoisier sign).

Special Tests

Virchow node: Palpable left supraclavicular lymph node is suggestive of an abdominal malignancy.

Digital rectal examination: Palpable mass in the rectal shelf is a nonspecific sign of peritoneal carcinomatosis (Blumer shelf).

> ● **CLINICAL PEARL**
>
> Five eponymous medical signs of GI malignancy may be appreciated on physical examination:
>
> 1. Palpable left supraclavicular lymph node (Virchow node)
> 2. Palpable left axillary lymph node (Irish node)
> 3. Lymph node that bulges into the umbilicus (Sister Mary Joseph node)
> 4. Palpable mass on DRE may indicate metastases to the pouch of Douglas (Blumer shelf).
> 5. Metastases to the ovaries (Krukenberg tumor)

What tests should be ordered?

Laboratory tests: CBC (anemia), metabolic panel (elevated bilirubin, ALP, GGT, AST, ALT, lipase, amylase, and glucose as pancreatic cancer can cause new-onset diabetes), and other serology (elevation of CA19-9 is suggestive of pancreatic cancer; however, CA19-9 is also elevated in liver failure, biliary obstruction, and hyperbilirubinemia. CA19-9 is useful for monitoring recurrence of disease postoperatively). IgG4 level should be assessed as autoimmune pancreatitis may masquerade as pancreatic cancer.

Imaging: Abdominal ultrasound is often the initial test to evaluate obstructive jaundice. An abdominal CT scan is the best modality to diagnose pancreatic cancer (**Fig. 3.63**), and MRCP is sometimes useful for staging.

Special Tests

Biopsy: suspicious masses are best biopsied using endoscopic ultrasound (EUS), ERCP, or image-guided biopsies.

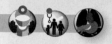

COLORECTAL CANCER

Presentation

A 65-year-old male presents with 2 weeks of intermittent blood loss per rectum. He also reports that his stool has become very thin and that he has lost 20 lb over the past 2 months.

Definition

CRC is a primary adenocarcinoma of the colon or rectum. Approximately 90% of patients are over age 50 years at the time of diagnosis.

What are common causes?

Sporadic mutations account for 70% of CRCs; adenomas progress to carcinoma with the accumulation of multiple gene mutations. Up to 20% of patients will have a positive family history[1] of CRC. Hereditary nonpolyposis colorectal cancer (HNPCC), or Lynch syndrome, is the most common hereditary colon cancer resulting from a heritable mutation in DNA mismatch repair genes. There is a predilection for right-sided colon cancers and increased risk of other cancers (e.g., ovarian, small bowel, gastric, and endometrial). Familial adenomatous polyposis (FAP) is caused by a mutation in the adenomatous polyposis coli (APC) tumor suppressor gene, resulting in the development of thousands of polyps at a young age with 100% chance of developing colon cancer unless a total colectomy is performed.

What is the differential diagnosis?

Rectal bleeding: The differential diagnosis includes diverticulosis (see Diverticular Disease Clinical Case), colitis (see Colitis Clinical Case), angiodysplasia, hemorrhoids, anal fissure, postpolypectomy, and vasculitis.

Colonic mass: The differential diagnosis includes Kaposi sarcoma, lymphoma, carcinoid tumors, and metastases from other malignancies such as ovarian cancer.

What symptoms might be observed?

Symptoms of CRC include changes in bowel habits including thinning in the caliber of the stool or constipation, abdominal pain, weight loss, hematochezia, iron deficiency anemia, and fatigue.

> ● **CLINICAL PEARL**
>
> Adults aged 50 years and older with new iron deficiency anemia should be investigated for CRC.

What are the possible findings on examination?

Vital signs: Typically normal.

Inspection: General cachexia, with temporal and proximal muscle wasting in advanced disease. In the setting of ascites or peritoneal carcinomatosis, a distended abdomen may be present.

Auscultation: Absent or high-pitched bowel sounds may be present in a bowel obstruction.

Percussion: Dullness in the RUQ may be present in hepatomegaly secondary to metastases; flank dullness may be present with ascites or peritoneal carcinomatosis.

Palpation: Abdominal mass or an enlarged and nodular liver edge.

Special Tests

Digital rectal examination: Palpable mass or presence of blood.

What tests should be ordered?

Laboratory tests: CBC (iron deficiency anemia with low mean corpuscular volume), metabolic panel (elevated liver enzymes may occur with liver metastasis), and other serology (CEA[2] is not used for diagnosis but may be helpful in quantifying the patient's response to therapy or to detect recurrence. Postoperative CEA >5 ng/mL is associated with worse prognosis[2]).

● **CLINICAL PEARL**

Streptococcus gallolyticus (subtype bovis) bacteremia and endocarditis are associated with colon cancer.

Imaging: CT colonography (CTC) can be the initial diagnostic test if screening by conventional colonoscopy is challenging or contraindicated. CTC has a similar diagnostic performance to endoscopy for cancers and polyps >6 mm. CTC can provide simultaneous staging of colon cancer in addition to colonic assessment for synchronous lesions. Alternatively, a CT scan of the abdomen is often used as a diagnostic and staging modality for colorectal cancer (**Fig. 3.64**).

Special Tests

Colonoscopy is the gold standard for diagnosing colorectal cancer and obtaining biopsies for pathology.

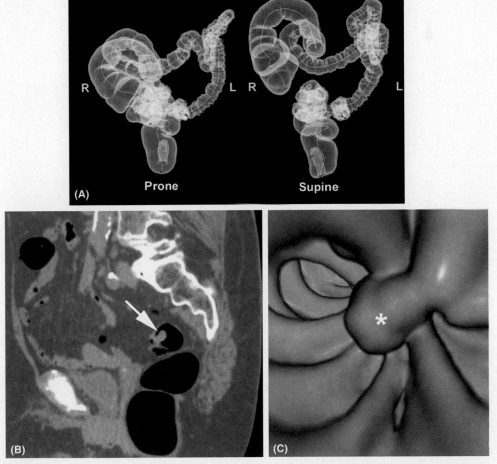

FIGURE 3.64. CT colonoscopy is performed by collecting images in both the supine and prone position and then using an algorithm to reconstruct the colon. **A.** Reconstructed colon in the prone and supine positions. **B.** Pedunculated polyp in the colon (*arrow*). **C.** The endoluminal view of the reconstructed colon (similar to what is seen on a colonoscopy) demonstrating a polyp (*asterisk*).

Pelvis

JOSHUA M. LIAO • R. PHELPS KELLEY • LAURA E. SMITH • SAGAR DUGANI • KELSEY E. MILLS • KENNETH B. CHRISTOPHER

4

The pelvis is the anatomical region that connects the abdomen to the lower extremities. The pelvis is surrounded by the bony pelvic girdle, abdomen, lower back, and gluteal region. The paired pelvic bones are formed by the fusion of the ilium, ischium, and pubis (**Fig. 4.1**). Anteriorly, the pelvic bones join at the pubic symphysis, and posteriorly, they articulate with the sacrum and coccyx. The ilium has three spines, whose names correspond to their anatomic position on the ilium: anterior superior iliac spine (ASIS), anterior inferior iliac spine (AIIS), and posterior superior iliac spine (PSIS). The space inside the bony pelvis is divided into two regions: false (or, greater) pelvis and true (or, lesser) pelvis. The false pelvis contains abdominal organs, and the true pelvis has foramina through which vessels, nerves, muscles and their tendons, and structures of the gastrointestinal (GI) and genitourinary (GU) organs traverse, allowing the pelvis to communicate with its surrounding compartments.

The perineum consists of the area between the thighs and buttocks, extending from the coccyx to the pubis, and to the shallow compartment superior to this area and inferior to the pelvic diaphragm. The perineum includes the anus and external genitalia: penis and scrotum in males and vulva in females (**Fig. 4.2**).

This chapter provides a comprehensive approach to the diagnosis of common disorders of the pelvis and perineum. An approach to examining the breast is also included, as some breast pathology may be related to pelvic pathology.

■ INITIAL EVALUATION AND ASSESSMENT

Pelvic and perineal diseases typically manifest with symptoms, including generalized or focal pain, fever, GU symptoms (e.g., dysuria, increased urinary frequency, and hematuria), rashes, vesicular lesions, vaginal bleeding, or purulent penile or vaginal discharge.

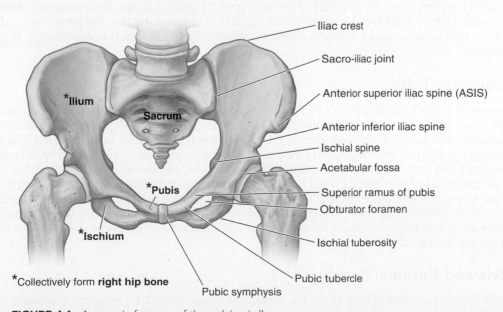

FIGURE 4.1. Anatomic features of the pelvic girdle.

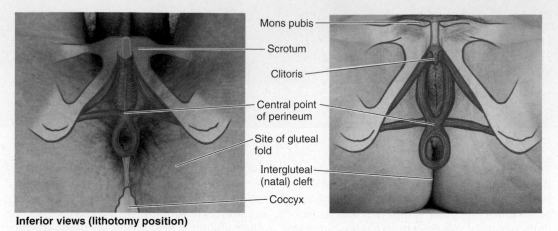

Mons pubis

Scrotum

Clitoris

Central point of perineum

Site of gluteal fold

Intergluteal (natal) cleft

Coccyx

Inferior views (lithotomy position)

FIGURE 4.2. Male and female perineal areas with associated superficial muscles.

General Pelvic and Perineal Examination

To evaluate pelvic and perineal pathology, a physical examination is performed with the patient in the supine or lithotomy position. A drape is placed across the abdomen and below, with only the examined areas being exposed. A systematic physical examination involves inspection, palpation, percussion, and auscultation.

The clinician stands in front of the patient and inspects the skin overlying the hip joint for signs of trauma, erythema, ecchymosis, or edema and for the presence of masses, obvious muscular atrophy, and bony protuberances. The lower extremities should be examined for symmetry in length and rotation, as these may be affected in a hip fracture or dislocation (Chapter 6). Further, the inguinal region is inspected for skin lesions and masses suggestive of hernia or lymphadenopathy. If the symptoms are related to the GU system, then the external genitalia should be inspected. A chaperone may be needed for the pelvic examination. The external genitalia should be inspected for obvious lesions, drainage, bleeding, skin conditions, or ecchymoses. The breast examination is discussed in a separate section.

After inspection, the pelvis is palpated in areas of reported pain or discomfort to determine the presence of masses, nodules, or lymphadenopathy. An internal pelvic examination (discussed separately) should also be performed to identify possible pelvic masses. Following palpation, the pelvic area may be percussed to assess pelvic fullness or bloating. Finally, the pelvic and abdominal areas may be auscultated to assess if abdominal pathology (Chapter 3) is contributing to pelvic symptoms.

Laboratory Tests

Common laboratory investigations to help diagnose pelvic and perineal diseases include a complete blood count (CBC) to diagnose infections, anemia, or hematological malignancy. Other markers of malignancy that could be checked include CA 125 (elevated in epithelial ovarian cancer and other pathology). A Pap test may be performed for cervical cancer screening. Serum electrolytes (sodium, potassium) and renal function (creatinine [Cr], bicarbonate, and blood urea nitrogen [BUN]) can also be measured to characterize renal function that can be impaired in pathology affecting the GU system. Urinalysis and urine sediment can also be evaluated for evidence of a urinary tract infection (UTI), hematuria, and proteinuria and for presence of casts or tumor cells. In the setting of a strong family history, mutations in the *BRCA1* and *BRCA2* genes can be assessed as a risk factor for ovarian and breast cancer.

Pelvic and Perineal Imaging

Typical imaging modalities include x-rays, computed tomography (CT), magnetic resonance imaging (MRI), and ultrasonography. In certain instance, positron emission tomography (PET) may be used to assess areas of increased metabolic activity seen in inflammation or malignancy. The type of initial investigation ordered depends on the region of interest.

Pelvic x-rays are a typical initial investigation to assess pelvic fractures and for the presence of surgical implants. These x-rays are typically obtained with the patient supine. If both sides are imaged, then the two sides can be compared for possible asymmetric changes. One approach to reading x-rays is as follows:

1. Determine the x-ray orientation (e.g., anteroposterior [AP], posterioanterior [PA], or lateral decubitis).
2. Assess bony structures for fractures or joint space disease.
3. Assess for the presence of surgical implants (e.g., screws or plates).
4. Assess soft tissue for obvious hematoma, nodularity, or other irregularities.

X-rays can also be used to identify renal calculi and breast pathology. CT scans generate high-resolution images of bones and can identify smaller fractures that may not be detected on x-rays. CT scans can also help to identify soft tissue pathology, be used for image-guided percutaneous biopsy, and be used to identify renal calculi (when used on nonintravenous contrast mode; contrast mode is not used as it may obscure visualization of renal calculi). MRI scans can be used to visualize pathology of soft tissue, hip joints, renal parenchymal pathology, and breast pathology.

■ FEMALE REPRODUCTIVE SYSTEM

Overview

The female reproductive organs are located in the pelvis and lie superior to the pelvic floor muscles and peritoneum. The female reproductive system is bordered by the pelvic brim and the ascending and descending/sigmoid colon. Organs of the female reproductive system include the clitoris, vagina, cervix, uterus, fallopian tubes, and ovaries. The fallopian tubes guide ova released from the ovaries toward the uterus. These structures are also the site of fertilization. The cervix extends inferiorly into the vaginal vault. At the center and distal aspect of the cervix lies the external os, which is the external opening of the conduit between the vagina and uterus (**Fig. 4.3**).

Physical Examination

For the female pelvic examination, the patient should be supine in the lithotomy position at the end of the examination table. The thighs should be flexed, abducted, and externally rotated at the hips, with feet in stirrups. The physical examination involves inspection of the external genitalia, internal examination of the vagina and cervix with a speculum, Pap test (when indicated), and the bimanual examination.

The external genitalia (collectively referred to as the *vulva*) include the labia minora, clitoris, urethral meatus, and vaginal introitus and should be inspected for changes in skin texture, presence of vaginal discharge, lesions, erythema, and swelling. For the internal examination, an appropriately sized speculum should be selected. The clinician wears gloves and with one hand separates

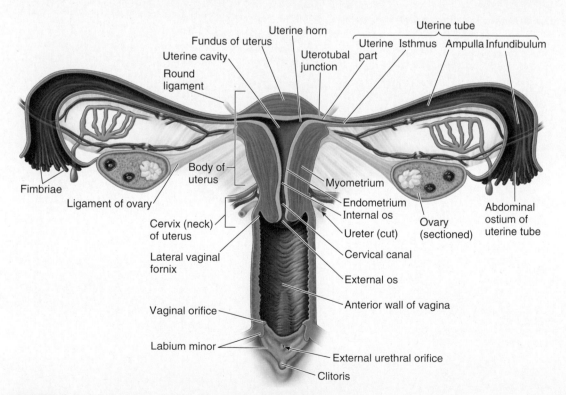

FIGURE 4.3. Coronal section of the internal female genital organs.

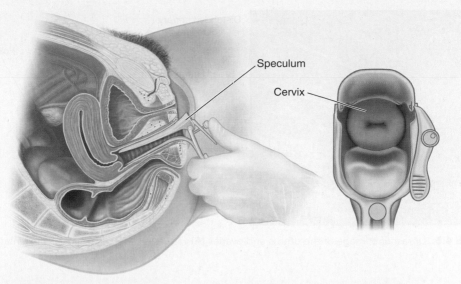

FIGURE 4.4. Inspection of speculum (A) to visualize the cervix and its os (B).

the labia majora to fully visualize the vaginal introitus. With the other hand, the clinician should insert the speculum and advance it slowly with gentle downward pressure into the vaginal vault. The vaginal vault and cervix should be inspected, and changes in color and presence of masses, bleeding, or discharge should be noted (**Fig. 4.4**). If discharge is noted, the appropriate cervical or vaginal swabs may be obtained. At this time and if indicated, a Pap test can be performed. After the sample is collected, the clinician should close the speculum and slowly withdraw it, observing the vaginal walls for any abnormalities.

The bimanual examination helps to assess the uterus, cervix, and adnexae (the ovaries and fallopian tubes) as shown in **Figure 4.5**. To perform this examination, the patient is asked about any points of tenderness or discomfort. The clinician then applies lubricating gel to the tip of

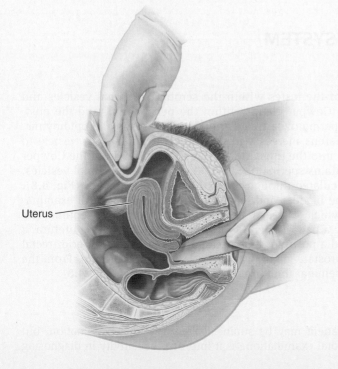

FIGURE 4.5. Bimanual examination to palpate the uterus shape, size, consistency, and possible masses.

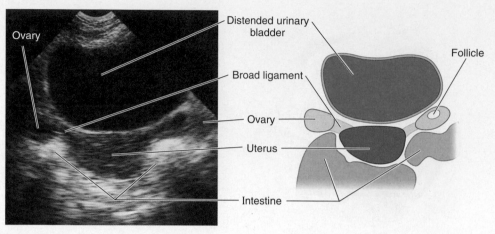

FIGURE 4.6. Ultrasound image of the uterus and ovaries (**A**) with associated graphical representation (**B**).

the second and third digits of the dominant hand and inserts them gently into the vagina at a downward angle. The cervix can be palpated for irregularities in size or consistency. The clinician can palpate the uterus by placing the nondominant hand on the abdomen between the pubis and umbilicus and elevating the cervix with the dominant hand. The size, shape, mobility, and orientation (e.g., anteversion, retroversion, or military position) of the uterus should be noted. The adnexae may be palpated between the clinician's abdominal and vaginal fingers in the left (LLQ) and right lower quadrants (RLQ), respectively. Here, pain, size, and mobility are noted. A rectovaginal examination is useful in certain circumstances to evaluate the posterior cul-de-sac for the presence of nodularity, which may be seen in malignancy or endometriosis.

Imaging

Ultrasonography and MRI scans can enhance assessment of the female reproductive system and are demonstrated in **Figures 4.6 and 4.7**

■ MALE REPRODUCTIVE SYSTEM

Overview

The male reproductive organs consist of the testes within the scrotum, seminal vesicles and prostate gland within the pelvic cavity, Cowper glands within the peritoneum, and the post-prostatic urethra. During ejaculation, spermatozoa travel from the testis, via the epididymis, to the ductus deferens. The ductus deferens merges with the duct of the seminal vesicle to form the ejaculatory duct, which drains into the prostatic urethra. Secretions from the Cowper glands merge to form seminal fluid (contains spermatozoa and fluid from the seminal vesicles, prostate, and Cowper glands) that is ejaculated through the external urethral orifice (**Fig. 4.8**).

The prostate gland lies inferior to the bladder and—significantly for the physical examination—just anterior to the rectum, from which it is separated by a thin rectovesical septum. The prostate gland is composed of five lobes: a pair of lateral lobes, a lobe anterior to the urethra, a median lobe posterior to the urethra, and a posterior lobe juxtaposed against the anterior rectal wall. The many exocrine glands of the prostate gland drain into the prostatic urethra. From the prostatic urethra onward, the course of seminal fluid is similar to that of urine (**Fig. 4.8**).

Physical Examination

For the male genital examination, the patient may be supine for most of the examination, but should be in standing position for the scrotal examination, as it improves sensitivity in diagnosing

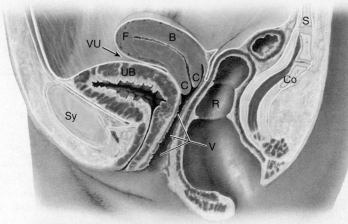

(A) Median anatomical section

Key	
B	Body of uterus
C	Cervix of uterus
CC	Cervical canal
Co	Coccyx
E	Endometrium
F	Fundus of uterus
M	Myometrium
R	Rectum
RA	Rectus abdominis
RU	Recto-uterine pouch
S	Sacrum
Sy	Pubic symphysis
UB	Urinary bladder
UC	Uterine cavity
V	Vagina
VU	Vesico-uterine pouch

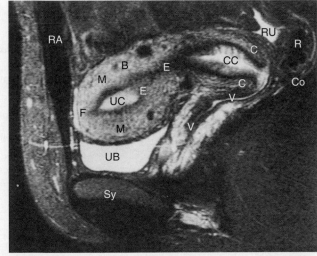

(B) Median MRI

FIGURE 4.7. Female pelvis structures as visualized by **(A)** median anatomical section and **(B)** MRI scan.

varicoceles and hernias. The physical examination involves inspection of the external genitalia for evidence of masses, erythema, excoriations, penile drainage, and other abnormalities. The clinician should inspect the penis and ask the patient to retract the prepuce, if present.

● CLINICAL PEARL

Inability to retract the prepuce is termed *phimosis*, and inability to return the retracted prepuce to its original position is termed *paraphimosis*.

Retraction of the prepuce may reveal smegma, a benign oily substance that helps lubricate movement of the prepuce over the glans penis. The glans may also be the site of skin lesions from sexually transmitted infections (STIs), such as a syphilitic chancre or papillomatous wart. The urethral meatus should be located in the middle of the glans; in the congenital condition of hypospadias, however, it is ventrally displaced and borders the edge of the glans penis. Following inspection, the penile shaft is palpated for masses or nodules. Palpating the glans widens the urethra and will express any discharge that is present.

Following this, the scrotum should be inspected for lesions and for asymmetric changes such as an empty hemiscrotum (may reflect cryptorchidism) or enlarged hemiscrotum (may be due

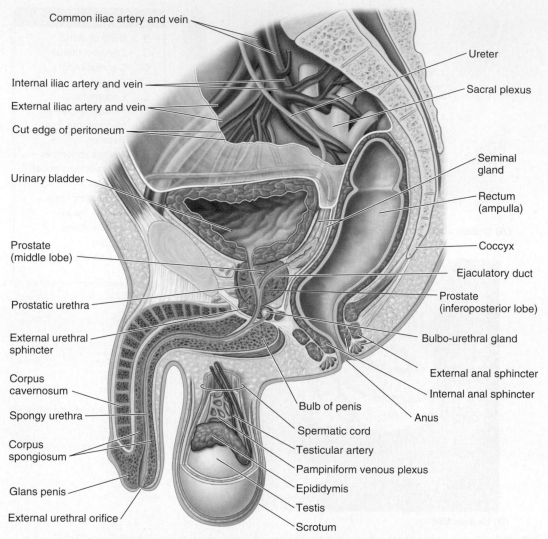

Common iliac artery and vein

Ureter

Internal iliac artery and vein

Sacral plexus

External iliac artery and vein

Cut edge of peritoneum

Seminal gland

Urinary bladder

Rectum (ampulla)

Prostate (middle lobe)

Coccyx

Ejaculatory duct

Prostatic urethra

Prostate (inferoposterior lobe)

External urethral sphincter

Bulbo-urethral gland

Corpus cavernosum

External anal sphincter

Internal anal sphincter

Spongy urethra

Bulb of penis

Corpus spongiosum

Anus

Spermatic cord

Testicular artery

Glans penis

Pampiniform venous plexus

Epididymis

External urethral orifice

Testis

Scrotum

Schematic medial section of male pelvis and penis, stepped dissection of scrotum and coverings of testis

FIGURE 4.8. Internal structures of male pelvis and perineum.

to fluid, blood, or mass effect). The clinician should palpate the testes, epididymis, and spermatic cords, assessing for irregularities in size, shape, and firmness. The digital rectal examination (Chapter 3) can help assess the prostate.

Imaging

CT and MRI scans to enhance assessment of the male reproductive system are demonstrated in **Figures 4.9 and 4.10**. Ultrasound can also be used to assess the scrotum and prostate.

■ URINARY SYSTEM

Overview

The urinary system consists of the kidneys, urethra, and bladder (**Fig. 4.11**). The kidneys are deep retroperitoneal structures and less amenable to palpation unless the patient has a lean frame, or the

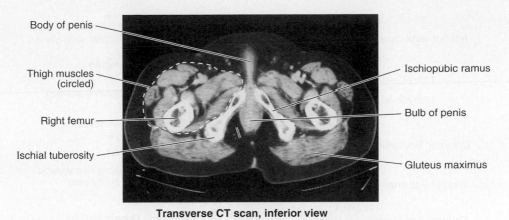

Transverse CT scan, inferior view

FIGURE 4.9. CT scan of male pelvis at the level of the superficial pouch.

kidneys are significantly enlarged (Chapter 3). Ureters emerge from the kidneys, course over the bifurcating iliac vessels, and drain into the posterior aspect of the base of the bladder. The urethra emerges from the bladder and leads to an external orifice. The female urethra is very short. The male urethra is longer and courses through the prostate gland and the penis. The male urethra is divided into four segments: preprostatic, prostatic, membranous, and spongy. From the prostatic

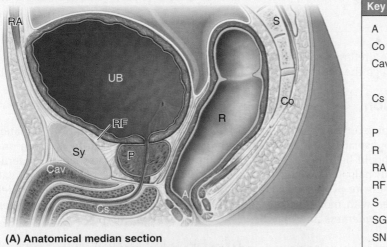

(A) Anatomical median section

Key	
A	Anus
Co	Coccyx
Cav	Corpus cavernosum of penis
Cs	Corpus spongiosum of penis
P	Prostate
R	Rectum
RA	Rectus abdominis
RF	Retropubic fat
S	Sacrum
SG	Seminal gland
SN	Sacral nerves
Sy	Pubic symphysis
UB	Urinary bladder

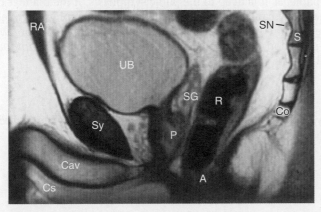

(B) Median MRI

FIGURE 4.10. Male pelvis and perineum as visualized anatomically (A) and by MRI scan (B).

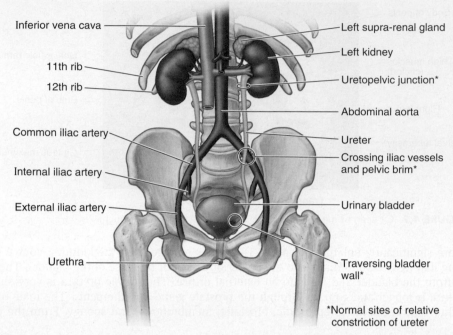

Inferior vena cava

11th rib

12th rib

Common iliac artery

Internal iliac artery

External iliac artery

Urethra

Left supra-renal gland

Left kidney

Uretopelvic junction*

Abdominal aorta

Ureter

Crossing iliac vessels
and pelvic brim*

Urinary bladder

Traversing bladder
wall*

*Normal sites of relative
constriction of ureter

FIGURE 4.11. Anterior view of genitourinary viscera with three areas of relative constriction of the uterus (*asterisk*).

urethra onward, the male urethra serves both a urinary and reproductive function. The spongy urethra then courses through the penis until it reaches its external orifice at the urethral meatus.

Physical Examination

The patient should be supine on the examination table. The clinician should stand by the patient's side and use one hand to displace the kidney anteriorly and the other hand to push down on the abdomen. The kidneys should be assessed for their firmness, shape, and presence of tenderness. The left kidney is less easily palpated owing to the presence of the spleen. The physical examination should also be used to assess for pyelonephritis. With the patient seated upright, the costovertebral angle should be percussed with moderate pressure. Pain elicited with this maneuver is referred to as *costovertebral angle tenderness* and may be seen with pyelonephritis (Figs. 3.21 and 3.22 in Chapter 3).

An empty bladder is not easily palpable, as it is deep to the pubic symphysis. If the bladder contains at least 500 mL of urine, its round dome can be palpable above the pubic symphysis while the patient lies supine. Further enlargement of the bladder manifests as dullness to percussion above the pubic symphysis. Tenderness on palpation of the dome of the bladder, known as *suprapubic tenderness*, is suggestive of a bacterial cystitis.

Imaging

Radiographic images, ultrasonography, and CT scans to enhance assessment of the male reproductive system are demonstrated in Figure 3.23 (Chapter 3).

■ BREAST

Overview

The breasts are part of the anterior thoracic wall and are more prominent in women than in men. Breasts consist of glandular and supporting fibrous tissue; the greatest prominence of the breast is

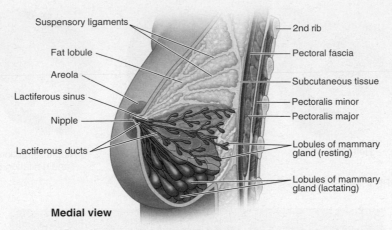

FIGURE 4.12. Sagittal section of the female breast with depiction of resting and lactating mammary glands. The anatomic relation of the breast and deeper thoracic structures is also depicted.

the nipple, which is surrounded by a circular pigmented area of skin called the *areola* (**Fig. 4.12**). Visually, the breast can be divided into four quadrants. The superior lateral quadrant has the most glandular tissue and, consequently, is the site of most breast tumors (**Fig. 4.13**).

Physical Examination

The patient should be seated on the examination table with arms by the side, and a female chaperone should be present in the room during the examination. Only areas being examined should be exposed, while the rest of the chest area should remain covered with a drape. The clinician stands in front of the patient and inspects the breasts for their color; size and symmetry; irregularities in the nipple or areola region; and the presence of obvious masses, skin retraction, nodularity, or spontaneous nipple discharge (**Fig. 4.14**). The inspection can be repeated with the patient's arms over the head, with hands pressed against the hips, and with leaning forward.

Following inspection, the patient should be in the supine position for palpation. One method of breast palpation is the vertical strip pattern demonstrated in **Figure 4.15**. This will help to identify superficial or deeper irregularities in the breast tissue. Finally, the nipples should be palpated for their elasticity. Reduced elasticity is seen in underlying cancer. Although the breast examination is more frequently done in women as part of health maintenance, the breast examination can also be performed in males.

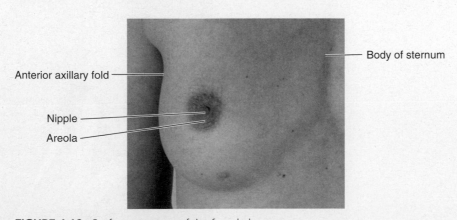

FIGURE 4.13. Surface anatomy of the female breast.

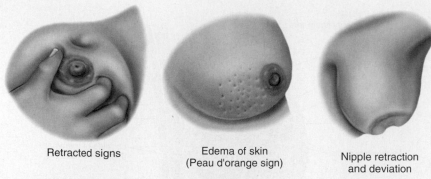

Retracted signs

Edema of skin
(Peau d'orange sign)

Nipple retraction
and deviation

FIGURE 4.14. Superficial signs of underlying breast cancer.

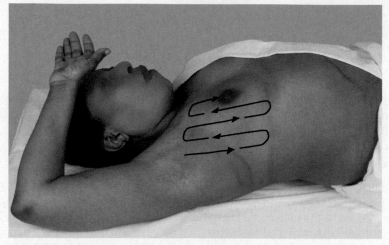

FIGURE 4.15. Vertical strip technique to examine the breast for underlying tenderness and masses. The examiner starts in one area and systematically palpates the breast to detect underlying abnormalities.

FIGURE 4.16. Technique to examine axillary lymph nodes.

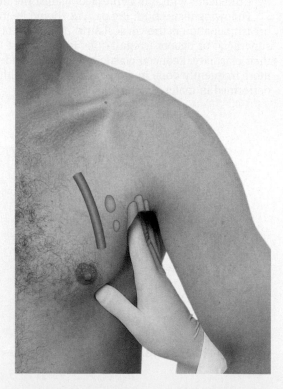

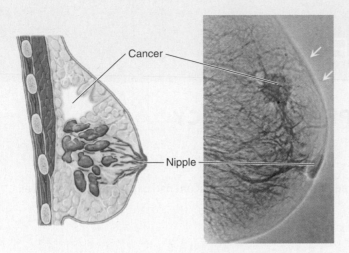

FIGURE 4.17. Anatomic and radiographic depiction of underlying breast cancer.

After inspecting and palpating the breast tissue, the lymph nodes are evaluated. To evaluate the axillary nodes, the patient should be seated with arms by the side. The clinician should palpate as high as possible in the apex of the axilla directed toward the midclavicle. The nodes should be assessed for size, shape, regularity, mobility, and texture (**Fig. 4.16**).

Imaging

Radiographic images, ultrasonography, MRI scans, and CT scans to enhance assessment of the breast are demonstrated in **Figures 4.17 and 4.18**.

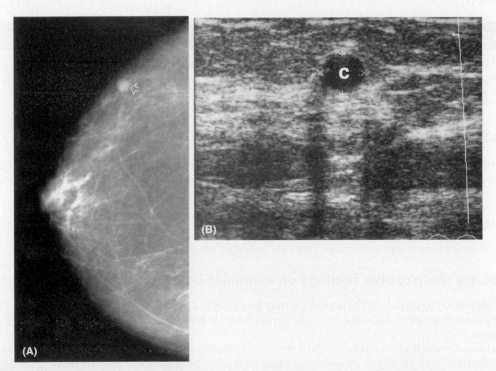

FIGURE 4.18. Benign breast cyst (**A**) with well-defined mass (*arrow*) and corresponding ultrasound (**B**) depicting well-defined boundaries (*C*).

CLINICAL CASES

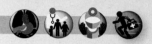 **ECTOPIC PREGNANCY**

Presentation

A 25-year-old female presents with severe RLQ pain. Her last menstrual period was 6 weeks ago.

Definition

Ectopic pregnancy is defined as implantation of the embryo outside of the uterine cavity. In 98% of cases, ectopic implantation takes place in the fallopian tubes.

What are common causes?

The most common causes are prior ectopic pregnancy and pelvic inflammatory disease (PID). Women who have undergone conservative surgical treatment for prior ectopic pregnancies have up to 15% risk of recurrence, whereas prior medical therapy typically confers < 10% risk of recurrence. PID is typically caused by *Chlamydia trachomatis* or *Neisseria gonorrhea* and is often related to the number of prior sexual partners.

Other etiologies, including tubal factor infertility, prior surgery on the fallopian tubes, history of abdominal surgery, presence of fibroids, and in vitro fertilization, are associated with ectopic pregnancy.

> ● **CLINICAL PEARL**
>
> A life-threatening complication of an ectopic pregnancy is rupture, and the following factors are associated with an increased risk: previous tubal damage and infertility, induction of ovulation, and a serum β-HCG level above 10,000 mIU/mL.

What is the differential diagnosis?

Abdominal pain: The differential diagnosis includes appendicitis, nephrolithiasis, ovarian torsion, ruptured ovarian cyst, exacerbation of inflammatory bowel disease, irritable bowel disease, and iliopsoas strain.

What symptoms might be observed?

Symptoms include lower abdominal pain, presyncope, amenorrhea, and vaginal bleeding.

What are the possible findings on examination?

Vital signs: Tachycardia and hypotension may be present.
Inspection: Speculum examination may reveal vaginal bleeding, but typically the cervical os is closed.
Palpation: Lower abdominal pain and exquisite tenderness to palpation accompanied by rebound tenderness and guarding. An adnexal mass may also be palpable. Cervical motion tenderness may be appreciated on bimanual examination.

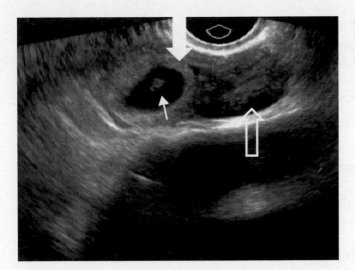

FIGURE 4.19. Ultrasound image of ectopic pregnancy depicting the thick-walled gestational sac (*solid large arrow*), near the ovary (*open arrow*). The embryonic pole is seen within the gestational sac (*thin arrow*).

What tests should be ordered?

Laboratory tests: CBC (leukocytosis suggests infection, and anemia may be consistent with significant blood loss) and metabolic panel (BUN:Cr > 20:1 suggests hypovolemia). If thrombocytopenia, consider disseminated intravascular coagulation (DIC) and check coagulation panel (elevated international normalized ratio [INR], elevated partial thromboplastin time [PTT], reduced fibrinogen) and peripheral blood smear (schistocytes). A blood group and screen should be performed to allow for the administration of Rho (D) immune globulin (RhIg) if needed and for a cross-match for transfusion if necessary. Urine qualitative β-human chorionic gonadotropin (HCG) assay can be used to screen for pregnancy, and serum quantitative β-HCG levels can be assessed.

Imaging: Transvaginal ultrasound (TVUS) is the main imaging modality to assess for presence of an ectopic pregnancy (**Fig. 4.19**). The ability of TVUS to detect an intrauterine pregnancy depends on the serum level of β-HCG. With a serum β-HCG level higher than 1,500–2,000 mIU/mL, TVUS has a specificity higher than 90% for visualizing an intrauterine pregnancy. When levels are lower, the specificity, sensitivity, and positive predictive value are also lowered.

> **● CLINICAL PEARL**
>
> In females of childbearing age, always perform a qualitative urine β-HCG test to assess for pregnancy. If necessary, a quantitative serum β-HCG test can also be measured.

 PLACENTA PREVIA

Presentation

A 30-year-old female at 32 weeks' gestational age presents with painless vaginal bleeding.

Definition

Placenta previa is the presence of placental tissue covering or in close proximity to the internal cervical os.

What are common causes?

The major risk factors for placenta previa are previous placenta previa, previous cesarean section, previous uterine surgery, spontaneous or induced abortion, and prior treatment for infertility.

What is the differential diagnosis?

Vaginal bleeding in pregnancy: The differential diagnosis includes vasa previa, abruptio placenta, and uterine rupture.

What symptoms might be observed?

Placenta previa typically presents as painless vaginal bleeding, most often around 32 weeks' gestation, with potential life-threatening maternal and neonatal consequences from hemorrhage.

What are the possible findings on examination?

Vital signs: Hypotension, depending on the extent of blood loss.
Inspection: Vaginal bleeding may be present. Internal examination should be avoided, depending on risk stratification for placenta previa with ultrasound. If performed, it would likely reveal bright red blood.
Palpation: The abdominal examination is typically normal with a nontender, soft uterus. The presentation of the fetus may be nonvertex (e.g., breech or transverse) in a woman with a placenta previa.

What tests should be ordered?

Laboratory tests: CBC (leukocytosis suggests infection, and anemia may be consistent with significant blood loss) and metabolic panel (BUN:Cr > 20:1 suggests hypovolemia). If thrombocytopenia, consider DIC and check coagulation panel (elevated INR, elevated PTT, reduced fibrinogen) and peripheral blood smear (schistocytes). A blood group and screen should be performed to allow for the administration of RhIg if needed, and for a cross-match for transfusion if necessary. In the case of antepartum bleeding, a Kleihauer-Betke test may be used to evaluate the maternal serum for the presence of fetal blood cells.
Imaging: Transabdominal and transvaginal ultrasonography are typically performed to determine location of the placenta, with the latter being superior to the former (**Fig. 4.20**).

FIGURE 4.20. Ultrasound image of placenta previa depicting the placenta (*P*), partially visualized urinary bladder (*B*), and the internal cervical os (*arrow*).

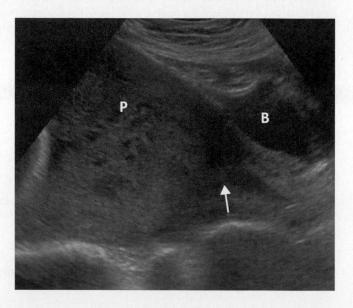

ABRUPTIO PLACENTA

Presentation

A 36-year-old female presents at 33 weeks' gestation with painful uterine contractions and vaginal bleeding.

Definition

Abruptio placenta refers to premature separation of the placenta from the uterine wall.

What are common causes?

Clinical risk factors include severe fetal growth restriction, prolonged rupture of membranes, hypertension, amniotic fluid disorders, cigarette smoking, advanced maternal age (age > 35 years), trauma, cocaine use, and male fetal gender. The presence of twins makes placental abruption approximately twice as likely to occur.

What is the differential diagnosis?

Abdominal pain and vaginal bleeding in pregnancy: The differential diagnosis includes active labor, chorioamnionitis, placenta previa, and uterine rupture.

What symptoms might be observed?

In contrast to placenta previa, abruptio placenta typically presents with acute-onset painful vaginal bleeding. Placental separation induces labor, resulting in uterine contractions. In < 20% of patients, the predominant presenting complaint involves uterine contractions as the majority of hemorrhage is retained behind the placenta. This scenario is termed "concealed abruption."

What are the possible findings on examination?

Vital signs: Hypotension, depending on extent of blood loss. The fetal heart rate is often abnormal.
Inspection: Bright red vaginal bleeding.
Palpation: Uterine contractions, decreased fetal movements, lower abdominal tenderness are felt.

> ● **CLINICAL PEARL**
>
> If clinical suspicion for placental abruption exists, an internal exam should not be performed prior to ultrasound as this could result in catastrophic hemorrhage.

What tests should be ordered?

Laboratory tests: CBC (leukocytosis suggests infection, and anemia may be consistent with significant blood loss). If thrombocytopenia, consider DIC and check coagulation panel (elevated INR, elevated PTT, reduced fibrinogen). Fibrinogen, in particular, is extremely helpful in anticipating the possibility of postpartum hemorrhage. Serum fibrinogen < 200 mg/dL has nearly 100% positive predictive value for postpartum hemorrhage, whereas fibrinogen > 400 mg/dL has nearly 80% negative predictive value for hemorrhage. A blood group and screen should be performed to

FIGURE 4.21. Abruptio placenta. Abdominal Doppler scan shows blood (*B*) between the placental tip (*P*) and uterine wall (*U*).

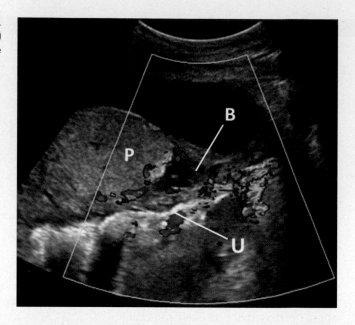

allow for the administration of RhIg, if needed, and for a cross-match for transfusion if necessary. In the case of antepartum bleeding, a Kleihauer-Betke test may be used to evaluate maternal serum for the presence of fetal blood cells.

Imaging: Ultrasound is typically thought to be of limited value (Sn 0.25), but classically shows radiolucency between the placenta and the uterine wall. To improve diagnostic yield, MRI could be considered if ultrasonography is negative, but there is high clinical suspicion for potential abruption (**Fig. 4.21**). However, placental abruption is considered an obstetrical emergency and is typically managed clinically without imaging.

 # URINARY STONES

Presentation

A 35-year-old female presents with intense, paroxysmal shooting LLQ pain along her left inguinal canal with associated nausea and vomiting. For several hours prior to presentation, she noticed painful micturition with red-tinged urine.

Definition

Urinary stones, or *nephroliths*, are stones in the urinary tract formed from various minerals. They can obstruct the ureteral lumen and urinary flow anywhere along their course from the kidney through the ureteropelvic junction inferiorly toward the bladder (**Fig. 4.22**).

What are common causes?

The most common causes include the following:

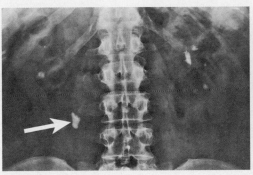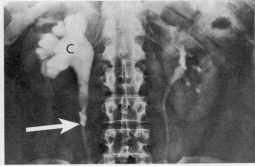

FIGURE 4.22. A. Abdominal x-ray depicting multiple renal calculi, the largest (*arrow*) of which is at the L3 level. **B.** Renal collecting system (*C*) and hydroureteronephrosis from a large calculus (*arrow*).

Type of stone	Characteristics
Calcium stones	Majority of cases (80%) of symptomatic stones, in the form of either calcium oxalate or, less frequently, calcium phosphate
Struvite stones (magnesium ammonium phosphate)	Associated with elevated urine pH and infections from urease-producing organisms, such as those from the *Proteus* and *Klebsiella* genera (**Fig. 4.23**)
Uric acid stones	Associated with low urine pH and result from precipitation of uric acid in the urinary system; predisposing factors include gout, diabetes, and metabolic syndrome
Cystine stones	Result from genetic mutations that predispose to urinary stones; patients frequently present with their first episode at younger ages, during childhood or adolescence

What is the differential diagnosis?

Lower abdominal pain: The differential diagnosis for acute lower abdominal pain includes appendicitis, diverticulitis, gallstones, and ectopic pregnancy and ovarian cyst rupture (in women).

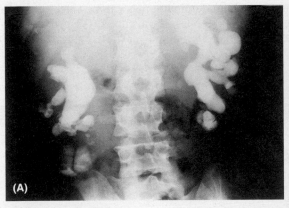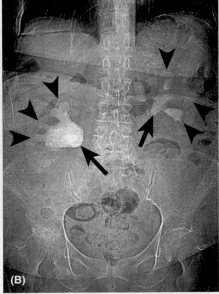

FIGURE 4.23. A. X-ray of staghorn calculi. **B.** CT x-ray in another patient showing staghorn calculi in the renal pelvis (*arrow*) and calyces (*arrowhead*).

What symptoms might be observed?

Symptoms include flank or lower quadrant pain (usually unilateral and paroxysmal) with radiation toward the groin, nausea, vomiting, dysuria, and urinary urgency.

> ● CLINICAL PEARL
>
> Pain related to a ureteric stone may range from dull discomfort and ache to intense and sharp; it may sometimes mimic acute abdomen or arterial dissection.

What are the possible findings on examination?

Vital signs: Tachycardia and tachypnea may be seen in the setting of pain; fever and other changes (tachycardia, hypotension) may also be seen in the setting of UTI secondary to an obstructing stone.

Inspection: Patients may be in mild distress (due to dull aching pain or between paroxysms of pain) or in acute distress (unable to lie still); the abdomen typically appears normal without obvious lesions or scars.

Palpation: Pain on palpation either around the kidney (Sn 0.86, Sp 0.76, positive LR 3.6, negative LR 0.2) or in the loin region (flank tenderness [Sn 0.15, Sp 0.99, positive LR 27.7, negative LR 0.9]; rebound tenderness and involuntary guarding are typically not observed.

Auscultation: Bowel sounds are typically present and normal.

Special Tests

CVA tenderness: Percussion of the flank over the area of the kidney (CVA) with the patient in sitting position; extreme discomfort or pain is consistent with potential acute pyelonephritis. Although there are no specific tests to elicit pain from ureteric stones, other tests (e.g., Rovsing sign, psoas sign, obturator sign; Chapter 3) and exams (pelvic exam, digital rectal exam) are important to rule out other etiologies of pain.

What tests should be ordered?

Laboratory tests: CBC (leukocytosis, if infection), urinalysis, urine sediment, urine qualitative β-HCG (women of childbearing age). If necessary, a serum quantitative β-HCG can also be measured.

Imaging: Helical CT scan of the abdomen without contrast is the gold standard. Ultrasound can be used to avoid radiation (e.g., pregnant women). Abdominal x-rays can be used but can miss small stones and will not detect radiolucent uric acid stones. Intravenous (IV) pyelogram is no longer used in view of large radiation exposure, risk of contrast reactions, and availability of newer imaging modalities.

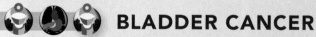

BLADDER CANCER

Presentation

A 68-year-old male presents with painless, intermittently red-tinged urine over the course of several weeks. He also notes urinary urgency during this period.

Definition

Bladder cancer, or malignancy affecting bladder tissue, is a common urologic cancer. It most commonly arises from the bladder urothelium, although the frequency of cancer types varies, depending on the layer from which the cancer originates.

What are common causes?

The most common causes include the following:

Type of malignancy	Characteristics
Transitional cell carcinoma	Most common histological type of bladder cancer in the developed world (accounts for >90% of bladder cancer in these regions) and can arise from anywhere in the urinary tract (e.g., renal pelvis, ureter, urethra, in addition to the bladder)
Squamous cell carcinoma	Most common bladder cancer in the developing world; its development has been associated with parasitic infection by *Schistosoma haematobium* as well as chronic bladder stones
Other (less common) types	Adenocarcinomas, sarcomas, lymphomas, and small cell carcinoma

What is the differential diagnosis?

Hematuria: The differential diagnosis includes urinary stones, UTIs (bacterial, parasitic), benign prostatic hyperplasia ([BPH] men), iatrogenic (instrumentation), congenital (polycystic kidney disease [PKD]), vascular (renal infarction), glomerulonephritis, and false positives (menstrual bleeding interpreted as hematuria, pigments mimicking hematuria).

What symptoms might be observed?

Frequently, bladder cancer presents as painless bleeding, and the presence of flank or suprapubic pain frequently signifies invasive or metastatic disease, causing obstruction and damage to surrounding structures. Other symptoms that may be present include increased urinary frequency, urgency, dysuria, decreased strength of urinary stream, sensation of incomplete voiding, and constitutional symptoms (weight loss, anorexia, fatigue).

What are the possible findings on examination?

Vital signs: Typically unremarkable.
Inspection: Frequently appear well, although in advanced cancer, the patient may appear cachectic or malnourished.
Palpation: Pain with palpation suggests invasive or metastatic disease involving surrounding structures; palpable solid masses or palpable metastatic liver lesions are observed in advanced disease.
Auscultation: Bowel sounds are typically normal.

What tests should be ordered?

Laboratory tests: CBC (leukocytosis if infection, anemia if blood loss), urinalysis, urine sediment, and urine cytology and culture.
Imaging: Direct visualization with cystoscopy is the gold standard for initial evaluation of suspected bladder cancer, and more recent adjunctive therapies with fluorescence cystoscopy have further increased the sensitivity of cystoscopy, especially in cases of carcinoma in situ (**Fig. 4.24**). Although ultrasound may have benefit in evaluating upper urinary tract disease, it is suboptimal for evaluating bladder cancer (cannot accurately assess extension, invasion, or staging). On the other hand, a CT scan of the abdomen and pelvis is helpful for staging and may reveal other obstructive masses (**Fig. 4.25**). IV pyelogram can be useful in detecting small lesions compared to ultrasound or CT scan. Nuclear imaging with PET or bone scan can be helpful in metastatic or advanced disease.

FIGURE 4.24. Cystoscopy to visualize the urinary bladder.

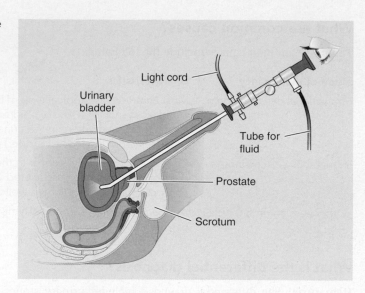

FIGURE 4.25. Bladder tumor resulting in obstructive uropathy. **A.** noncontrast CT scan shows the dilated collecting system (*C*) with bilateral hydronephrosis. Also noted is associated abdominal ascites (*asterisk*). **B.** The distal ureters (*arrowhead*) are obstructed by a mass due to transitional cell carcinoma (*t*). A Foley catheter (*f*) is placed in the bladder.

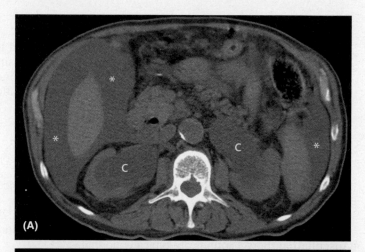

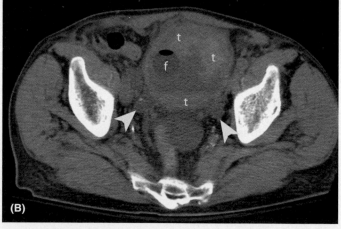

POLYCYSTIC KIDNEY DISEASE

Presentation

A 27-year-old male presents with RLQ pain and a fever of 38.3°C (101°F) with associated nausea and vomiting. Ten hours prior to his presentation, he developed low-grade periumbilical pain.

Definition

PKD is an inherited, autosomal dominant condition that results from mutations in either *PKD1* or *PKD2* genes, leads to alteration in nephron development, and ultimately causes progression to renal dysfunction due to cyst formation, enlargement, compression, and rupture. It is marked by phenotypic heterogeneity and, consequently, patients with the same mutations may have different disease courses.

What are common causes?

A *PKD1* mutation (located on chromosome 16) comprises ~85% of cases and is the more severe phenotype than a *PKD2* mutation (located on chromosome 4), which comprises ~15% of cases and features later onset and slower progression.

What is the differential diagnosis?

Hematuria: The differential diagnosis includes urinary stones, UTIs (bacterial, parasitic), glomerular disease, BPH (men), iatrogenic (instrumentation), malignant (urothelial tumors), vascular (renal infarction), glomerulonephritis, and false positives (menstrual bleeding interpreted as hematuria, pigments mimicking hematuria).

What symptoms might be observed?

Symptoms include flank pain, polyuria, nocturia, early satiety (mass effect), and right upper quadrant pain (in the setting of hepatic cysts, which are the most common extrarenal finding in PKD).

What are the possible findings on examination?

Vital signs: Hypertension may be seen in some cases.
Inspection: Bulging or prominent flank masses may be present.
Palpation: Bilateral flank masses can sometimes be palpated.
Percussion: Typically normal.
Auscultation: Bowel sounds are typically present and normal.

What tests should be ordered?

Laboratory tests: CBC (anemia may be present), basic metabolic panel (elevated BUN and Cr), genetic linkage analysis testing for *PKD1* and *PKD2* mutations, and urinalysis (proteinuria and hematuria may be present).
Imaging: Screening imaging is frequently done, particularly in patients with a positive family history for cysts. The sensitivity of ultrasound to identify renal cysts is reportedly higher than 90%; however, there is significant variability based on patient age and cyst size. As such, CT (**Fig. 4.26**) and T2-weighted MRI scans are more sensitive in identifying asymptomatic, younger patients.

FIGURE 4.26. CT image shows multiple cysts (*C*) consistent with PKD. The cysts are heterogeneous with increased proteinaceous or hemorrhagic contents (*arrowhead*) and calcification (*arrow*).

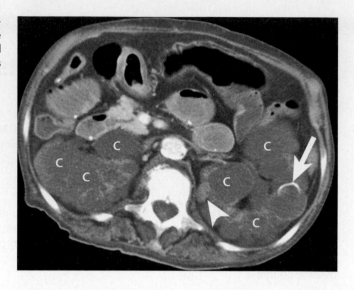

Special Tests

Genetic testing can be used when imaging is equivocal, and screening imaging for extrarenal manifestations (e.g., intracranial aneurysms) should be limited to patients at high risk or with a positive personal or family history of these complications.

 # HYDRONEPHROSIS

Presentation

A 65-year-old male presents with subacute onset of right flank pain, fluctuating but decreased urine output, and suprapubic fullness.

Definition

Hydronephrosis is the distension of the renal calyces and pelvis due to distal obstruction in the GU tract, although it can sometimes be present without evidence of obstruction (**Fig. 4.27**). *Hydroureter* is a related and analogous term that relates to the distension of the ureter.

What are common causes?

The most common etiologies include the following:

Type	Etiologies
Intrinsic obstruction	Tumors, calculi, polyps, blood clots, strictures, valves, infections (e.g., tuberculosis) at the levels of the ureter, bladder, and urethra
Extrinsic obstruction	Tumors (e.g., retroperitoneal lymphoma or sarcoma, cervical cancer, prostate cancer), reproductive organs (e.g., tubo-ovarian abscess, uterine prolapse, ovarian cysts), primary retroperitoneal or pelvic processes (e.g., retroperitoneal hemorrhage, pelvic lipomatosis, retroperitoneal fibrosis), and vascular disease (e.g., aortic aneurysm)
Nonobstructive causes	Pregnancy and large-volume diuresis (e.g., significant nephrogenic diabetes insipidus)

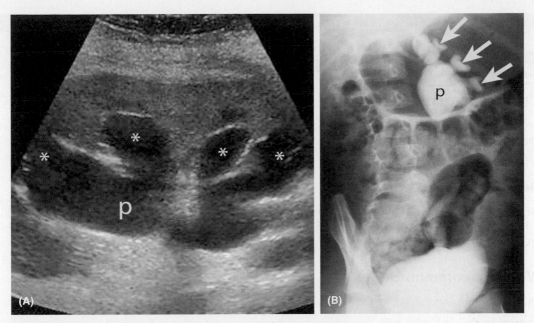

FIGURE 4.27. A. Sagittal ultrasound section with distension of the renal pelvis (*p*) and calyces (*asterisk*). **B.** Intravenous urography image with a dilated renal pelvis (*p*) and calyces (*arrow*).

What is the differential diagnosis?

Pelvic pain: The differential diagnosis includes renal calculi, gallstones, acute appendicitis, ruptured ovarian cyst, and UTI.

What symptoms might be observed?

Hydronephrosis alone is frequently asymptomatic; however, other possible symptoms include flank pain or discomfort and suprapubic fullness.

What are the possible findings on examination?

Vital signs: Typically unremarkable.
Inspection: Typically unremarkable.
Palpation: Suprapubic fullness may be present. In addition, flank tenderness may be present, but this is nonspecific.
Percussion: Typically unremarkable.
Auscultation: Bowel sounds are typically normal.

What tests should be ordered?

Laboratory tests: CBC (leukocytosis, if infection), basic metabolic panel (elevated BUN and Cr), urinalysis, urine sediment, and urine qualitative β-HCG (women of childbearing age). If necessary, a serum quantitative β-HCG can also be measured.
Imaging: Ultrasound is the imaging modality of choice for evaluating hydronephrosis and hydroureter. CT scan of the abdomen is an alternative, particularly if there is clinical suspicion of a cause that can be evaluated by CT scan (e.g., urinary stone or mass effect) (**Fig. 4.27**). IV pyelogram can also be used, although it is limited by radiation exposure and risk of contrast reactions.

 # PELVIC INFLAMMATORY DISEASE

Presentation

A 22-year-old female presents to the Emergency Department with 1 day of worsening lower abdominal pain and fever.

Definition

PID refers to inflammation of the uterus, fallopian tubes, and ovaries. It is often caused by STIs. If left untreated, PID can lead to pelvic adhesions and is a major cause of infertility and ectopic pregnancy.

What are common causes?

The most common causes include the following:

Organism	Etiologies
Chlamydia trachomatis	Common STI; many women are asymptomatic and therefore may not be diagnosed or treated; if untreated, up to 30% will develop PID
Neisseria gonorrhoea	Common STI; ~10%–20% of infected women will develop PID if they do not receive adequate treatment
Vaginal flora	Normally occurring bacteria in the vagina or GI tract that may ascend the lower genital tract and result in PID
Other	May develop during childbirth, after procedures such as endometrial biopsy or insertion of an intrauterine device, or after a spontaneous or therapeutic abortion

What is the differential diagnosis?

Lower abdominal pain: The differential diagnosis includes acute appendicitis, ovarian torsion, ectopic pregnancy, septic abortion, ruptured ovarian cyst, and acute enteritis.

What symptoms might be observed?

Symptoms include abdominal pain, dyspareunia, abnormal vaginal bleeding, malodorous vaginal discharge, dysuria, and dyschezia.

What are the possible findings on examination?

Vital signs: Typically normal, although the patient may present with fever, tachycardia, or hypotension if septic.
Inspection: External examination may reveal purulent vaginal discharge or vaginal bleeding. Internal examination may reveal purulent discharge or blood at the cervical os, with cervical erythema. The internal examination may also be normal in asymptomatic PID.
Palpation: On bimanual examination, symptomatic patients typically have tenderness with palpation and motion of the cervix. The clinician may also note firmness in the adnexal regions in the case of a tubo-ovarian abscess. The bimanual examination may be normal in asymptomatic PID.
Percussion: Typically unremarkable.
Auscultation: Bowel sounds are typically normal.

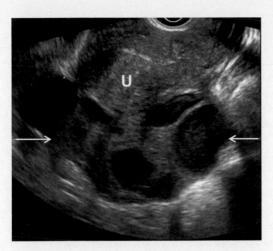

FIGURE 4.28. Ultrasound image with tubo-ovarian abscess depicted by heterogeneous mass between *arrows* and behind the uterus (*U*).

● CLINICAL PEARL

Infections with *Chlamydia* can cause reactive arthritis. *Neisseria* can cause disseminated infection that presents with tenosynovitis, dermatitis, and polyarthralgias.

What tests should be ordered?

Laboratory tests: CBC (leukocytosis with infection) and qualitative urine β-HCG to rule out pregnancy. Microbiology includes endocervical swab specimens may reveal demonstrate polymorphonuclear leukocytes and Gram-negative diplococci. Nucleic acid amplification tests (NAATs) should be sent to detect *C. trachomatis* and *N. gonorrhea.*

● CLINICAL PEARL

Qualitative urine β-HCG should be checked in women of childbearing age to rule out pregnancy. If necessary, a serum quantitative β-HCG can also be measured.

Imaging: TVUS may show a tubo-ovarian abscess (**Fig. 4.28**) or evidence of salpingitis.

 # OVARIAN CYST

Presentation

A 24-year-old female presents for a periodic physical examination and is noted to have fullness in the LLQ.

Definition

An ovarian cyst is a collection of fluid within the ovary and may be benign or malignant. Cysts are further classified by their features on histology and imaging. Malignant ovarian tumors are discussed in a later section.

What are common causes?

Type of cyst	Characteristics
Follicular cyst	Generally noted if the ovum is not released during ovulation
Corpus luteum cyst	Appears during ovulation as a remnant of the follicle and generally resolves 5–9 days after ovulation unless conception occurs, but may rupture and cause intraperitoneal hemorrhage
Theca lutein cyst	A cyst made of theca cells, which surround the developing ovum
Polycystic ovary syndrome (PCOS)	Multiple ovarian cysts often with a classic "string of pearls" sign
Endometriod cyst	Caused by ovarian endometriosis and are known as *chocolate cysts* due to the hemorrhagic appearance on laparoscopy
Dermoid cyst	Cystic structure arising from the germ cell layer of the ovary, with mature tissue derived from ectoderm, endoderm, and mesoderm
Serous cystadenoma	Simple cyst associated with a benign ovarian tumor
Mucinous cystadenoma	Thicker-walled cyst made up of mucin

What is the differential diagnosis?

Abdominal fullness or pain: The differential diagnosis includes pregnancy, ovarian tumor, tubo-ovarian abscess, endometriosis, ectopic pregnancy, fibroid, appendicitis, and ovarian torsion.

What symptoms might be observed?

Symptoms include abdominal pain or pressure, pain associated with ovulation, abnormal uterine bleeding, and midmenstrual cycle pain localizing to one side of the abdomen. However, benign ovarian cysts are most frequently asymptomatic.

What are the possible findings on examination?

Vital signs: Typically normal.
Inspection: External and internal examinations are typically normal.
Palpation: Bimanual examination may reveal tender or nontender fullness in the adnexa. In the case of a ruptured hemorrhagic cyst, the patient may exhibit peritoneal tenderness.
Auscultation: Bowel sounds are typically normal.

What tests should be ordered?

Laboratory tests: CBC (leukocytosis, if inflammation, infection, or malignancy); serum CA 125 may be elevated in epithelial ovarian cancer, but can also be elevated in other causes of benign ovarian pathology. Qualitative urine β-HCG should be checked to rule out pregnancy in women of childbearing age. If necessary, a serum quantitative β-HCG can also be measured.
Imaging: TVUS is the gold standard method for diagnosis. Transabdominal ultrasound may show large ovarian cysts (**Fig. 4.29**), but may not adequately show the adnexa. If small, ovarian cysts are rarely seen on CT imaging.

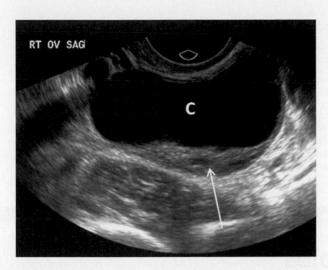

FIGURE 4.29. Simple ovarian cysts (*C*) arising from the surface of the ovary (*arrow*).

 POLYCYSTIC OVARY SYNDROME

Presentation

A 24-year-old female presents to her health care provider with a chief complaint of acne and irregular, heavy periods.

Definition

PCOS is an endocrine disorder involving anovulation, excess androgens, and development of polycystic ovaries.

What are common causes?

The primary cause of PCOS is not well understood. The hallmark features of PCOS include anovulation, excess androgens, and polycystic ovaries. PCOS is thought to have a multifactorial etiology, but also is thought to have a hereditary component. Anovulation leads to amenorrhea and/or infrequent menstrual cycles, whereas excess androgens lead to acne and hirsutism. The syndrome is also associated with obesity, hyperinsulinemia, and infertility.

What is the differential diagnosis?

Heavy, irregular menstruation: The differential diagnosis includes ovarian cyst, metabolic syndrome, hypothyroidism, Cushing syndrome, adult-onset congenital adrenal hyperplasia, adrenal tumor, acromegaly, insufficiency of the hypothalamic–pituitary axis, and pregnancy.

What symptoms might be observed?

Symptoms include irregular menses, heavy menstrual bleeding, acne, excess hair growth, and infertility.

What are the possible findings on examination?

Vital signs: Typically normal.

Inspection: Male pattern hair loss, increased body hair, obesity, acanthosis nigrans, and cystic acne.
Palpation: Typically unremarkable.

What tests should be ordered?

Laboratory tests: Basic metabolic panel (hyperglycemia), serum lipids (hyperlipidemia), thyroid-stimulating hormone (TSH), prolactin,17-hydroxyprogesterone, DHEAS, and total testosterone levels will help to rule out other causes of excess androgens.
Imaging: TVUS may show polycystic ovaries in one or both ovaries. Criteria include > 12 follicles measuring 2–9 mm and increased ovarian volume (> 10 cm³).

 # UTERINE FIBROIDS

Presentation

A 35-year-old female presents to her health care provider complaining of heavy periods and chronic pelvic pain. She and her husband have been unable to conceive for the past year.

Definition

A uterine fibroid is a benign smooth muscle tumor (or, *leiomyoma*) that develops from the muscle wall of the uterus.

> ● CLINICAL PEARL
>
> Fibroids are very common tumors in females. In one study, 51% of premenopausal women were found to have evidence of fibroids on ultrasound. There is a higher incidence in African American women.

What are common causes?

The common risk factors associated with developing uterine fibroids are ethnicity (higher in African Americans), diet (alcohol and red meat intake associated with higher risk, and fruits/vegetables associated with lower risk), and hereditary predisposition through unclear mechanisms.

What is the differential diagnosis?

Pelvic pain: The differential diagnosis includes uterine leiomyosarcoma, adenomyosis, endometrial polyps, endometrial hyperplasia, endometrial carcinoma, ovarian cancer, and pregnancy.

What symptoms might be observed?

Symptoms include heavy and painful menses, abdominal bloating, pelvic pain, backache, urinary retention, dysuria, and infertility. Patients may also be asymptomatic.

What are the possible findings on examination?

Vital signs: Typically normal.
Inspection: External examination is typically normal. On internal examination using a speculum, pedunculated cervical fibroids may be visualized within the cervical os.
Palpation: An enlarged or boggy uterus may be palpated on bimanual examination.
Auscultation: Typically normal bowel sounds.

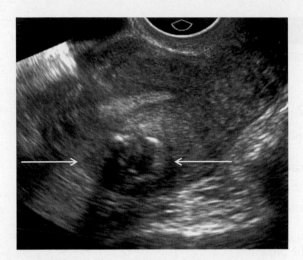

FIGURE 4.30. Ultrasound image shows uterine fibroid depicted by echogenic mass with internal shadowing from the calcifications (*arrows*).

What tests should be ordered?

Laboratory tests: CBC (anemia if significant bleeding).

Imaging: TVUS is the typical modality used to diagnose fibroids, which appear as echodense, well-circumscribed masses within the uterus (**Fig. 4.30**). Pelvic MRI can also be used to characterize pelvic fibroids, but this modality is not frequently used due to cost. MRI may be useful in distinguishing fibroids from sarcoma. Sonohysterography or a hysterosalpingogram can also demonstrate submucosal fibroids.

 # ENDOMETRIAL CARCINOMA

Presentation

A 65-year-old female presents with new-onset vaginal bleeding.

Definition

Endometrial carcinoma is a malignancy that arises from the endometrium (or inner lining) of the uterus.

What are common causes?

Approximately 75% of endometrial cancer is due to endometrioid adenocarcinoma, a tumor of the endometrial glands of the uterus. These tumors are generally estrogen dependent and develop in the setting of endometrial hyperplasia. The remaining 25% of endometrial cancers are made up of high-grade malignancy, such as serous and clear cell tumors. These malignancies tend to be more aggressive and are less related to estrogen stimulation.

> ● **CLINICAL PEARL**
>
> A strong association exists between body-mass index and endometrial hyperplasia, which can lead to endometrial cancer.

What is the differential diagnosis?

Uterine mass: The differential diagnosis includes endometrial hyperplasia, adenomyosis, endometriosis, ovarian cancer, cervical cancer, uterine fibroids, and leiomyosarcoma.

What symptoms might be observed?

Symptoms include abdominal pain/cramping and vaginal bleeding.

What are the possible findings on examination?

Vital signs: Typically unremarkable.
Inspection: External examination may be unremarkable, and internal examination may reveal presence of blood in the vaginal vault.
Palpation: Bimanual examination may reveal an enlarged uterus.
Auscultation: Typically normal bowel sounds are present.

What tests should be ordered?

Laboratory tests: CBC (anemia if ongoing blood loss).

Special Tests

Endometrial biopsy to assess for the presence of endometrial hyperplasia or cancer can be performed during a speculum exam with an endometrial pipelle.

Imaging: TVUS is the imaging test of choice to evaluate for endometrial hyperplasia. Endometrial thickness > 3 mm may indicate endometrial cancer in women with postmenopausal bleeding (Sn 0.98, Sp 0.35). Endometrial carcinoma can also be visualized by MRI (**Fig. 4.31**).

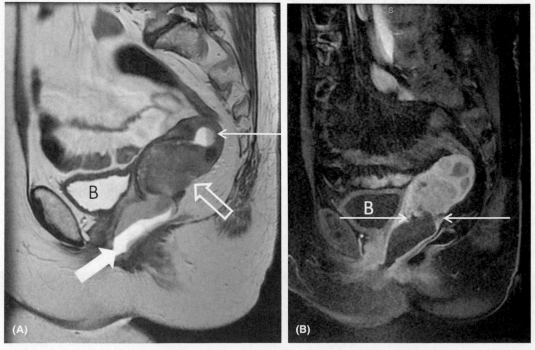

FIGURE 4.31. A. MRI scan shows a hyperintense mass (*open arrow*) and retained fluid (*thin arrow*) near the urinary bladder (*B*). The hyperintense fluid in the vagina (*closed arrow*) reflects gel used to facilitate evaluation of the mass. **B.** MRI scan shows extension of mass into the cervical stroma (*between arrows*).

OVARIAN CANCER

Presentation

A 55-year-old female presents with increasing abdominal distension and bloating.

Definition

Ovarian cancer is a malignancy that arises from the ovary.

What are common causes?

Most ovarian tumors are epithelial carcinomas. There are eight subtypes of epithelial ovarian carcinoma, including serous, endometrioid, clear cell, mucinous, transitional cell, mixed epithelial, undifferentiated, and unclassified. Ovarian germ cell and sex cord stromal tumors have lower malignant potential and are described elsewhere. The exact cause of ovarian cancer remains unknown, but risk factors include early menarche, late menopause, nulliparity, endometriosis, PCOS, obesity, family history of ovarian cancer, and *BRCA1* and *BRCA2* mutations. Oral contraceptives have a protective effect against ovarian cancer.

What is the differential diagnosis?

Abdominal distension and bloating sensation: The differential diagnosis includes liver cirrhosis, ovarian cyst, uterine fibroids, endometrial carcinoma, adenomyosis, germ cell tumor, and Krukenberg tumor.

What symptoms might be observed?

Symptoms include abdominal discomfort, abdominal bloating, abdominal distension, back pain, constipation, vaginal bleeding, and dysuria.

What are the possible findings on examination?

Vital signs: Typically unremarkable.
Inspection: Abdominal distension may be present. Ascites with fluid wave may be noted on abdominal examination.
Palpation: A palpable abdominal mass should raise concern for ovarian malignancy. External examination is typically unremarkable. Bimanual exam may reveal the presence of adnexal masses or an enlarged uterus. A rectovaginal exam may reveal the presence of nodularity in the cul-de-sac.
Auscultation: Bowel sounds are typically normal.

What tests should be ordered?

Laboratory tests: CBC (leukocytosis), serum CA 125 levels may be elevated in epithelial ovarian carcinoma, but may also be elevated in pregnancy, ovarian cysts, PID, endometriosis, cirrhosis, and liver disease. *BRCA1* and *BRCA2* testing may be indicated if a strong family history of breast or ovarian cancer exists.
Imaging: TVUS is the diagnostic test of choice in the primary care clinic and a rapid way to assess for ovarian cancer (Sn 0.79–0.91, Sp 0.63–0.92). CT scan can show evidence of ovarian masses, but may be of lower yield (Sn 0.87, Sp 0.84), as smaller masses and carcinomatosis are not as easily visualized. MRI is also a sensitive and specific modality for detecting malignant ovarian tumors (Sn 0.92, Sp 0.88), but is more time consuming and expensive (**Fig. 4.32**).

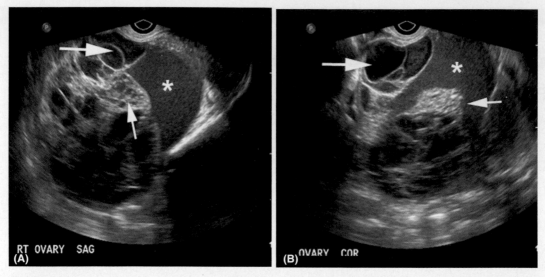

FIGURE 4.32. Right ovarian mucinous cystadenocarcinoma. Sagittal (**A**) and Coronal (**B**) sections show a heterogeneous solid (*small arrow*) with typical areas of increased (*asterisk*) and decreased (*large arrow*) echogenicity.

 # CERVICAL CANCER

Presentation

A 55-year-old female who has had no medical care for several decades presents with vaginal bleeding after intercourse and pelvic discomfort.

Definition

Cervical cancer is a malignant neoplasm that arises from cells in the cervix.

What are common causes?

The majority of cervical cancers are squamous cell carcinomas, the epithelial cells that line the cervix. Cervical adenocarcinoma arises in glandular epithelial cells of the cervix. Infection with human papillomavirus (HPV) is the greatest risk factor for cervical cancer. Classically, HPV types 16 and 18 are most frequently associated with cervical cancer.

Risk factors for cervical cancer include infection with HPV, human immunodeficiency virus (HIV), prior STIs, smoking, having multiple sex partners, and having sex with men who have had multiple sex partners.

What is the differential diagnosis?

Abnormal vaginal bleeding: The differential diagnosis includes PID, cervical polyps, fibroid tumors, cervical lymphoma, endometrial carcinoma, ovarian carcinoma, and endometriosis.

What symptoms might be observed?

Symptoms include dyspareunia, dysuria, and changes in vaginal discharge.

What are the possible findings on examination?

Vital signs: Typically unremarkable.
Inspection: External pelvic examination is typically unremarkable. Internal pelvic examination may reveal an ulcerating, fungating, or bleeding mass associated with the cervix.
Palpation: A firm, fungating, often friable mass may be palpated in the cervix. The extent of cancer involvement may be appreciated on exam, with more invasive cancer extending from the walls of the cervix to the pelvic side wall and parametrium.
Auscultation: Typically unremarkable bowel sounds.

> ● **CLINICAL PEARL**
>
> Pap test is the screening test of choice for cervical cancer and can show evidence of dysplastic or neoplastic cells.

What tests should be ordered?

Laboratory tests: CBC (leukocytosis may be present).
Imaging: Pelvic MRI is the diagnostic test of choice in radiographic staging of cervical cancer and often helpful to characterize the depth of invasion into surrounding soft tissues (**Fig. 4.33**). Although CT and MRI scans can be helpful in radiographic staging, cervical cancer is staged clinically.

> ● **CLINICAL PEARL**
>
> Colposcopy is a magnified visual inspection of the cervix aided by acetic acid preparation that can highlight abnormal cells on the surface of the cervix.

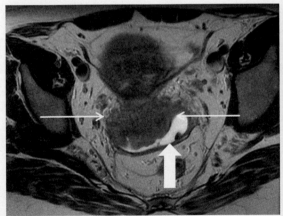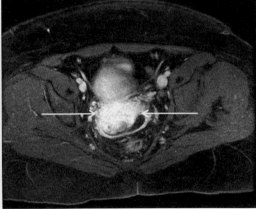

FIGURE 4.33. Cervical carcinoma. MRI scan shows a hypointense mass (*thin arrows*) replacing the fibrous cervical stroma and extending into the vagina (*closed arrow* shows ultrasound gel).

Back

5

JANICE WONG • SHAMIK BHATTACHARYA •
SAGAR DUGANI • JOSHUA P. KLEIN

The back consists of the posterior portion of the trunk, which lies inferior to the neck and superior to the buttocks. This complex region contains skin, subcutaneous tissue, muscles, posterior aspect of the ribs, the vertebral column, spinal cord and nerves, and blood vessels. Because the back is continuous with the head, neck, and extremities, it plays an important role in maintaining stance, posture, gait, upper extremity and trunk mobility, and balance. The scapulae are also located in the back; however, they are considered part of the appendicular skeleton of the upper extremities and are discussed in Chapter 6.

■ INITIAL EVALUATION AND ASSESSMENT

When a patient presents with a chief complaint related to the back, the clinician usually develops a differential diagnosis to identify the most likely etiology (Chapter 1). Typically, back pain is caused by primary back-related pathology including congenital, degenerative, traumatic, neoplastic, infectious, or inflammatory etiologies; however, back pain may be secondarily referred from other regions such as the thorax (Chapter 2), abdomen (Chapter 3), or pelvis (Chapter 4). Further, nerve roots innervating the extremities emerge from the spine, and back-related pathology may also manifest as weakness, pain, or numbness in the extremities.

As described in Chapter 1, initial evaluation begins with observing the patient's general appearance, behavior, expression, posture, and gait, the latter of which provides important information on primary back-related pathology.

General Back Examination

After obtaining consent to carry out a physical examination, the patient should be draped with a gown to completely expose the back (described in Chapter 1). The patient stands with feet together and hands by the side. A systematic physical examination involves the IPPA approach—that is, inspection, palpation, percussion, and auscultation. The clinician stands behind and then to the side of the patient and inspects the skin for discoloration, bruises, scars, or rashes, with an emphasis on visualizing bony landmarks including spinous processes, paravertebral muscles, iliac crests, and the posterior superior iliac spine. When observed in lateral view, the back will reveal four curves: cervical lordosis, thoracic kyphosis, lumbar lordosis, and sacral kyphosis (**Fig. 5.1**). Lordosis refers to inward (anterior) curvature of the spine, whereas kyphosis refers to outward (posterior) curvature of the spine. These normal curvatures reflect the contour of the underlying vertebral column (**Fig. 5.2**).

The clinician should assess the curvature and posture of the back, symmetry of shoulder height, and symmetry of the iliac crests and posterior inferior iliac spines, as well as note the presence of excessive kyphosis or scoliosis or other abnormalities (**Fig. 5.3**).

After inspection, the midline of the back is palpated. Vertebrae may not be easily visualized on surface anatomy; however, on neck flexion, the most superior prominent spinous process (vertebra prominens), typically the C7 vertebra, can be palpated (**Fig. 5.4A**). Starting at the neck, the C2–C7 vertebrae and their facet joints (located 1 inch from the midline) are palpated for underlying tenderness or pain, a process continued caudally toward the sacroiliac joints. Inferior to the neck, the facet joints cannot be readily palpated as they are located deep to the underlying muscles. Important landmarks include the T3 spinous process at the level of the scapular spine and the L4 vertebral body at the most superior portion of the iliac crest (**Fig. 5.4B**).

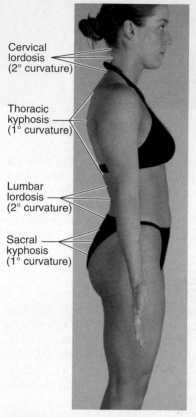

FIGURE 5.1. Surface anatomy of curvature of the vertebral column with normal typical lordosis and kyphosis.

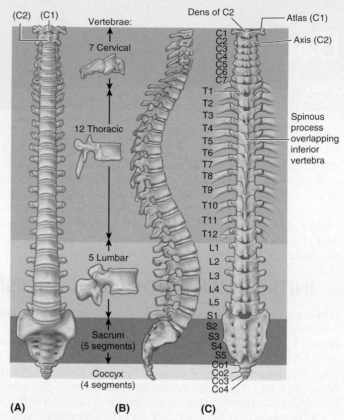

FIGURE 5.2. The vertebral column with its five regions: cervical, thoracic, lumbar, sacral, and coccygeal segments. Depicted are the **(A)** anterior view, **(B)** right lateral view, and **(C)** posterior view with vertebral ends of ribs.

After inspection, palpation, and percussion, special maneuvers can be performed to reveal information on the functional capacity of joints and regions of the back. Depending on the symptoms, the neck may be examined along with the back. Typical maneuvers include testing range of motion (ROM) of the back on flexion, extension, rotation, and lateral bending (**Figs. 5.5 and 5.6**).

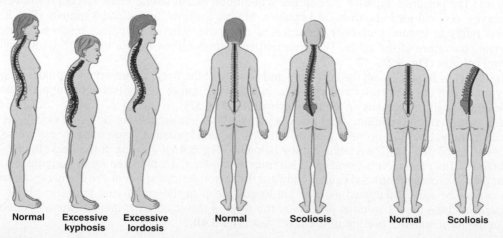

FIGURE 5.3. Abnormal curvatures of the vertebral column.

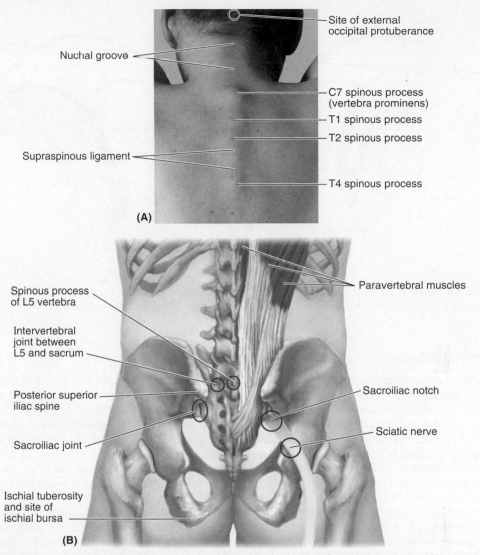

FIGURE 5.4. **A.** Posterior view with neck and back flexed and scapulae protracted. **B.** Location of major landmarks in the lower back.

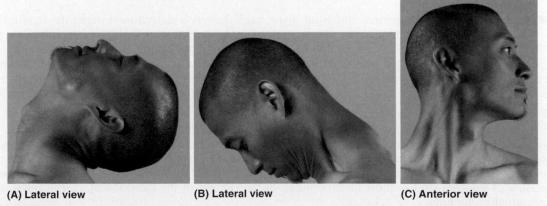

(A) Lateral view **(B) Lateral view** **(C) Anterior view**

FIGURE 5.5. Surface anatomy of selected movements of the cervical spine. **A.** Extension of the neck. **B.** Flexion of the neck. **C.** Head rotated to the left.

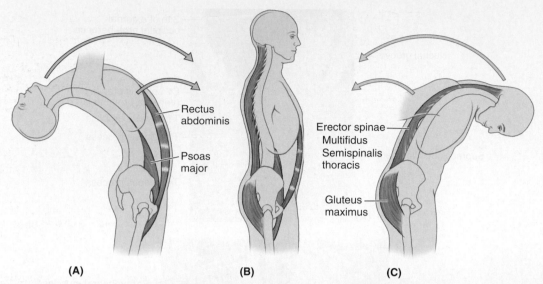

Rectus
abdominis

Psoas
major

Erector spinae
Multifidus
Semispinalis
thoracis

Gluteus
maximus

(A)   **(B)**   **(C)**

FIGURE 5.6. Major muscles producing movement of the thoracic and lumbar intervertebral joints for **(A)** flexion from an extended position, **(B)** neutral position, and **(C)** extension from a flexed position.

Several additional maneuvers can be performed depending on symptoms:

- Cervical intervertebral foraminal stenosis: Cervical foraminal stenosis can result in nerve root impingement that produces upper extremity pain, weakness, and numbness. In the cervical spine, the Spurling maneuver and the shoulder abduction test are used to assess for stenosis. In the Spurling maneuver, the neck is slightly extended and laterally flexed toward the affected side, followed by application of vertical downward pressure on the patient's head. Reproduction of symptoms is considered a positive result for foraminal stenosis. In the shoulder abduction test, the patient abducts the shoulder by placing his or her hand (on the symptomatic side) on the head. Resolution of symptoms is considered a positive result for foraminal stenosis.

- Lumbosacral intervertebral foraminal stenosis: Foraminal stenosis can result in nerve root impingement and lower extremity weakness, pain, and cramping. A commonly used maneuver to assess for stenosis at the L5 or S1 level is the straight leg raise maneuver (also known as *Lasègue test*). In this maneuver, the patient is placed in the supine position with the hip flexed and lower extremity extended passively on the affected side. Reproduction of symptoms is considered a positive result for foraminal stenosis (Lasègue sign). A variation of this test is the crossed straight leg raise test, in which raising the lower extremity contralateral to the affected side elicits symptoms.

- Impaired lower back flexion: Impaired lower back flexion is determined using the modified Schober test. In this maneuver, the patient stands upright, and the L5 vertebral level is marked; then, levels 5 cm below (point A) and 10 cm above (point B) this mark are made, thus marking a 15-cm distance. The patient is instructed to flex the hips without flexing the knees. In normal instances, the distance between points A and B should increase by at least 5 cm, and failure to achieve this is considered a positive result for impaired lower back flexion.

Physical examination maneuvers have limited specificity and sensitivity. If there is suspicion of underlying pathology or when physical examination findings do not correlate with symptoms, medical imaging may be considered to identify the underlying cause. Importantly, many incidental abnormalities (without associated pathology) may be detected on imaging studies; therefore, the results of imaging studies must be interpreted in the context of the clinical history and physical examination findings.

Laboratory Tests

Common laboratory investigations to help diagnose back-related diseases include a complete blood count (CBC) to diagnose infections, anemia, or hematological malignancy. Inflammatory markers including erythrocyte sedimentation rate (ESR) and C-reactive protein (CRP) may be elevated in the setting of inflammatory diseases affecting the musculoskeletal systems. Renal function (creatinine, bicarbonate, and blood urea nitrogen [BUN]) may be impaired in conditions affecting the retro-peritoneal spaces and the kidneys. The cerebrospinal fluid (CSF) may also be tested for cytology (leukocytosis may be present with infection or inflammation), malignancy, and infection (bacteria, viruses, and fungi).

Back Imaging

The most common imaging modalities for the back are conventional radiography (x-ray), computed tomography (CT), magnetic resonance imaging (MRI), and, less commonly now, CT myelography. An introduction and general approach to these imaging modalities is provided in Chapter 1.

One approach to reading an x-ray is as follows:

1. Identify vertebrae and assess the anterior and posterior alignment of vertebral bodies and the spinolaminar line.
2. Evaluate the extent of overlap of facet or zygapophysial joints.
3. Assess the distance between spinous processes, between laminae, and between disc and joint spaces.
4. Assess for possible fractures or abnormal changes in bone density, fluid collections (suggestive of an infection or abscess), and other suspicious masses in the paravertebral region.

With this approach, x-rays can be a useful first step in evaluating the vertebral column (**Figs. 5.7 and 5.8**).

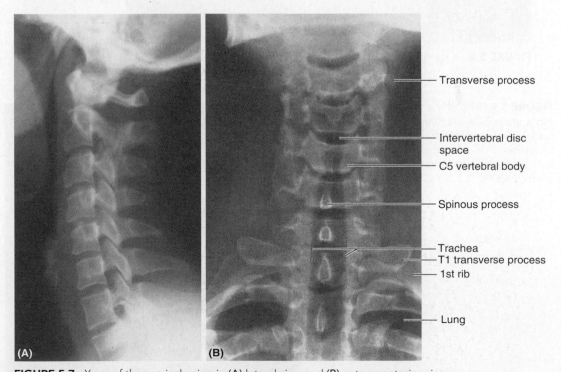

FIGURE 5.7. X-ray of the cervical spine in (**A**) lateral view and (**B**) anteroposterior view.

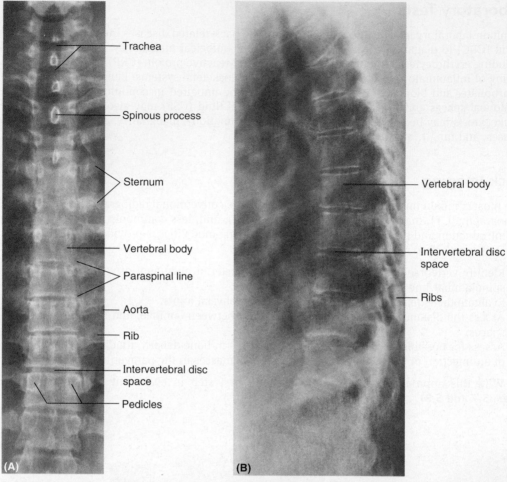

FIGURE 5.8. X-ray of the thoracic spine in AP (**A**) and lateral (**B**) views.

FIGURE 5.9. MRI of the thoracic spine revealing compression fracture at the level of T10 (*asterisks*) secondary to Langerhans cell histiocytosis. This compression fracture is not to be mistaken for a posttraumatic fracture of the thoracic spine.

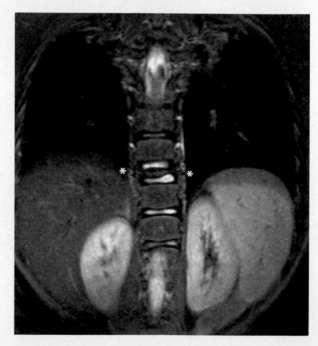

Although x-rays provide important information, they have limited sensitivity in identifying subtle structural changes. Compared to x-rays, CT scans have a higher sensitivity for assessing fractures. One approach to reviewing CT scans is the "ABCS system": alignment abnormalities, bone integrity abnormalities, cartilage abnormalities, and soft tissue abnormalities. In the nonemergent setting, or in instances in which MRI scans are contraindicated, CT scans can be used to visualize bony structures and the foramina, though they have limited sensitivity for soft tissue changes (such as disc herniation) compared to MRI scans.

MRI scans have higher sensitivity for soft tissue changes and are the preferred modality for assessing spinal cord injury, epidural hematoma or abscess, and ligamentous injury. MRI scans also provide detailed imaging of soft tissue structures (**Fig. 5.9**), including ligaments. Findings on MRI scans, however, must be correlated with clinical symptoms as many asymptomatic individuals may have incidentally discovered abnormal imaging findings.

With both CT and MRI scans, intravenous (IV) contrast can be used to enhance lesions, especially when there is concern for tumor, infection (or, abscess), or demyelinating diseases such as multiple sclerosis. CT scans performed with intrathecal contrast (CT myelography) have similar accuracy to MRI in demonstrating compressive lesions of the spinal cord, though its use is limited by the invasive nature of the test (the need to access the intrathecal space) and exposure to ionizing radiation. Finally, CT or MR angiography can help visualize vascular injuries such as arterial dissections or arteriovenous malformations (AVMs) and fistulae.

SYSTEMS OVERVIEW

▪ CERVICAL, THORACIC, LUMBAR, AND SACRAL SPINE

Overview

The adult vertebral column consists of 33 vertebrae, although the number can range from 32 to 35, depending on the number of coccygeal segments. The 24 individual vertebrae and 9 fused vertebrae are linked by ligaments, fibrocartilaginous joints, and synovial facet (zygapophysial) joints. The sacral and coccygeal segments fuse to form the sacrum and coccyx, respectively. The anterior aspect of a typical vertebra consists of a large vertebral body (**Fig. 5.10**). Bodies of the vertebrae are joined by intervertebral discs (fibrocartilaginous joints or symphyses) that facilitate weight bearing and by fibrous longitudinal ligaments that are located anteriorly and posteriorly. The intervertebral discs consist of an inner gelatinous mass (nucleus pulposus) encircled by a fibrous structure (anulus fibrosus), as shown in **Figure 5.11**.

The vertebral arch lies posterior to the vertebral body and consists of two (right and left) pedicles and laminae. The vertebral arch and posterior surface of the vertebra surround the vertebral foramen. Seven processes arise from the vertebral arch: a single median spinous process projecting posteriorly; two transverse processes projecting posterolaterally; and four articular processes projecting superiorly and inferiorly, that form the zygapophysial (facet) joints. The laminae of adjacent vertebral arches are joined by the strong, elastic ligamenta flava (**Fig. 5.12**).

The series of vertebral foramina collectively forms the vertebral canal, which contains the spinal cord, dural sac, and associated vasculature. Spinal nerves from the spinal cord exit the vertebral canal laterally via intervertebral foramina, which are located between pedicles (**Fig. 5.13**). The mobility of the vertebral column results from compressibility and elasticity of the intervertebral discs and movement of the zygapophysial (facet) joints.

The adult spinal cord is ~45 cm long, extending from the medulla oblongata of the brainstem to the L1–L2 intervertebral disc level. The inferior end of the spinal cord terminates via the tapering conus medullaris, from which a strand of connective tissue, the filum terminale, extends inferiorly to attach to the distal end of the coccyx (**Fig. 5.14**). The meninges covering the spinal cord are continuous with the meninges of the brain and extend inferiorly to the level of the S2 vertebra, which is well beyond the level at which the spinal cord terminates.

▪ SPINAL CORD AND NERVES

Overview

Each segment of the spinal cord gives rise to bilateral pairs of anterior and posterior *spinal roots*. The anterior root consists of motor (efferent) fibers that extend peripherally from nerve cell bodies in the anterior horn of spinal cord gray matter to effector organs (e.g., muscles and glands). The posterior root consists of sensory (afferent) neurons with cell bodies in the spinal sensory (dorsal root) ganglia that receive peripheral processes from sensory endings (e.g., from the skin, muscle spindles, and articular capsules) and send central processes into the posterior horn of the spinal cord gray matter (**Fig. 5.15**). The anterior and posterior roots of a particular spinal cord level merge to form a pair of spinal nerves. In total, there are 31 pairs of spinal nerves: 8 cervical, 12 thoracic, 5 lumbar, 5 sacral, and 1 coccygeal. Because the spinal cord ends at the L1–L2 intervertebral disc space, most of the lumbosacral nerve roots descend in the subarachnoid space until they reach the intervertebral foramina through which they exit. This collection of spinal nerve roots descending from the inferior end of the spinal cord is called the *cauda equina*.

Internally, the spinal cord includes central *gray matter* that contains nerve cell bodies and surrounding white matter that contains nerve axons. When viewed in transverse section, the gray

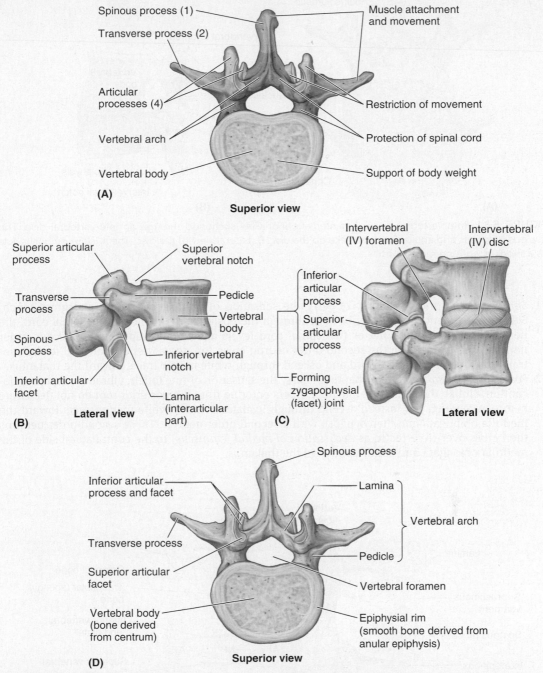

Parts:

Spinous process (1)

Transverse process (2)

Articular processes (4)

Vertebral arch

Vertebral body

Functions:

Muscle attachment and movement

Restriction of movement

Protection of spinal cord

Support of body weight

(A)

Superior view

Superior articular process

Transverse process

Spinous process

Inferior articular facet

Superior vertebral notch

Pedicle

Vertebral body

Inferior vertebral notch

Lamina (interarticular part)

(B) **Lateral view**

Intervertebral (IV) foramen

Intervertebral (IV) disc

Inferior articular process

Superior articular process

Forming zygapophysial (facet) joint

(C) **Lateral view**

Spinous process

Inferior articular process and facet

Transverse process

Superior articular facet

Vertebral body (bone derived from centrum)

Lamina

Vertebral arch

Pedicle

Vertebral foramen

Epiphysial rim (smooth bone derived from anular epiphysis)

(D) **Superior view**

FIGURE 5.10. Typical vertebra, depicted by the L2 vertebra. **A.** Vertebral body, vertebral arch (*red*), and vertebral processes (*blue* and *yellow*). **B, D.** The vertebral arch and vertebral body form the boundary of the vertebral foramen. **C.** The intervertebral foramen is formed by the superior and inferior processes of adjacent vertebrae and the intervertebral disc.

matter reveals a "butterfly-" (or, "H-") shaped structure with four symmetrically placed horns (**Fig. 5.16**).

The two major ascending pathways for afferent sensory fibers are the spinothalamic tracts and posterior columns:

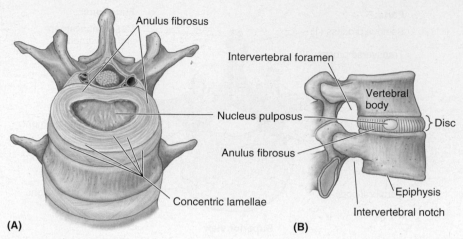

FIGURE 5.11. Intervertebral discs. **A.** Anterosuperior view sectioned through an intervertebral disc. The nucleus pulposus and anulus fibrosus make up the disc. **B.** Lateral view of the disc. The nucleus pulposus acts as a shock-absorbing mechanism.

1. *Spinothalamic tracts* (Chapter 7) carry the sensation of pain, temperature, and gross touch. Sensory fibers enter the posterior horn through the posterior root. Once in the spinal cord, the nerve fibers ascend for one or two spinal cord levels and then synapse with a second-order neuron. The axons from the second-order neuron cross (or, *decussate*) at that level to the contralateral side of the spinal cord and ascend through white matter tracts toward the thalamus.

2. *Posterior or dorsal columns* (Chapter 7) carry the sensation of fine touch, vibration, and proprioception. Unlike the spinothalamic tract, fibers entering from the posterior root do not decussate before ascending, but instead ascend through ipsilateral dorsal white matter tracts toward the medulla oblongata and then synapse with a second-order neuron. These second-order neurons then cross over (referred to as *decussation of medial lemniscus*) to the contralateral side of the medulla oblongata and continue toward the thalamus.

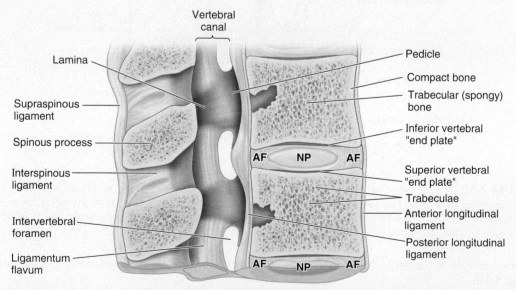

FIGURE 5.12. Medial view of adjacent lumbar vertebrae and associated intervertebral discs. Herniation of nucleus pulposus (*NP*) through the anulus fibrosus (*AF*) between L1 and L2. The ligamentum flavum extends across vertebrae and continues with the fibrous capsule of the zygapophysial joint.

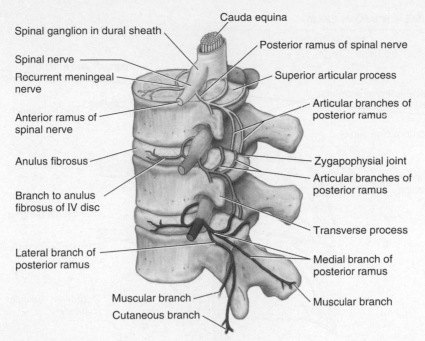

FIGURE 5.13. Zygapophysial joint innervation. The posterior rami emerge from the spinal nerves and divide into medial and lateral branches.

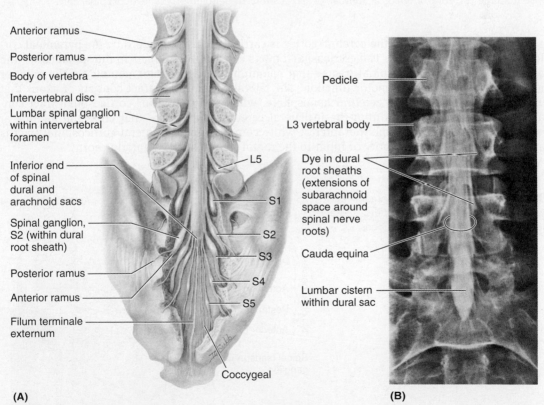

(A)

(B)

FIGURE 5.14. Inferior end of spinal dural sac. **A.** Posterior view. Laminectomy has been performed to expose the inferior end of the dural sac, which encloses the lumbar cistern containing CSF and the cauda equina. In the lumbar region, the nerves exiting the intervertebral foramina pass superior to the intervertebral discs at that level; consequently, herniation of the nucleus pulposus tends to impinge on nerves passing to lower levels. **B.** AP view. CT myelogram of the lumbar region, obtained by injection of contrast medium into the lumbar cistern.

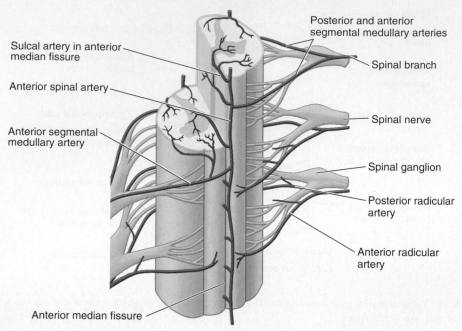

FIGURE 5.15. Blood supply of spinal cord with segmental medullary and radicular arteries. Spinal branches arise from the vertebral, intercostal, lumbar, or sacral artery, depending on the level of spinal cord.

Motor information from the cerebral cortex is carried to the spinal cord by the pyramidal corticospinal tracts (Chapter 7). The corticospinal tracts consist of two tracts in the spinal cord—the lateral and anterior corticospinal tracts—that communicate with motor neurons in the anterior horn to regulate peripheral motor function. The lateral corticospinal tract consists of axons that cross from the contralateral cerebral hemisphere, whereas the anterior corticospinal tract contains some uncrossed fibers from the ipsilateral cerebral hemisphere that cross the midline at each spinal cord level through the anterior white commissure. The lateral corticospinal tract is larger and provides the majority of input to the motor neurons in the anterior horn.

FIGURE 5.16. Spinal cord, anterior and posterior nerve roots and rootlets, spinal ganglia, spinal nerves, and meninges.

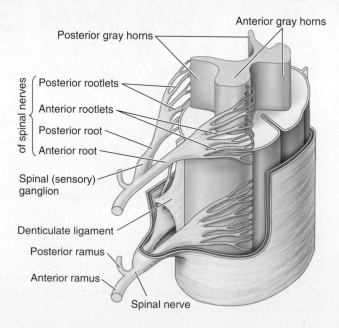

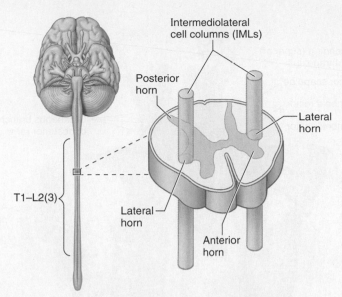

FIGURE 5.17. Intermediolateral cell columns. Each IML or nucleus constitutes the lateral horn of gray matter of spinal cord segments T1–L2 or L3 and consists of the cell bodies of the presynaptic neurons of the sympathetic nervous system.

In the thoracic and lumbar spinal cord, the intermediolateral cell column contains cell bodies of presynaptic sympathetic neurons. The intermediolateral cell column extends from T1 to L2 or L3 and forms the lateral horn of the gray matter seen in cross sections of the spinal cord at those levels (**Fig. 5.17**). Similarly, in the sacral spinal cord, the S2–S4 segments have a cluster of cells in the lateral aspect of the gray matter that are part of the autonomic nervous system and predominantly composed of presynaptic parasympathetic neurons.

■ MUSCLES

Overview

Discomfort in the area adjacent to the vertebral column could represent paravertebral muscular pain. There are two major groups of muscles in the back: extrinsic back muscles (which include superficial and intermediate muscles) and intrinsic (deep) back muscles.

The superficial extrinsic back muscles, including the trapezius, latissimus dorsi, levator scapulae, and rhomboids, produce and control movement of the extremities. The intermediate extrinsic back muscles, including the serratus posterior muscles, aid in respiration and proprioception.

The intrinsic back muscles consist of three layers:

- The superficial layer, consisting of splenius cervicis and splenius capitis, holds the deep neck muscles in place and aids in extension of the cervical spine and head (**Fig. 5.18**).
- The intermediate layer, erector spinae or sacrospinal muscles, consists of three main columns: iliocostalis, longissimus, and spinalis. Their main function is to extend and laterally flex the vertebral column and to extend the head (**Fig. 5.19**).
- The deep layer of transversospinales muscles consists of three main muscle groups: semispinalis, multifidus, and rotatores. Their main function is to extend the head and cervical, thoracic, and lumbar regions of the vertebral column; stabilize vertebrae during local movement; and facilitate rotator movement of the vertebral column. The rotatores muscle also helps in proprioception (**Fig. 5.20**).

Inspection of the paravertebral region may reveal reduced muscle bulk (or, *atrophy*), swelling, or fasciculations. Then, starting at the inferior aspect of the neck and descending toward the coccygeal region, palpation and percussion of the paravertebral region may reveal underlying tenderness.

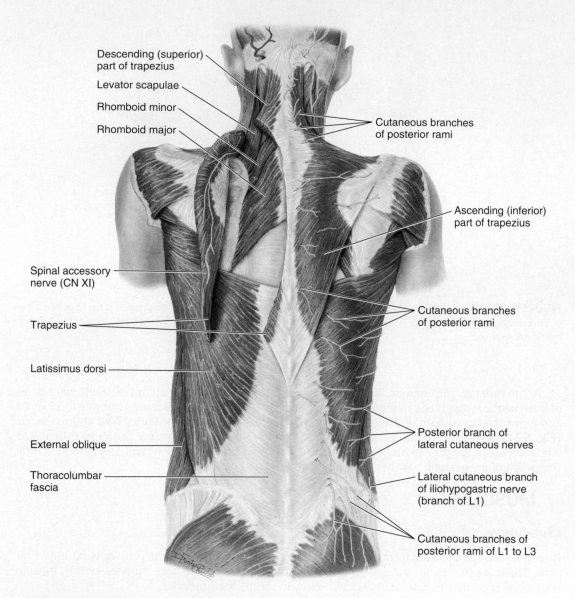

FIGURE 5.18. Superficial extrinsic muscles of the back.

Labels in figure:
- Descending (superior) part of trapezius
- Levator scapulae
- Rhomboid minor
- Rhomboid major
- Cutaneous branches of posterior rami
- Ascending (inferior) part of trapezius
- Spinal accessory nerve (CN XI)
- Cutaneous branches of posterior rami
- Trapezius
- Latissimus dorsi
- Posterior branch of lateral cutaneous nerves
- External oblique
- Lateral cutaneous branch of iliohypogastric nerve (branch of L1)
- Thoracolumbar fascia
- Cutaneous branches of posterior rami of L1 to L3

▦ CIRCULATORY SYSTEM OF THE SPINAL CORD

Overview

The circulatory system of the spinal cord and back cannot be assessed by auscultation but can be visualized using imaging modalities. Arterial supply to the spinal cord is dependent on the variable contributions of the anterior spinal artery, posterior spinal arteries, anterior medullary arteries, posterior medullary arteries, and their branches. The anterior spinal artery, formed by the union of arteries branching from the vertebral arteries, runs in the anterior median fissure of the spinal cord. The posterior spinal arteries (pair of arteries) are branches of the vertebral artery or the posterior inferior cerebellar artery and descend along the posterior aspect of the spinal cord. The anterior and posterior spinal arteries form anastomoses with the anterior and posterior segmental medullary arteries (**Fig. 5.21**).

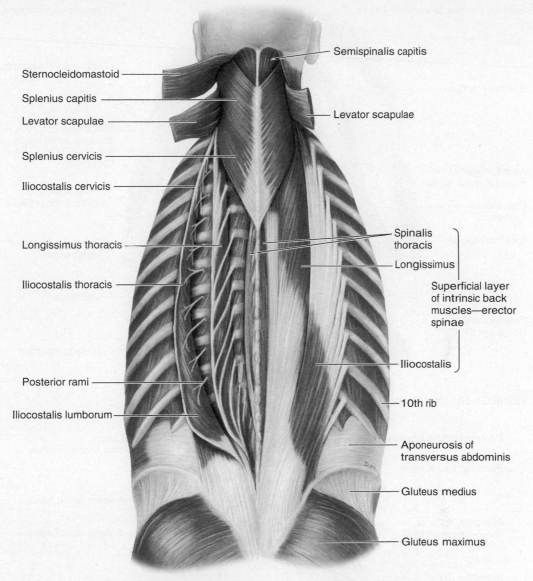

Semispinalis capitis

Sternocleidomastoid

Splenius capitis

Levator scapulae

Levator scapulae

Splenius cervicis

Iliocostalis cervicis

Spinalis thoracis

Longissimus thoracis

Longissimus

Iliocostalis thoracis

Superficial layer of intrinsic back muscles—erector spinae

Iliocostalis

Posterior rami

Iliocostalis lumborum

10th rib

Aponeurosis of transversus abdominis

Gluteus medius

Gluteus maximus

FIGURE 5.19. Intermediate muscles of the back.

The radicular arteries supply the nerve roots at most levels. However, they do not reach the anterior and posterior spinal arteries. Segmental medullary arteries replace the radicular arteries at the irregular levels at which they occur, supplying both roots and the spinal cord. A prominent segmental medullary artery is the great segmental medullary artery of Adamkiewicz, which typically arises on the left between T9 and T11; compromise of this artery can produce sufficient hypoperfusion to cause infarction of the anterior part of the caudal spinal cord.

The venous drainage of the spinal cord is organized around six longitudinal venous channels. The anterior median vein runs in the anterior median fissure and drains the central gray matter. These venous channels communicate segmentally with intervertebral veins and superiorly with intracranial dural venous sinuses.

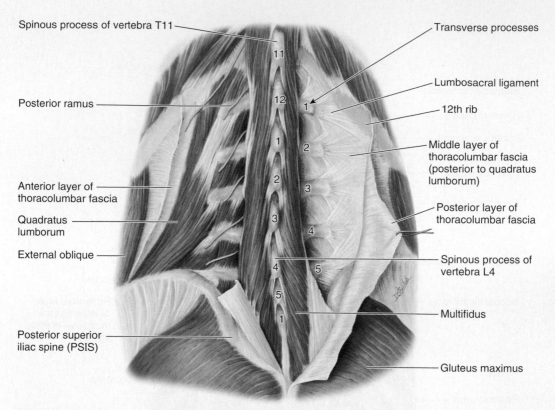

Spinous process of vertebra T11

11

12

1

1

2

2

3

3

4

4

5

5

1

Posterior ramus

Anterior layer of
thoracolumbar fascia

Quadratus
lumborum

External oblique

Posterior superior
iliac spine (PSIS)

Transverse processes

Lumbosacral ligament

12th rib

Middle layer of
thoracolumbar fascia
(posterior to quadratus
lumborum)

Posterior layer of
thoracolumbar fascia

Spinous process of
vertebra L4

Multifidus

Gluteus maximus

FIGURE 5.20. Deep muscles of the back.

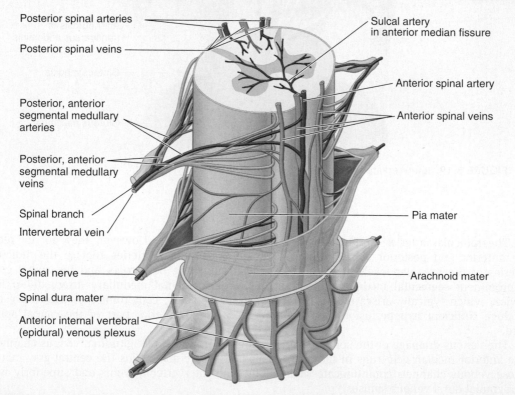

Posterior spinal arteries

Posterior spinal veins

Posterior, anterior
segmental medullary
arteries

Posterior, anterior
segmental medullary
veins

Spinal branch

Intervertebral vein

Spinal nerve

Spinal dura mater

Anterior internal vertebral
(epidural) venous plexus

Sulcal artery
in anterior median fissure

Anterior spinal artery

Anterior spinal veins

Pia mater

Arachnoid mater

FIGURE 5.21. Anterolateral view of blood supply to the spinal cord. Spinal branches arise from the vertebral, intercostal, lumbar, or sacral artery, depending on the level of spinal cord.

CLINICAL CASES

 ## RADICULOPATHY

Presentation

A 57-year-old male presents with back pain after lifting heavy boxes. He reports pain radiating from his right lower back down the posterior aspect of the right lower extremity and to his ankles.

Definition

Radiculopathy is the compression of a spinal nerve or nerve root and typically leads to pain, paresthesia, numbness, or weakness.

What are common causes?

The most common causes are herniated disc, osteophyte formation, spinal stenosis, tumor, and infection or abscess.

> ● **CLINICAL PEARL**
>
> Risk factors for lumbosacral radiculopathy include age (peak onset between ages 45 and 64 years), upper range of height, history of smoking, and strenuous activity such as lifting and prolonged driving.

What is the differential diagnosis?

Back pain: The differential diagnosis includes vertebral fracture, musculoskeletal pain, herpes zoster infection (if pain tracks along a dermatome), and abscess or fluid collection.

What symptoms might be observed?

The most common symptoms include upper or lower extremity pain, neck or back pain, numbness or paresthesia, muscle hypotrophy, and muscle weakness.

What are the possible findings on examination?

Vital signs: Typically normal.
Inspection: Asymmetric changes including reduced ROM and lower muscle bulk may be observed on the affected side.
Neurologic examination: Impaired sensation, motor strength, deep tendon reflexes, and coordination and gait (Chapter 6) may be seen on the affected side. Typical findings in cervical and lumbosacral radiculopathy are listed in **Tables 5.1 and 5.2**.

Special Tests

Spurling maneuver, shoulder abduction test, and straight leg raise test may be positive on the affected side.

TABLE 5.1. Findings in cervical radiculopathy

Nerve Root	Decreased Sensation	Decreased Muscle Strength	Decreased Deep Tendon Reflexes
C5	Shoulder, lateral proximal upper extremity	Shoulder abduction Shoulder external rotation	Biceps and brachioradialis
C6	Lateral forearm, thumb, second digit	Elbow joint flexion Forearm supination Wrist joint extension	Biceps and brachioradialis
C7	Third digit, posterior forearm	Elbow joint extension Wrist joint flexion Finger joint extension	Triceps
C8	Fifth digit, distal medial forearm	Intrinsic hand muscles	Finger flexor
T1	Medial forearm	Intrinsic hand muscles	Finger flexor

What tests should be ordered?

Laboratory tests: Typically not required; if red flag symptoms are present, then CBC (leukocytosis may reveal infection), metabolic panel (hypercalcemia), and other serology (elevated ESR for infection or inflammation).

Imaging: MRI spine is the preferred modality to detect nerve root compression (**Fig. 5.22**). CT spine is the preferred modality to detect skeletal pathology, such as osteophytes and fractures.

> ● **CLINICAL PEARL**
>
> Cervical and lumbosacral regions, typically at C7 and S1 nerve levels, are common sites of radiculopathy. Cervical radiculopathy typically presents as unilateral neck and upper extremity pain that is exacerbated by rotating or bending the head toward the symptomatic site. Lumbosacral radiculopathy typically presents as low back pain that radiates in a dermatomal distribution (**Fig. 5.23**). Radiculopathy may also present as weakness in a myotomal distribution.

> ● **CLINICAL PEARL**
>
> What is the difference between disc herniation and bulge? Herniation occurs, by definition, when more than 50% of the disc circumference is displaced beyond the epiphyseal rim (ring apophyses). When <50% is displaced, the displacement is called a *bulge*.

TABLE 5.2. Findings in lumbosacral radiculopathy

Nerve Root	Decreased Sensation	Decreased Muscle Strength	Decreased Deep Tendon Reflexes
L4	Medial calf	Knee joint extension Hip joints adduction Ankle joint extension	Patellar
L5	Lateral calf and dorsal surface of foot	Foot extension, eversion, and inversion Toe joint extension Hip joint abduction	
S1	Plantar and lateral surface of foot	Ankle, metatarsophalangeal, and phalangeal joint plantar flexion Hip joint extension	Achilles tendon (ankle jerk)

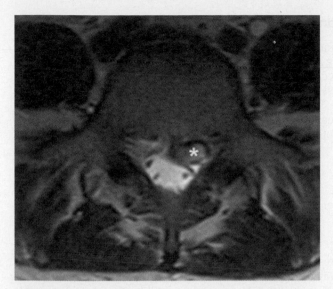

FIGURE 5.22. Disc extrusion. Axial T2-weighted image shows extrusion in the left paracentral location (*asterisk*) with consequent mass effect on the L5 nerve root.

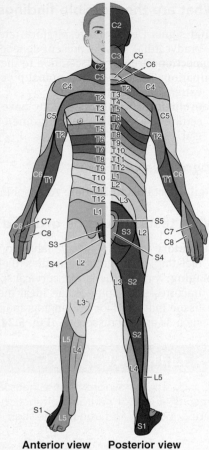

Anterior view   Posterior view

FIGURE 5.23. Dermatome map.

TRAUMATIC COMPRESSIVE MYELOPATHY VERTEBRAL FRACTURE

Presentation

A 41-year-old female is brought to the Emergency Department following a motor vehicle accident (MVA) in which she was an unrestrained passenger.

Definition

Traumatic compressive myelopathy vertebral fracture is a traumatic injury that results in a fracture of one or more vertebrae and causes compression of the spinal cord.

What are common causes?

The most common causes are falls, MVAs, and sports injuries.

What symptoms might be observed?

Symptoms include back pain, numbness or paresthesia, weakness, bladder or bowel incontinence, and urinary retention.

What are the possible findings on examination?

Vital signs: Depressed respiratory rate and oxygen saturation, hypotension, and tachycardia (or, bradycardia) may be present depending on severity of the collision.
Inspection: Bruises or laceration to the neck and back may be present.
Palpation: Tenderness over spinal processes and paraspinal muscles and decreased muscle tone in extremities may be present.
Neurological examination: May have decreased sensation (particularly saddle anesthesia in the setting of cauda equina syndrome), motor strength, deep tendon reflexes, and coordination and gait.

Special Tests

Digital rectal examination: Anal sphincter tone may be reduced in spinal cord injury.

What tests should be ordered?

Laboratory tests: No specific laboratory tests are necessary to make the diagnosis. CBC (anemia if bleeding) or coagulation studies (if elevated, may reflect impairment in clotting) may be obtained.
Imaging: X-ray of the lateral cervical spine along with CT scan of spine will help to identify possible fractures. MRI spine is the ideal modality to assess for spinal cord, ligamentous, or other soft tissue injury. CT or MR angiography should be performed if there is concern for vascular injury such as arterial dissection (**Fig. 5.24**).

● **CLINICAL PEARL**

Cauda equina syndrome is a neurologic emergency, in which damage to the cauda equina results in loss of neurologic function. It may manifest with back pain, saddle anesthesia, gait abnormalities, and urinary retention.

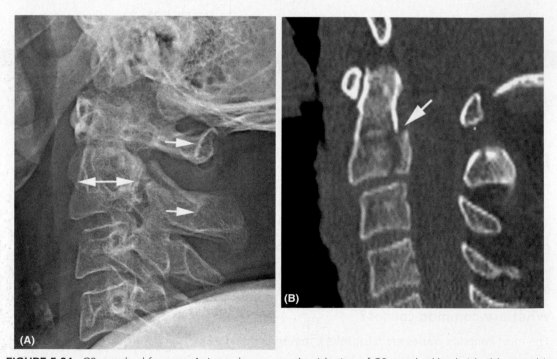

FIGURE 5.24. C2 vertebral fracture. **A.** Lateral x-ray reveals widening of C2 vertebral body (*double arrow*) in relation to C3. Also note the disruption of the spinolaminar line (*single arrows*). **B.** Sagittal reconstructed CT image reveals coronal fracture (*arrow*) in the posterior body of C2.

SPINAL EPIDURAL ABSCESS

Presentation

A 34-year-old male with a history of intravenous drug use presents with back pain and fever.

Definition

A spinal epidural abscess is an infectious collection in the epidural space. The epidural space is the area between the dura and vertebrae, which normally contains fat tissue, nerve roots, lymphatics, and blood vessels.

What are common causes?

The most common risk factors include diabetes mellitus, obesity, end-stage renal disease, sepsis, human immunodeficiency virus (HIV) infection, malignancy, long-term steroid use, intravenous drug use, alcohol use, or instrumentation of the spine.

What is the differential diagnosis?

Back pain and fever: The differential diagnosis includes infection (fluid collection, abscess, septic emboli, and osteomyelitis), inflammation (arthritis, especially spondyloarthropathies), and malignancy.

What symptoms might be observed?

Symptoms include back pain, numbness or paresthesia, weakness, bladder or bowel incontinence, and urinary retention.

What are the possible findings on examination?

Vital signs: Fever, tachycardia, hypotension, and tachypnea.
Inspection: Asymmetric changes including reduced ROM and lower muscle bulk may be observed on the affected side. The skin may reveal injection track marks consistent with intravenous drug use.
Palpation: Tenderness over spinal processes and paraspinal muscles may be present.
Neurologic examination: Decreased sensation, motor strength, deep tendon reflexes, and coordination and gait may be present.

Special Tests

Digital rectal examination: Anal sphincter tone may be reduced.

What tests should be ordered?

Laboratory tests: CBC (leukocytosis), other serology (elevated ESR, elevated CRP), urine profile (presence of recreational drugs), and microbiology (blood culture, urine culture).
Imaging: MRI spine with gadolinium is the study of choice and should be obtained emergently. CT myelography may be obtained if MRI spine is contraindicated or unavailable but has lower specificity (**Fig. 5.25**).

Special Tests

Transthoracic echocardiogram (TTE) can be obtained if suspicion for endocarditis exists.

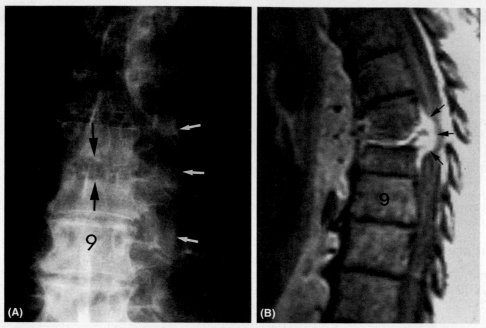

FIGURE 5.25. C2 vertebral fracture. Disc space infection at T7–T8 level. **A.** Frontal x-ray shows erosion of T7–T8 disc space (*black arrows*) and increased width of prevertebral soft tissues (*white arrows*). **B.** Gradient echo MRI shows an epidural abscess (*arrows*) compressing the thecal sac at T7–T8.

● **CLINICAL PEARL**

Red flags of back pain include fever, chills, unexplained weight loss, unremitting pain at night, previous cancer, immunosuppression, intravenous drug use, bowel or bladder dysfunction, and saddle anesthesia.

 METASTATIC DISEASE TO THE SPINE

Presentation

A 70-year-old male with metastatic prostate cancer presents with worsening lower back and right lower extremity pain.

Definition

Metastatic disease to the spine is spread of a primary cancer to the vertebral column.

What are common causes?

Common malignancies associated with bony metastases include prostate cancer, breast cancer, multiple myeloma, thyroid cancer, renal cancer, and pulmonary cancer.

What is the differential diagnosis?

Back pain: The differential diagnosis includes vertebral fracture, degenerative changes (osteopenia, osteoporosis), radiculopathy, and infection (abscess, fluid collection, and osteomyelitis).

What symptoms might be observed?

Symptoms include night sweats, back pain, fatigue, constipation, gait instability or imbalance, bladder or bowel incontinence, and urinary retention.

What are the possible findings on examination?

Vital signs: Fever.
Inspection: Asymmetric changes including reduced ROM and lower muscle bulk may be observed on the affected side.
Palpation: Tenderness over spinal processes and paraspinal muscles may be present.
Neurologic examination: May have decreased sensation, motor strength, deep tendon reflexes, and coordination and gait.

Special Tests

Digital rectal examination: Anal sphincter tone may be reduced.

What tests should be ordered?

Laboratory tests: CBC (anemia, leukocytosis, thrombocytopenia may be present), metabolic panel (hyponatremia, hypercalcemia), and coagulation (elevated international normalized ratio [INR] may be present).
Imaging: MRI spine with gadolinium is the modality of choice to assess for metastatic disease and for suspected disruption of bone, soft tissue, or spinal cord/canal. Reduction in brightness of normal bone marrow on T1-weighted MRI spine may reflect a marrow replacement process as seen in metastatic disease (**Fig. 5.26**).

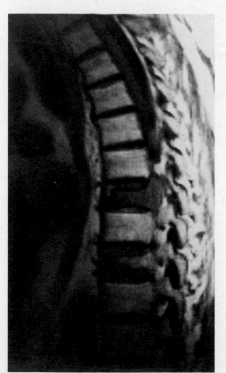

FIGURE 5.26. Metastatic disease of the spine. Sagittal T1-weighted image shows areas of low signal (*dark*) as well as compression in two vertebrae.

OSTEOPOROSIS OF THE BACK

Presentation

A 90-year-old female presents to her health care provider with worsening lower back pain.

Definition

Osteoporosis results from loss of bone density. When vertebrae become osteoporotic, they are more likely to develop other nonpathological fractures.

What are common causes?

The most common risk factors for osteoporosis-related fractures include prior fractures, post-menopausal status, older age, low dietary calcium, vitamin D deficiency, smoking, alcohol use, steroid use, being under- or overweight, and family history of fractures in a first-degree relative.

What is the differential diagnosis?

Back pain: The differential diagnosis includes vertebral fracture, degenerative changes (osteope-nia, osteoporosis), radiculopathy, infection (abscess, fluid collection, and osteomyelitis), and malignancy.

What symptoms might be observed?

Symptoms include back pain, weakness, numbness, and gait instability or imbalance.

What are the possible findings on examination?

Vital signs: Typically normal.
Inspection: Asymmetric changes including reduced ROM and lower muscle bulk may be observed on the affected side.
Palpation: Tenderness over spinal processes and paraspinal muscles may be present.
Neurologic examination: Decreased sensation, motor strength, deep tendon reflexes, and coordination and gait may be present.

Special Tests

Please see Chapter 6.

What tests should be ordered?

Laboratory tests: The tests are described in Chapter 6.
Imaging: MRI may reveal osteoporosis of the lumbar spine with fat replacement of the marrow (hyperintensity on T1 images) (**Fig. 5.27**). Osteoporosis screening is recommended in women of age 65 years or older and in younger women with high-risk factors. Fracture risk can be assessed using an online FRAX (fracture risk assessment) calculator. Bone density is measured with dual energy x-ray absorptiometry scanning.

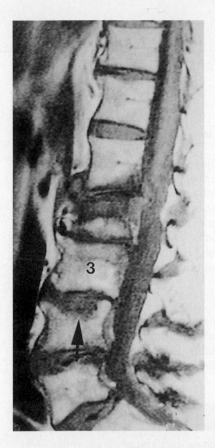

FIGURE 5.27. T1-weighted image revealing osteoporotic collapse of L2 vertebral body. There is low signal in a linear distribution, typical of nonpathologic collapse. Note the central Schmorl node of L4 vertebra (*arrow*).

INTRINSIC MYELOPATHY AND TRANSVERSE MYELITIS

Presentation

A 21-year-old female presents to the Emergency Department with a 3-day history of deep back pain, difficulty ambulating, and numbness in her feet. She comes in today because she is unable to urinate.

Definition

Transverse myelitis is inflammation of the spinal cord causing symptoms of myelopathy in the absence of a compressive lesion.

What are common causes?

The most common etiologies include multiple sclerosis, neuromyelitis optica, systemic autoimmune disorder, vitamin deficiency (e.g., vitamin E), and paraneoplastic conditions.

What is the differential diagnosis?

Back pain: The differential diagnosis includes vertebral fracture, degenerative changes (osteopenia, osteoporosis), radiculopathy, infection (abscess, fluid collection, and osteomyelitis), and malignancy.

What symptoms might be observed?

Symptoms include weakness, numbness, gait instability or imbalance, bladder or bowel incontinence, and urinary retention.

What are the possible findings on examination?

Vital signs: Typically normal.

Inspection: Asymmetric changes including reduced ROM, and lower muscle bulk may be observed on the affected side.

Palpation: Tenderness over spinal processes and paraspinal muscles may be present.

Neurologic examination: Decreased sensation, motor strength, deep tendon reflexes, and coordination and gait may be present. Distinguishing signs of myelopathy are diminished sensation of pain and temperature below the affected dermatome level; weakness in lower extremities consistent with an upper motor neuron lesion (flexors are weaker than extensors); Babinski reflex (pathologic extension of the big toe with abduction of other toes when the sole of the foot is stroked); decreased anal sphincter tone; and L'hermitte sign (paresthesia in the spine upon neck flexion). Acutely, deep tendon reflexes may be diminished; however, with time, they are typically increased.

What tests should be ordered?

Laboratory tests: CSF (leukocytosis; glucose and protein level may be increased, decreased, or unchanged, depending on etiology). Additional tests are based on the differential diagnosis (**Table 5.3**).

Imaging: MRI spine with contrast is the preferred imaging modality. Lesions are typically identified by T2 hyperintensity in that segment of the spinal cord. Enhancement is indicative of active inflammation (**Fig. 5.28**).

● CLINICAL PEARL

Weakness due to myelopathy typically involves lower extremities and, depending on the level of myelopathy, may also involve the upper extremities. Sensory symptoms in myelopathy often respect a "level," and patients typically develop decreased sensation below a sensory dermatome.

TABLE 5.3. Diagnostic tests associated with various back-related pathologies

Condition	Test
Multiple sclerosis	MRI brain with contrast; presence of oligoclonal bands in the CSF
Neuromyelitis optica (NMO)	Serum and CSF tests for IgG antibodies against NMO (aquaporin 4)
Systemic autoimmune disorder	Serum tests (antinuclear antibody, anti-dsDNA, anti-Sm antibodies for systemic lupus erythematosus (SLE); anti-Ro and anti-La for Sjögren syndrome); serum and CSF tests for angiotensinogen-converting enzyme levels for sarcoidosis Chest x-ray to assess for bilateral hilar lymphadenopathy typically seen in sarcoidosis
Toxins	Serum copper levels
Vitamin deficiency	Serum vitamin B_{12} levels
Infection	Serum tests for antibodies against mycoplasma and varicella; serum varicella polymerase chain reaction; additional testing will depend on exposure history
Paraneoplastic	Serum and CSF paraneoplastic panel, and consider age-appropriate cancer screening
Postinfectious or postvaccination	No specific laboratory testing
Idiopathic	By definition, no laboratory tests, and constitutes ~15%–30% of cases

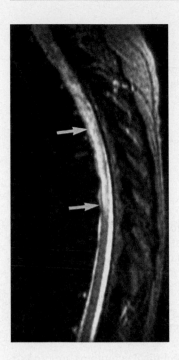

FIGURE 5.28. Transverse myelitis. T2-weighted MRI scan revealing subtle intramedullary mass effect and abnormal T2 signal (*arrows*) in a long segment of the upper and mid thoracic spinal cord.

DEGENERATIVE DISEASE OF THE SPINE AND ANKYLOSING SPONDYLITIS

Presentation

A 35-year-old male presents with 5 months of low back pain that is worse in the morning but improves later in the day.

Definition

Ankylosing spondylitis is a chronic inflammatory autoimmune disease of the vertebral column and sacroiliac joint characterized by back pain and stiffness.

What are common causes?

Ankylosing spondylitis is associated with a positive human leukocyte antigen (HLA) B27 haplotype.

What is the differential diagnosis?

Back pain: The differential diagnosis includes vertebral fracture, degenerative changes (osteopenia, osteoporosis), radiculopathy, infection (abscess, fluid collection, and osteomyelitis), and malignancy.

What symptoms might be observed?

Symptoms include chronic back pain (3 months or longer), stiffness (usually worse in the morning or after rest), enthesitis (particularly of Achilles tendon), and arthritis.

What are the possible findings on examination?

Vital signs: Typically normal.

Inspection: Asymmetric changes in posture and ROM of the back may be present. In particular, presence of increased thoracic kyphosis or loss of lumbar lordosis, decreased chest expansion, joint pain or swelling, pupil asymmetry or unresponsiveness to light, and pitted nails should be assessed.

Palpation: Tenderness over spinal processes and paraspinal muscles.

Neurologic examination: May have deficiencies in sensation, motor strength, deep tendon reflexes, and coordination and gait.

Special Tests

Modified Schober test: Described in the introductory section.

FABER (flexion, abduction, external rotation) test: Used to assess for tenderness in the sacroiliac joint. With the patient supine, the knee is flexed with the ankle resting on the contralateral knee. Downward pressure is applied to the flexed knee, and reproduction of pain in the groin or buttock on the tested side is considered a positive finding.

What tests should be ordered?

Laboratory tests: CBC (leukocytosis, anemia), other serology (elevated ESR, elevated CRP; consider HLA-B27 antigen).

Imaging: Hip x-ray to assess for sacroiliac joint sclerosis (**Fig. 5.29**). If clinical symptoms are present without findings on plain x-ray, then obtain MRI scan of lumbosacral spine.

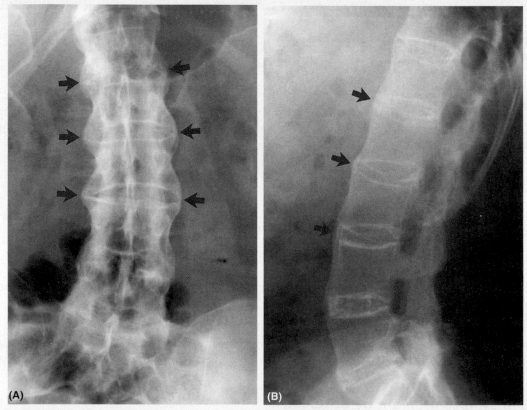

(A)   **(B)**

FIGURE 5.29. Ankylosing spondylitis. **A.** Frontal lumbar x-ray shows typical syndesmophytes bridging the intervertebral disc spaces (*arrows*), giving a characteristic "bamboo" appearance. **B.** Lateral lumbar x-ray shows the anterior syndesmophytes (*arrows*).

RHEUMATOID ARTHRITIS OF THE CERVICAL SPINE

Presentation

A 71-year-old male with rheumatoid arthritis (RA) presents with vertigo and pain at the back of his head.

Definition

RA (Chapter 6) involves chronic inflammation of synovial membranes with damage to cartilage, bones, ligaments, and tendons. At least 50% of patients with RA have abnormalities of the cervical spine. Although most have asymptomatic cervical spine involvement, the major risks of such arthritis are atlantoaxial subluxation and craniovertebral ligamentous deformation (also known as *craniovertebral settling*). In atlantoaxial subluxation, the C1 and C2 vertebrae become misaligned, and in craniovertebral ligamentous deformation, inflammatory infiltrates lead to loss of stability in the supporting ligamentous structures.

What are common causes?

The etiology of c-spine involvement in RA is not fully understood and may involve the same mechanisms that affect other joints.

What is the differential diagnosis?

Back pain: The differential diagnosis includes vertebral fracture, degenerative changes (osteopenia, osteoporosis), radiculopathy, infection (abscess, fluid collection, and osteomyelitis), and malignancy.

What symptoms might be observed?

Symptoms include neck or head pain, vertigo, lack of coordination, gait instability or imbalance, weakness, numbness, bladder or bowel incontinence, and urinary retention.

What are the possible findings on examination?

Vital signs: Typically normal.
Inspection: Asymmetric changes in posture and ROM of the back may be present. The presence of skin nodules, rashes or other lesions, and joint deformities should be assessed.
Palpation: Tenderness over joints, spinal processes, and paraspinal muscles.
Neurologic examination: May have deficiencies in sensation, motor strength, deep tendon reflexes, and coordination and gait.

Special Tests

May have reduced neck ROM (flexion, extension, and lateral flexion).

What tests should be ordered?

Laboratory tests: CBC (leukocytosis, anemia), other serology (elevated ESR, elevated CRP). If suspicion for RA, then could check serum rheumatoid factor and anti–cyclic citrullinated peptide (CCP) antibodies as these are relatively specific for RA.
Imaging: Lateral x-rays may show abnormalities in cervical vertebral placement, which can be confirmed on CT imaging. For example, in atlantoaxial subluxation, lateral x-rays may reveal subluxation of C1 on C2, with widening of predental space and misalignment of spinolaminar

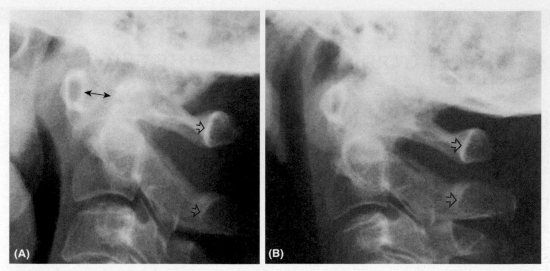

FIGURE 5.30. Atlantoaxial subluxation in rheumatoid arthritis. **A.** Lateral x-ray in flexion shows anterior sub-luxation of C1 on C2, with widening of the predental space (*double arrow*) and malalignment of the spinol-aminar lines of C1 and C2 (*open arrows*). **B.** Lateral x-ray in extension shows subluxation with near complete resolution. The spinolaminar line (*open arrows*) is still not automatically aligned.

lines of C1 and C2 (**Fig. 5.30**). In craniovertebral ligamentous injury, sagittal CT scans may reveal the tip of the dens protruding through the foramen magnum. Sagittal MRI scans further delineate impingement of the dens on the brainstem. MRI scans can better delineate impingement of the brainstem or cervical cord (**Fig. 5.31**).

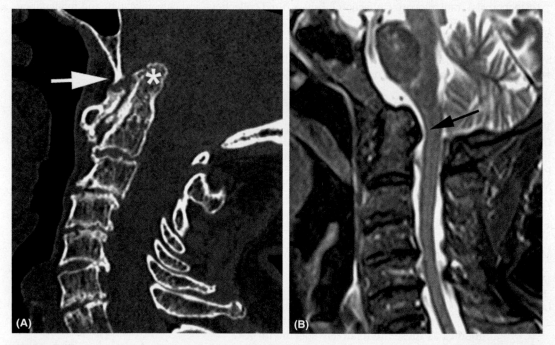

FIGURE 5.31. Craniovertebral settling in rheumatoid arthritis. **A.** Sagittal reconstructed CT images in two different patients show the tip of the dens (*asterisk*) protruding through the foramen magnum. The dens should normally be 12 mm below the basion (*arrow*). **B.** Sagittal MRI shows impingement of the dens on the medulla (*arrow*).

Upper and Lower Extremities

6

SEBASTIAN HEAVEN • TRI NYUGEN • SARAH M. TROSTER
JEFFREY E. ALFONSI • NICKOLAUS BIASUTTI • MARILYN HENG

The upper and lower extremities are composed of a network of bones (axial skeleton), muscles, tendons, ligaments, nerves, and blood vessels that work together to produce movements. The upper extremities allow for movements such as reaching, grasping, and performing fine motor tasks. The lower extremities are extensions of the trunk and serve to support the body while standing and ambulating (**Fig. 6.1**).

■ INITIAL EVALUATION AND ASSESSMENT

Pathology of the upper or lower extremity can manifest with a variety of symptoms, including pain or inability to perform a movement (**Table 6.1**). Recognizing symptom patterns can assist the clinician in localizing the pathology to an anatomical region or tissue type. If pain is the presenting symptom, it is important to characterize the pain based on location, onset (acute or chronic), alleviating factors (e.g., rest or activity), aggravating factors (e.g., movement), quality (e.g., sharp, dull, or aching), radiation, severity, and progression.

General Extremity Examination

For the upper extremity examination, the patient is typically sitting upright with a drape tied under the axilla, wrapping around the thorax. For the lower extremity, the patient is typically supine with both legs exposed ensuring that the groin is covered. A systematic examination involves inspection, palpation, and special maneuvers. Percussion and auscultation are typically not relevant. Special maneuvers are used to assess joint motion and integrity, nerve function (i.e., sensation, power, reflexes, and coordination), and blood flow. The joints above and below the joint of interest should be examined too because the joints of the extremities are closely linked, and pain can be referred throughout the extremity. When describing the findings on examination, internationally accepted anatomical terms (Chapter 1) should be used.

Observations on inspection and palpation of the extremities are summarized in **Tables 6.2 and 6.3**, respectively.

The range of motion (ROM; expressed in degrees) of each joint is assessed actively (patient moves the joint) and passively (clinician moves the joint). Most joints of the upper and lower extremities are synovial joints. In synovial joints, contacting portions of the bones are covered in articular cartilage (**Fig. 6.2**). Synovial joints are contained within a joint capsule lined with a synovial membrane that covers all nonarticular surfaces, and they are filled with synovial fluid to provide nutrients to the joint. Loss of active and passive ROM along with pain and swelling is indicative of articular (joint) pathology. Loss of active but not passive ROM suggests an extra-articular problem (e.g., pathology related to muscle, tendon, ligament, bursa, and/or the nervous system). Closely related to ROM testing are the vascular and neurological examinations (neurovascular examination).

● CLINICAL PEARL

Evidence of vascular pathology can be determined by examining for the 6Ps:

Pallor: skin paleness
Polar: cold extremity (on palpation)
Paresthesia: decreased sensation (Chapter 7)
Paralysis: decreased power (Chapter 7)
Pain: worsening with palpation and movement
Pulse: decreased pulse strength

In the upper extremities, pulses are palpated in the brachial and radial arteries (**Fig. 6.3**). In the lower extremities, pulses are palpated in the femoral, popliteal, posterior tibial, and dorsalis pedis arteries. It is important to note that 2% to 3% of healthy individuals have an absent dorsalis pedis artery.

Arterial perfusion can be assessed by pulse strength and capillary refill. The pulse strength is graded using a 5-point scale: 0 = absent pulse, 1 = barely palpable, 2 = easily palpable,

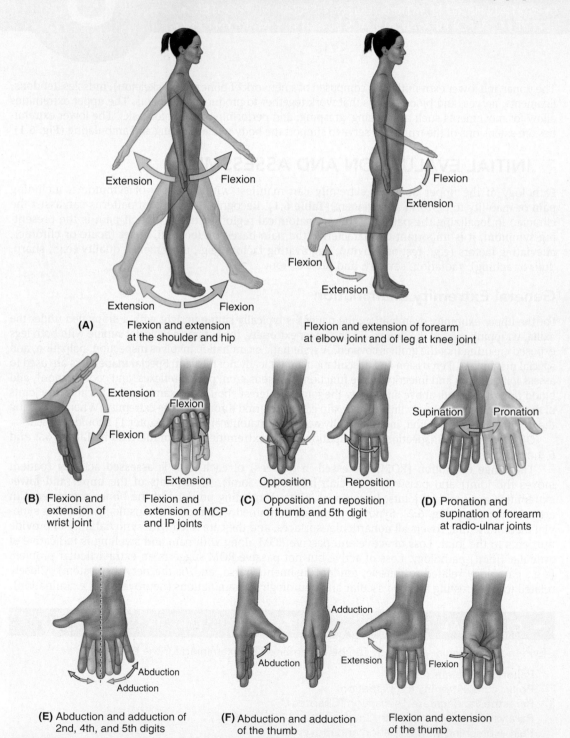

(A) Flexion and extension at the shoulder and hip

Flexion and extension of forearm at elbow joint and of leg at knee joint

(B) Flexion and extension of wrist joint

Flexion and extension of MCP and IP joints

(C) Opposition and reposition of thumb and 5th digit

(D) Pronation and supination of forearm at radio-ulnar joints

(E) Abduction and adduction of 2nd, 4th, and 5th digits

(F) Abduction and adduction of the thumb

Flexion and extension of the thumb

FIGURE 6.1. A–I. Anatomical terms to assess joint motions in the upper and lower extremities. *IP,* interphalangeal joints; *MCP,* metacarpophalangeal.

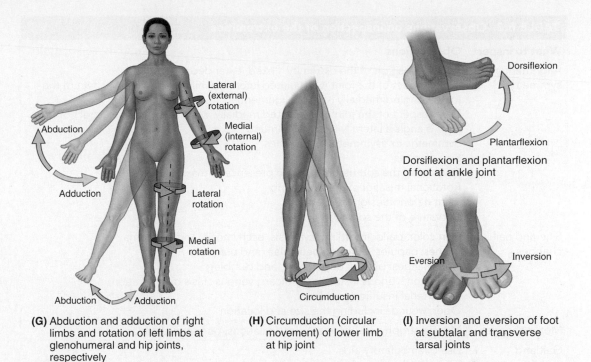

(G) Abduction and adduction of right limbs and rotation of left limbs at glenohumeral and hip joints, respectively

(H) Circumduction (circular movement) of lower limb at hip joint

(I) Inversion and eversion of foot at subtalar and transverse tarsal joints

FIGURE 6.1. (*Continued*)

3 = full pulse, and 4 = aneurysmal or bounding pulse. Capillary refill is assessed by applying pressure to the nail bed to occlude blood flow and cause blanching. Once the tissue is blanched, pressure is released, and the amount of time it takes for color to return to the nail is noted. A normal capillary refill is 2–3 seconds. The ankle–brachial index (ABI) is a more objective noninvasive screening tool used to evaluate blood flow in the lower extremity. To perform this test, the blood pressure is measured in both arms and legs. The ABI is calculated by dividing the highest systolic blood pressure for each leg by the highest systolic blood pressure in either arm. For example, if the systolic blood pressure is 140 mmHg in the left arm and 145 mmHg in the right arm, 145 mmHg will be used when calculating the ABI for each leg. A normal ratio is between 0.9 and 1.4. ABI

TABLE 6.1. Symptoms by tissue type	
Symptom Category	**Symptoms**
Joint symptoms	Pain with active or passive movement, swelling, erythema, stiffness (which should be further characterized as stiffness that is worse in the morning or after activity), joint locking or clicking, joint instability, or a joint "giving out"
Soft tissue (muscles, bursae, and tendons)	Tenderness, pain with movement, swelling, weakness, or muscle wasting
Neurologic symptoms	Paresthesia, numbness, paralysis, burning or neuropathic pain, weakness, or muscle wasting
Vascular symptoms	Calf or leg pain brought on by exercise; ischemic symptoms that manifests as a combination of the 6Ps: pain, pallor, polar (cold limb), paresthesia, paralysis, and pulselessness; ulcers; or skin changes
Associated symptoms	Constitutional: fever, unintended weight loss, or night sweats Dermatologic: rashes, skin nodules, hair loss, or pitted nails Gastroenterologic: diarrhea (especially bloody), abdominal cramping, or oral ulcers Ophthalmologic: eye pain, red eyes, or dry eyes Genitourinary: dysuria or recent sexually transmitted infections

TABLE 6.2. Observations on inspection of the extremities	
What to Inspect	**Observations**
Alignment and symmetry	Resting position of the extremity: flexed, extended, neutral
	Distal aspect of the joint is angulated laterally, while the proximal aspect of the joint is angled medially (valgus alignment)
	Distal aspect of the joint is angulated medially, while the proximal aspect of the joint is angled laterally (varus alignment)
	Symmetric or asymmetric extremities
	Size of joints
	Contour of the soft tissues and the presence of masses or swelling
	Rotational misalignment of the limb
	Joint deformities or dislocations
	Curvature of the spine (Chapter 5)
Skin and nail changes	Skin color: pallor, mottling, cyanosis, ecchymosis, and erythema
	Rashes: papules, purpura, petechiae, and plaques
	Nail changes: pitting, onycholysis, and clubbing
	Ulceration: venous insufficiency ulcers, venous stasis discoloration, and arterial insufficiency ulcers
	Open wounds including the size and location
Motor changes	Muscle atrophy or asymmetry, fasciculations, poor coordination
Gait and mobility	Use of ambulatory aids
	Speed and cadence of gait
	Specific gait patterns: antalgic, ataxic, vaulting, steppage, Trendelenburg, parkinsonian

values (ratio < 0.9) are indicative of compromised vascular flow to the lower extremity, as seen in peripheral artery disease (PAD) or a vascular injury sustained during a knee dislocation. ABI values above 1.4 indicate calcification or vessel hardening.

The neurologic examination involves examining motor and sensory function and is covered in Chapter 7. The nerves that supply the upper extremity arise from a network of nerves called the *brachial plexus*. The brachial plexus is comprised of the anterior rami of the cervical spinal cord (C5–T1). The rami form three trunks and then split into six divisions, three cords, and five terminal branches (**Fig. 6.4**).

The major sensory (dermatomes) and motor (myotomes) nerve roots of the upper extremity are summarized in **Figures 6.5 and 6.6**, respectively.

The nerves of the lower extremity arise from the lumbar plexus. The major sensory and motor nerve roots of the lower extremity are summarized in **Figure 6.7**.

The major sensory (dermatomes) and motor (myotomes) nerve roots of the lower extremity are summarized in **Figures 6.8 and 6.9**, respectively.

● CLINICAL PEARL

Knowledge of dermatomes and myotomes helps localize lesions to a single peripheral nerve or to nerve roots (Table 6.4).

TABLE 6.3. Palpation of the extremities	
What to Palpate	**Findings**
Joints	Warmth, effusions, crepitus, joint line tenderness
Skin	Nodules, masses, warmth, indurations
Soft tissues (muscles, tendons, bursa) changes	Muscle bulk, strength, and tone, swollen and tender bursae, tenderness
Bones	Bony landmarks, localized tenderness, gaps, and step deformities

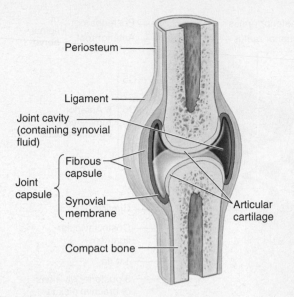

FIGURE 6.2. Structure of a synovial joint.

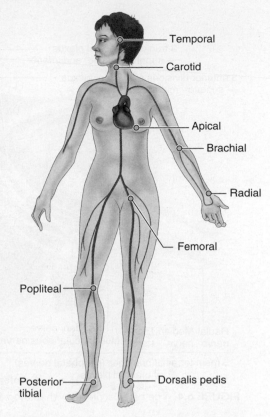

FIGURE 6.3. Pulses are palpable when arteries run close to the surface of the skin (*blue dots*).

Gait assessment helps to assess the neurologic and musculoskeletal components of the lower extremity. Abnormalities in gait may be a manifestation of pain, joint pathology, muscle weakness, or neurologic disorders. Gait is evaluated for fluidity and symmetry of arm and leg movements, step size, and for width between the feet. Some common abnormal gait patterns include:

Antalgic: Shortening of the time the affected leg bears weight.

Hemiparetic: A leg that is weak, spastic, and extended, with the elbow on the affected side being flexed. During ambulation, the patient circumducts the affected leg in order to clear the floor. By definition, only one side (either the right or left side) of the body is affected. This gait is observed following a stroke.

Parkinsonian: Gait characterized by slow, small, and shuffling steps with a hunched posture and decreased arm swing, as seen in Parkinson disease.

Ataxic: Uncoordinated and wide-based gait typically caused by cerebellar injury or sensory loss in the legs.

Vaulting: During the stance phase of the affected leg, the patient rises up on his or her toes. This gait is indicative of leg length discrepancy.

Steppage: Increased hip and knee flexion to allow the foot to clear the ground. Steppage is seen when the ankle is plantar flexed and cannot be returned to the neutral position (a 90° angle to the leg). This is termed *equinus ankle contracture*.

Trendelenburg: Downward tilting of the pelvis on the non–weight-bearing side during the stance phase and the leaning of the trunk in the opposite direction (toward the affected side) to compensate. This gait is caused by weakness of the hip abductor muscles (**Fig. 6.10**).

Laboratory Tests

Common laboratory investigations to help diagnose pathology of the extremities include a complete blood count (CBC) to assess for infection; bone pathology, indicated by elevated alkaline

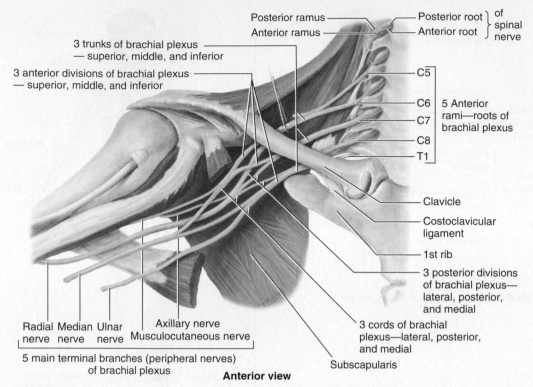

Posterior ramus — Posterior root ⎱ of
Anterior ramus — Anterior root ⎰ spinal nerve

3 trunks of brachial plexus
— superior, middle, and inferior

3 anterior divisions of brachial plexus
— superior, middle, and inferior

C5

C6 ⎱ 5 Anterior
C7 ⎰ rami—roots of
brachial plexus
C8
T1

Clavicle

Costoclavicular ligament

1st rib

3 posterior divisions of brachial plexus—lateral, posterior, and medial

Radial Median Ulnar Axillary nerve
nerve nerve nerve Musculocutaneous nerve

3 cords of brachial plexus—lateral, posterior, and medial

5 main terminal branches (peripheral nerves) of brachial plexus

Subscapularis

Anterior view

FIGURE 6.4. The brachial plexus with related anatomic structures.

phosphatase (ALP), may compromise the bone marrow and decrease one or more hematologic cell lines. Hypercalcemia may result from bone pathology, particularly in metastatic disease. Rheumatoid factor and antinuclear antibody (ANA) may help to diagnose inflammatory arthritis. Muscle pathology may present with elevated levels of creatine kinase (CK), aspartate aminotransferase (AST), and alanine aminotransferase (ALT). Abnormal blood glucose, high serum alcohol, and low serum vitamin B_{12} and folate may result in nerve damage. Erythrocyte sedimentation rate (ESR) and C-reactive

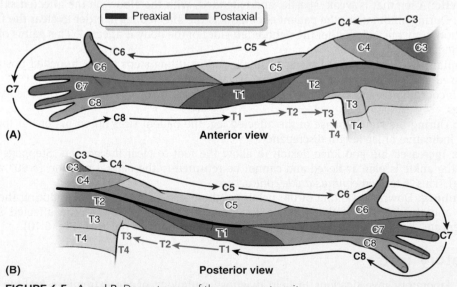

Preaxial Postaxial

(A) **Anterior view**

(B) **Posterior view**

FIGURE 6.5. A and B. Dermatomes of the upper extremity.

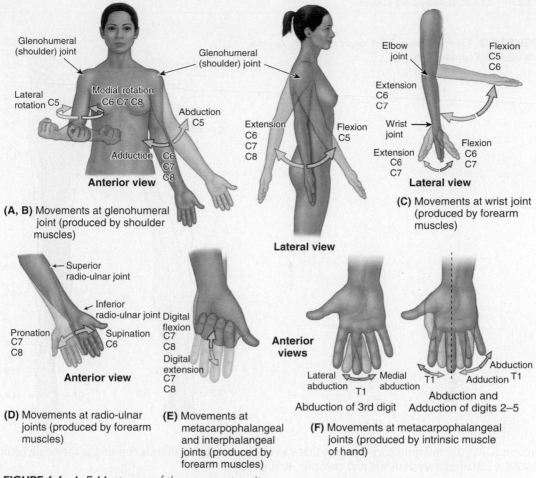

(A, B) Movements at glenohumeral joint (produced by shoulder muscles)

Glenohumeral (shoulder) joint

Glenohumeral (shoulder) joint

Lateral rotation C5

Medial rotation C6 C7 C8

Abduction C5

Adduction C6 C7 C8

Anterior view

Extension C6 C7 C8

Flexion C5

Lateral view

Elbow joint

Flexion C5 C6

Extension C6 C7

Wrist joint

Extension C6 C7

Flexion C6 C7

(C) Movements at wrist joint (produced by forearm muscles)

Lateral view

Superior radio-ulnar joint

Inferior radio-ulnar joint

Pronation C7 C8

Supination C6

Anterior view

(D) Movements at radio-ulnar joints (produced by forearm muscles)

Digital flexion C7 C8

Digital extension C7 C8

(E) Movements at metacarpophalangeal and interphalangeal joints (produced by forearm muscles)

Anterior views

Lateral abduction T1

Medial abduction T1

Abduction of 3rd digit

Abduction T1

Adduction T1

Abduction and Adduction of digits 2–5

(F) Movements at metacarpophalangeal joints (produced by intrinsic muscle of hand)

FIGURE 6.6. A–F. Myotomes of the upper extremity.

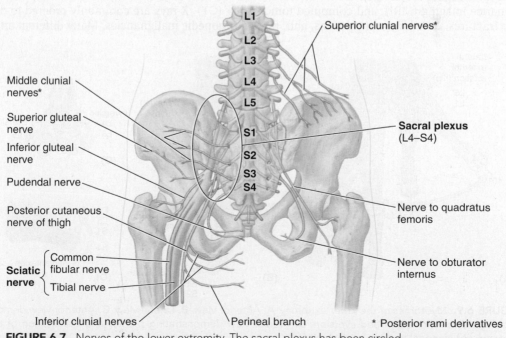

Middle clunial nerves*

Superior gluteal nerve

Inferior gluteal nerve

Pudendal nerve

Posterior cutaneous nerve of thigh

Sciatic nerve {Common fibular nerve, Tibial nerve}

Inferior clunial nerves

Perineal branch

Superior clunial nerves*

Sacral plexus (L4–S4)

Nerve to quadratus femoris

Nerve to obturator internus

L1 L2 L3 L4 L5 S1 S2 S3 S4

* Posterior rami derivatives

FIGURE 6.7. Nerves of the lower extremity. The sacral plexus has been circled.

FIGURE 6.8. Dermatomes of the lower extremity. **A.** Anterior view. **B.** Posterior view.

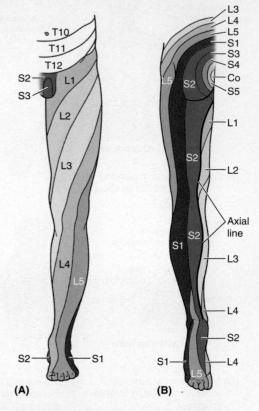

protein (CRP) are inflammatory markers that can be elevated in numerous conditions including osteomyelitis, inflammatory arthritis and myositis, and infection.

Extremity Imaging

Common imaging modalities for the extremities include conventional x-rays, ultrasound, magnetic resonance imaging (MRI), and computed tomography (CT). X-rays are commonly ordered to diagnose fractures, dislocations, infections, and, rarely, orthopedic malignancies. Many different angles

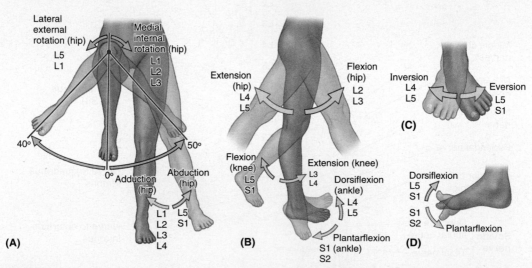

FIGURE 6.9. Myotomes of the lower extremity. **A.** Anterior view. **B.** Lateral view. **C.** Anterior view demonstrating subtalar inversion and eversion. **D.** Medial view demonstrating plantar and dorsiflexion of the metatarsophalangeal and phalangeal joints.

TABLE 6.4. Muscle groups, associated nerve roots, and peripheral nerves			
Muscle	**Action**	**Root**	**Nerve**
Upper Extremities			
Deltoid	Shoulder abduction and extension	C5, C6	Axillary
Biceps	Elbow flexion	C5, C6	Musculocutaneous
Triceps	Elbow extension	C6, C7, C8	Radial
Flexor carpi radialis	Wrist flexion	C6, C7	Median
Wrist extensors	Wrist extension	C6, C7	Radial
Finger flexors	Finger flexion	C7, C8, T1	Median, ulnar
Extensor digitorum	Finger extension	C7, C8	Posterior interosseous
First dorsal interossei	Index finger abduction	C8, T1	Ulnar
Lower Extremities			
Iliopsoas	Hip flexion	L1, L2, L3	Femoral
Gluteus maximus	Hip extension	L5, S1, S2	Inferior gluteal
Hamstrings	Knee flexion	L5, S1, S2	Sciatic
Quadriceps femoris	Knee extension	L2, L3, L4	Femoral
Tibialis anterior	Ankle dorsiflexion	L4, L5	Deep peroneal
Gastrocnemius and soleus	Ankle plantar flexion	S1, S2	Tibial
Extensor hallucis longus	Large toe extension	L5, S1	Deep peroneal

(e.g., anterior–posterior [AP], lateral, or oblique) are used to better view joints and bones. One approach to interpreting extremity x-rays is

1. Identify the x-ray type, body part imaged, and anatomic plane.
2. Analyze the bones and joints using ABCDS:
   A = anatomic appearance and alignment
   B = bony mineralization and texture

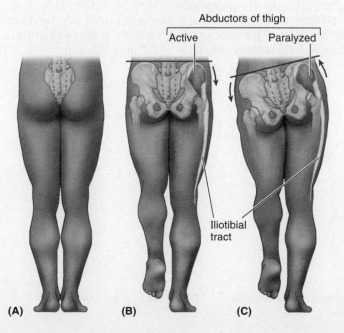

Abductors of thigh

Active   Paralyzed

Iliotibial tract

(A)   (B)   (C)

FIGURE 6.10. A–C. Trendelenburg gait. The weak hip abductors on the right side cannot stabilize the pelvis, which dips inferiorly to the left.

C = cartilage (joint space)
D = distribution of affected joints
S = soft tissue abnormalities

3. Assess the joint alignment and spacing. Note any misalignments, joint erosion, or joint space narrowing.
4. Assess the bone. Trace the bone noting the dense, outer cortical bone for discontinuities. Also, a thin cortex may be seen in osteopenia or osteoporosis.
5. Check the soft tissue for swelling.

Orthogonal x-ray views (e.g., AP and lateral) help to diagnose fractures and identify

1. The part of the bone (e.g., the epiphysis, metaphysis, or diaphysis, which is further divided into distal, middle, and proximal thirds) that is fractured. They also help to determine if the fracture crosses a joint (intra-articular) or not (extra-articular).
2. The fracture pattern (e.g., transverse, oblique, spiral, compression) as shown in **Figure 6.11**.
3. If the fracture is displaced. In displaced fractures, the anatomic position of the bone is not preserved. In undisplaced fractures, the anatomic position of the bone is preserved.
4. Changes in soft tissues for evidence of open fractures (protrusion of a bone fragment beyond the skin envelope or air within the soft tissue envelope) or effusions.

> ● **CLINICAL PEARL**
>
> Open fractures need urgent irrigation and debridement. Start appropriate antibiotics immediately and consider prophylaxis tetanus vaccination.

CT scans can identify fractures that may not appear on x-rays and help with operative planning. MRI scans are excellent at identifying soft tissue abnormalities, such as ligament or meniscal injuries of the knee, muscle inflammation, and injury to the spinal cord. Ultrasound is used for assessing blood vessels, muscle or tendon tears, and joint effusions.

Special Tests

Special investigations for the extremities include biopsies (bone, muscle, and nerve), electromyography and nerve conduction study (EMG/NCS), and arthrocentesis.

Diagnostic arthrocentesis is indicated to evaluate for monoarticular arthritis, suspected septic arthritis, or suspected crystal arthropathy. A therapeutic arthrocentesis may be performed to drain an effusion or deliver medications. To perform an arthrocentesis, a needle is placed into the joint and synovial fluid is aspirated; the fluid is analyzed for infection (with a Gram stain and culture), crystals with microscopy, and a cell count to help identify the cause of the joint effusion.

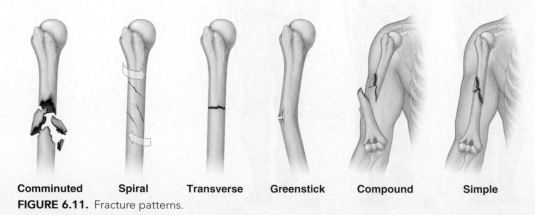

| Comminuted | Spiral | Transverse | Greenstick | Compound | Simple |

FIGURE 6.11. Fracture patterns.

SYSTEMS OVERVIEW

■ SHOULDER

Overview

The shoulder region is composed of three bones: clavicle, scapula, and humerus. The clavicle connects the upper extremity (the superior appendicular skeleton) to the trunk (the axial skeleton) (**Fig. 6.12**). There are three main joints in this region. The sternoclavicular joint is a saddle-type synovial joint between the clavicle and the manubrium. The acromioclavicular (AC) joint is a plane-type synovial joint between the clavicle and acromion of the scapula. The glenohumeral joint is a ball-and-socket synovial joint between the head of the humerus and the glenoid cavity of the scapula (**Fig. 6.13**).

The muscles that mobilize the shoulder joint can be organized into three muscle groups: the anterior axioappendicular, posterior axioappendicular, and scapulohumeral (**Table 6.5**).

Physical Examination

Both shoulders are inspected for swelling, erythema, scars, or deformities. Palpation is started at the sternoclavicular joint and continued laterally along the clavicle to the AC joint and head of the greater tuberosity of the humerus. The spine of the scapula is also palpated. Areas of tenderness and/or deformities are noted.

To assess ROM, a series of maneuvers are performed on both shoulders (**Fig. 6.1; Table 6.6**). Pain with external or internal rotation may indicate rotator muscle injury or adhesive capsulitis. Pain during adduction may indicate AC joint pathology.

The shoulder region contains four rotator cuff muscles to stabilize the joint (**Fig. 6.14**). Rotator cuff tears and impingement of the muscle tendons are common, debilitating injuries. Maneuvers to test the rotator cuff muscles are summarized in **Figure 6.16** and **Table 6.7**.

The Neer and Hawkins tests are used to detect impingement of the rotator cuff tendons against the acromion. Repetitive impingement of the rotator cuff tendon causes inflammation; therefore, reproduction of pain with these maneuvers is a positive finding.

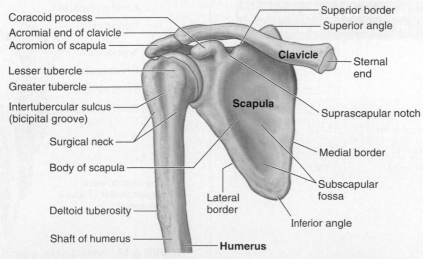

Coracoid process
Acromial end of clavicle
Acromion of scapula
Lesser tubercle
Greater tubercle
Intertubercular sulcus (bicipital groove)
Surgical neck
Body of scapula
Deltoid tuberosity
Shaft of humerus
Superior border
Superior angle
Clavicle
Sternal end
Scapula
Suprascapular notch
Medial border
Subscapular fossa
Lateral border
Inferior angle
Humerus

FIGURE 6.12. Bones of the shoulder region.

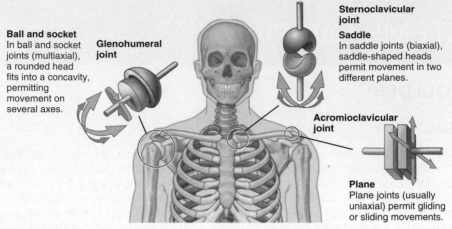

FIGURE 6.13. Synovial joints of the shoulder region.

TABLE 6.5. Muscle groups of the shoulder by anatomical group with peripheral nerve supply

Anterior Axioappendicular	Posterior Axioappendicular	Scapulohumeral
Pectoralis major and minor (medial and lateral pectoral n.) Serratus anterior (long thoracic n.) Subclavius (nerve to subclavius)	*Superficial:* Trapezius (accessory n.) Latissimus dorsi (thoracodorsal n.) *Deep:* Levator scapulae (dorsal scapular n.) Rhomboid major and minor (dorsal scapular n.)	*Rotator cuff:* Supraspinatus (suprascapular n.) Infraspinatus (suprascapular n.) Teres minor (axillary n.) Subscapularis (nerve to subclavius) Deltoid (axillary n.) Teres major (lower subscapular n.)

n., nerve.

TABLE 6.6. Normal values for the range of motion of the shoulder

Movement	Normal Range
Flexion	0°–180°
Extension	0°–60°
Abduction	0°–180°
Adduction, horizontal	0°–45°
Rotation, internal	0°–70°
Rotation, external	0°–90°

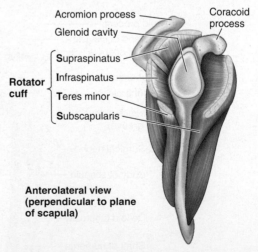

FIGURE 6.14. Anterolateral view of the rotator cuff muscles (SITS).

TABLE 6.7. Rotator cuff tests		
Area Tested	**Test Name**	**Technique**
Supraspinatus	Jobe or "empty can" test	The patient flexes both shoulders to 90° and abducts to 45° (scapular plane) while keeping the elbows straight. Next, the patient internally rotates the shoulders so the thumbs points downward. Instruct the patient to resist downward pressure applied simultaneously to both arms. If the patient cannot resist the downward pressure, supraspinatus pathology may be present.
Infraspinatus and Teres Minor	External rotation test	The patient's arms are placed at the side with elbows flexed to 90°. Instruct the patient to externally rotate both shoulders, while the clinician applies resistance to both forearms. Weakness indicates infraspinatus pathology.
Subscapularis	Gerber or Lift-off test	The patient places the dorsal aspect of their one hand over the middle of their lumbar spine. Instruct the patient to lift their hand off of their back. If they are not able to, this indicates subscapularis pathology.
Shoulder impingement	Neer test	The patient's shoulder is internally rotated with the elbow extended. The clinician stabilizes the scapula and then passively flexes the shoulder above the patient's head. Pain in the anterior or lateral aspect of the shoulder indicates a positive finding.
	Hawkins test	The patient's elbow and shoulder are flexed to 90°. Next, the clinician internally rotates the patient's shoulder. Pain in the superior or lateral aspect of the shoulder indicates a positive finding.

Imaging

The articular surface of the humerus is normally parallel with the glenoid cavity (**Fig. 6.15A**). A normal shoulder x-ray is shown in **Figure 6.15B**. A normal MRI of the shoulder is presented in **Figure 6.15C**.

▪ ELBOW AND RADIOULNAR JOINTS

Overview

The elbow is a hinge-type synovial joint located between the upper arm and forearm formed by the distal humerus (capitellum, trochlear notch, and olecranon fossa), proximal ulna (coronoid process and olecranon), and radial head (**Fig. 6.16**). The forearm consists of the radius and ulna, connected by an interosseous membrane. These bones form the pivot-type synovial joints (proximal and distal radioulnar joints) that allow the forearm to supinate and pronate.

The biceps brachii and brachialis muscles facilitate elbow flexion. The biceps brachii muscle has a short and long head and is innervated by the musculocutaneous nerve. The brachialis lies deep to the biceps muscle and is innervated by both the musculocutaneous and radial nerves. The triceps brachii facilitates elbow extension and is innervated by the radial nerve. The biceps brachii muscle facilitates forearm supination, while the pronator quadratus and pronator teres facilitate forearm pronation (**Fig. 6.17**).

Physical Examination

On examination, the elbow is inspected for deformities, scars, erythema, and swelling (**Table 6.2**). The distal humerus, proximal radius, and ulna are palpated for tenderness or deformities (**Table 6.3**).

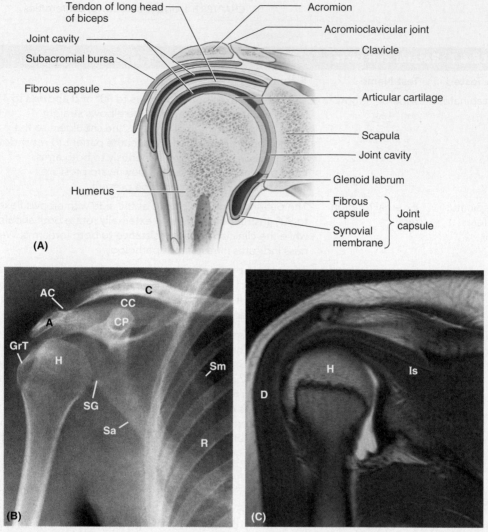

FIGURE 6.15. **A.** Coronal section of the shoulder joint. **B.** Normal AP x-ray of the right shoulder. *A*, acromion; *AC*, acromioclavicular joint; *C*, clavicle; *CC*, coracoclavicular joint; *CP*, coracoid process; *GrT*, greater tuberosity; *H*, humerus; *R*, rib; *Sa*, scapula axillary border; *SG*, scapula glenoid; *Sm*, medial scapula border. **C.** Normal coronal T1-weighted MR image of the right shoulder. *D*, deltoid; *H*, humerus; *Is*, infraspinatus ligament.

FIGURE 6.16. Elbow and proximal radioulnar joints.

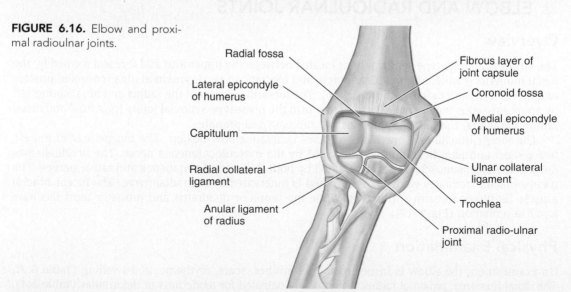

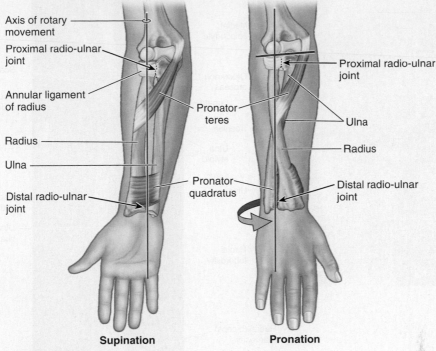

FIGURE 6.17. Supination and pronation of the forearm.

Tenderness at the insertion site of tendons on the medial epicondyle is seen in *golfer's* or *pitcher's elbow*, whereas tenderness on the lateral epicondyle is seen in *tennis elbow*.

ROM testing involves assessing elbow flexion, extension, supination (rotating the palm anteriorly), and pronation (rotating the palm posteriorly).

Imaging

In a normal elbow x-ray, the humerus runs along the same axis as do the ulna and radius in the AP view (**Fig. 6.18A**). The radial head articulates with the center of the capitellum of the humerus. The radius and ulna are in close proximity at their articulation in the proximal radioulnar joint and may even overlap. In a normal forearm x-ray, the radius and ulna run in the same plane and may overlap if the arm is pronated (**Fig. 6.18B**). The ulna is slightly shorter than the radius distally. The radiocarpal joint is congruent with equal spacing between the carpus and distal radius.

■ WRIST AND HAND

Overview

The bones of the hand consist of 8 carpal bones, 5 metacarpals, and 14 phalanges. The carpal bones are arranged in two rows. The radius and the proximal row of carpal bones form the radiocarpal (wrist) joint, which allows flexion, extension, radial and ulnar deviation, and circumduction (**Fig. 6.19**).

The muscles of the forearm responsible for hand and wrist movement can be grouped into the anteromedial (flexor-pronator) and posterolateral compartments. The 8 muscles of the flexor–pronator compartment are located on the anteromedial aspect of the forearm and facilitate flexion of the wrist, fingers, and thumb. The flexor–pronator muscles are innervated by the median nerve with the exception of flexor carpi ulnaris and the fourth and fifth digits of flexor digitorum profundus, which are innervated by the ulnar nerve. The posterolateral compartment

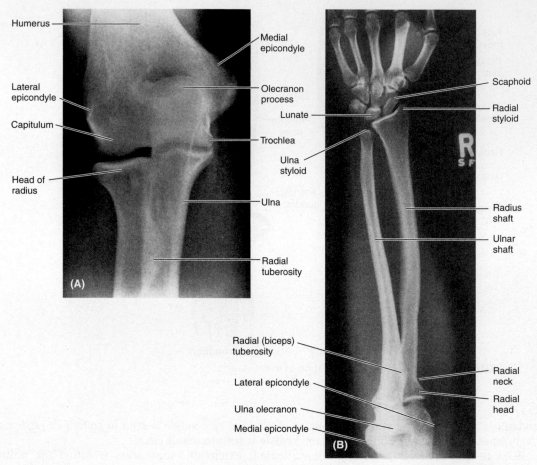

FIGURE 6.18. **A.** Normal AP x-ray of the right elbow joint. **B.** Normal AP x-ray of the right forearm.

contains 12 muscles that facilitate extension of the wrist and metacarpophalangeal (MCP) joints. The posterolateral muscles also supinate the forearm and abduct and extend the thumb and are innervated by the radial nerve. The intrinsic hand muscles are divided into five compartments (**Table 6.8**).

Physical Examination

On examination, the wrists, hands, and nails are inspected for deformities (**Table 6.2**). Next, the bones of the hand and wrist are palpated for tenderness or deformities (**Table 6.3**). Tenderness in the anatomic snuffbox (formed by the abductor pollicis longus and extensor pollicis longus tendons of the thumb) may indicate a scaphoid fracture. The MCP joints are palpated for effusions by flexing the finger to open up the joint and using the thumb and index fingers to ballot. This process is repeated for the proximal interphalangeal (PIP) and distal interphalangeal (DIP) joints.

The ROM of the wrist (flexion–extension, ulnar–radial deviation), MCP (flexion–extension, adduction–abduction), PIP (flexion–extension), and DIP (flexion–extension) joints should be approximated. Instructing the patient to make a fist and then extending the fingers assesses flexion and extension of the MCP, PIP, and DIP joints. To test the interossei muscles, ask the patient to spread the fingers wide (abduction) and push them together (adduction), noting any abnormalities in these movements (**Fig. 6.20**). A dynamometer can be used to measure total hand (grip) strength.

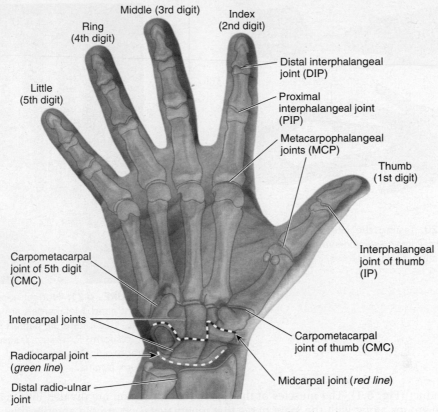

FIGURE 6.19. Surface anatomy of the palmar aspect of the hand.

Imaging

In a normal x-ray of the hand, all eight carpal bones are visible with preserved joint alignment and spaces between each bone (**Fig. 6.21**). The carpometacarpal (CMC) and interphalangeal joints are congruent.

▇ HIP AND FEMUR

Overview

The hip is a ball-and-socket synovial joint composed of the head of the femur and acetabulum of the pelvis (**Fig. 6.22**). The hip joint can flex–extend, abduct–adduct, internally–externally rotate,

TABLE 6.8. Intrinsic muscles of the hand, their function, and nerve supply		
Compartment	**Function**	**Nerve**
Thenar	Abduction, flexion, and opposition of the thumb	Median
Adductor	Adducts the thumb	Ulnar
Hypothenar	Adducts, flexes, and opposes the fifth digit	Ulnar
Central	Contains the lumbricals that flex the MCP and extend the interphalangeal joints	First and second lumbricals: Median Third and fourth lumbricals: Ulnar
Interosseous	Adduct and abduct the fingers depending on which are active	Ulnar

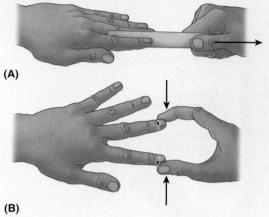

(A)

(B)

FIGURE 6.20. Testing the interossei muscles. **A.** Testing palmar interossei innervated by the ulnar nerve. **B.** Testing dorsal interossei innervated by the ulnar nerve.

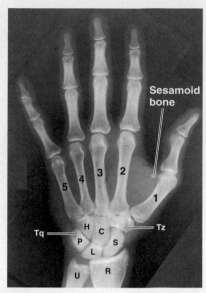

FIGURE 6.21. Normal x-ray of the right hand. Metacarpals are numbered 1–5. *C*, capitate; *H*, hamate; *L*, lunate; *P*, pisiform; *R*, radius; *S*, scaphoid; *Td*, trapezoid; *Tq*, triquetrum; *Tz*, trapezium; *U*, ulna.

and circumduct (**Fig. 6.1**). The muscles of the hip and femur region are divided into four groups. The muscle groups along with the main nerve that innervates each are the anterior thigh (femoral nerve), medial thigh (obturator nerve), posterior thigh (sciatic nerve), and gluteals (superior and inferior gluteal nerves).

Physical Examination

The hip and femur examination begins with the assessment of gait. Next, the hip is examined for swelling, erythema, or deformities (**Table 6.2**). The anterior superior iliac spine (ASIS), posterior superior iliac spine (PSIS), greater trochanter, and ischial tuberosity are palpated for tenderness (**Table 6.3**). Pain on palpation of the greater trochanter may indicate trochanteric bursitis, and pain over the ischial tuberosity may indicate ischiogluteal bursitis (**Fig. 6.23**).

FIGURE 6.22. Bones of the pelvis, hip joint, and proximal femur.

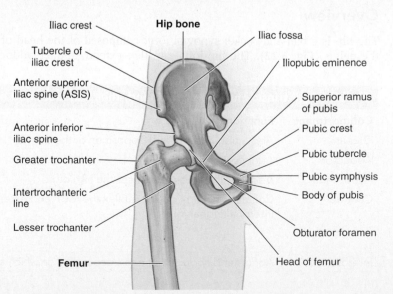

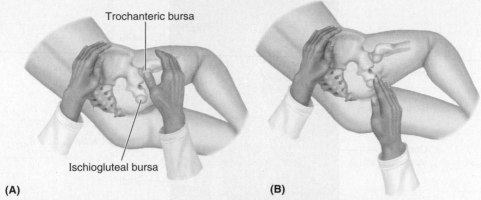

Trochanteric bursa

Ischiogluteal bursa

(A)   **(B)**

FIGURE 6.23. A–B. Examination of the trochanteric and ischiogluteal bursae.

> ● CLINICAL PEARL
>
> Hip joint pathology usually manifests as groin pain that worsens with rotation of the hip.

The movements of the hip joint are summarized in **Table 6.9**.

> ● CLINICAL PEARL
>
> There are two leg length measurements. True leg length is measured from the ASIS to the medial malleolus. Apparent leg length is measured from the umbilicus to the medial malleolus. Causes of leg asymmetry include hip fractures (short and externally rotated leg), scoliosis, and congenital abnormalities.

Imaging

In a normal x-ray of the hip, the femoral head articulates with the acetabulum, the joint space is present, and both hip joints are symmetrical (**Fig. 6.24**).

TABLE 6.9. Range of motion testing for the hip		
Hip Movement	**Primary Muscles Affecting Movement**	**Patient Instructions**
Flexion	Iliopsoas	"Bend your knee to your chest and pull it to your abdomen."
Extension	Gluteus maximus	"Lying face down, bend your knee and lift it up." Or "Lying flat, move your lower leg away from the midline and down over the side of the table."
Abduction	Gluteus medius and minimus	"Lying flat, move your lower leg away from the midline."
Adduction	Adductor brevis, adductor longus, adductor magnus, pectineus, gracilis	"Lying flat, bend your knee and move your lower leg toward the midline."
External rotation	Internal and external obturators, quadratus femoris, superior and inferior gemellus	"Lying flat, bend your knee and turn your lower leg and foot across the midline."
Internal rotation	Iliopsoas	"Lying flat, bend your knee and turn your lower leg and foot away from the midline."

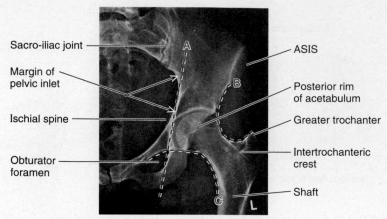

FIGURE 6.24. Normal AP x-ray of the left hip. Several different lines and curvatures are used in the detection of hip abnormalities. The Kohler line (*red A*) is normally tangential to the pelvic inlet and the obturator foramen. The acetabular fossa should lie lateral to this line. The Shenton line (*red B*) and the iliofemoral line (*red C*) should appear in a normal AP x-ray as smooth, continuous lines that are bilaterally symmetrical. *ASIS,* anterior superior iliac spine.

◼ KNEE

Overview

The knee is a hinge-type synovial joint composed of the distal femur, proximal tibia, and patella (**Fig. 6.25A**). The knee joint is stabilized by the medial collateral ligament (MCL), lateral collateral ligament (LCL), anterior cruciate ligament (ACL), and posterior cruciate ligament (PCL). The medial and lateral menisci are crescent-shaped fibrocartilage that cushions the joint (**Fig. 6.25B**). The quadriceps muscles are responsible for knee extension, and the hamstring muscles are responsible for knee flexion.

Physical Examination

The knee examination begins with the assessment of gait. Next, the joint is inspected for loss of infrapatellar indentations that may indicate an effusion (**Fig. 6.26**).

Tests used to detect a knee effusion are summarized in **Table 6.10**. The knee is also inspected for deformities or erythema.

The distal femur, patella, proximal tibia, and joint line are palpated for points of tenderness; the popliteal fossa is palpated for masses that may represent a popliteal cyst (Baker cyst).

ROM testing of the knee includes flexion and extension. Normal knee flexion is 120°–150°, and normal knee extension is 0°–5° hyperextended. After ROM is evaluated, the ligaments and menisci are tested, as discussed in the clinical cases.

Imaging

In a normal knee x-ray, the femur and tibia articulate symmetrically (**Fig. 6.27**), the joint space (knee) is visible, and the patella is proximal to the tibia.

◼ ANKLE AND FOOT

Overview

The ankle is a hinge-type synovial joint composed of the articulation between the tibial plafond (including the medial malleolus), distal fibula (lateral malleolus), and talus. The ankle joint is stabilized by the syndesmosis, medially by the deltoid ligament, and laterally by the anterior

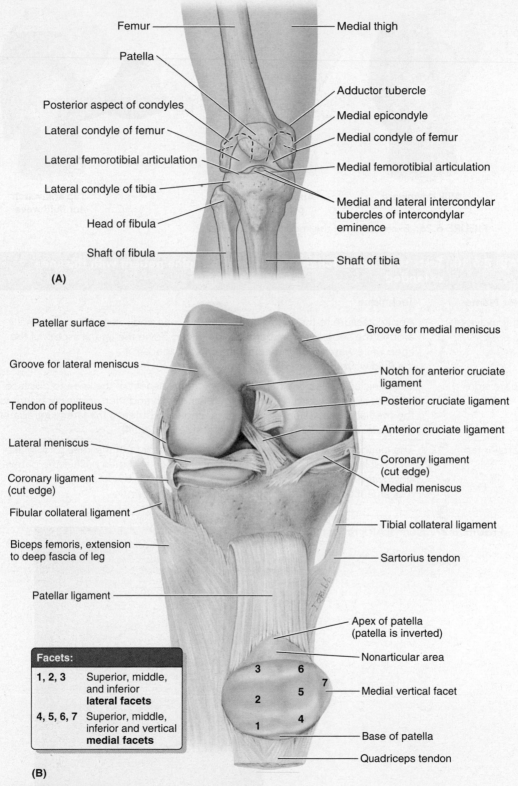

Femur — — Medial thigh

Patella

— Adductor tubercle

Posterior aspect of condyles — — Medial epicondyle

Lateral condyle of femur — — Medial condyle of femur

Lateral femorotibial articulation — — Medial femorotibial articulation

Lateral condyle of tibia — — Medial and lateral intercondylar tubercles of intercondylar eminence

Head of fibula —

Shaft of fibula — — Shaft of tibia

(A)

Patellar surface — — Groove for medial meniscus

Groove for lateral meniscus — — Notch for anterior cruciate ligament

— Posterior cruciate ligament

Tendon of popliteus — — Anterior cruciate ligament

Lateral meniscus — — Coronary ligament (cut edge)

Coronary ligament (cut edge) — — Medial meniscus

Fibular collateral ligament — — Tibial collateral ligament

Biceps femoris, extension to deep fascia of leg — — Sartorius tendon

Patellar ligament — — Apex of patella (patella is inverted)

— Nonarticular area

Facets:	
1, 2, 3	Superior, middle, and inferior **lateral facets**
4, 5, 6, 7	Superior, middle, inferior and vertical **medial facets**

3 6

2 5 7 — Medial vertical facet

1 4

— Base of patella

— Quadriceps tendon

(B)

FIGURE 6.25. **A.** Anterior view of the bones of the knee joint. **B.** Anterior view with knee flexed demonstrating the ligaments of the knee joint.

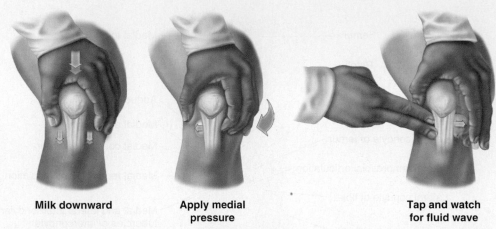

Milk downward   **Apply medial
                            pressure**

**Tap and watch
for fluid wave**

FIGURE 6.26. Examination of the knee for a joint effusion.

TABLE 6.10.	Tests to examine for knee effusion in a supine patient with the knee extended
Test Name	Technique
Fluid wave test	Apply pressure to the medial aspect of the knee and sweep hand proximally around the superior aspect of the patella and down the lateral aspect of the knee while watching the medial infrapatellar space. If a fluid wave appears, the test is positive.
Bulge sign	The clinician places one hand on the proximal aspect of the knee to displace synovial fluid down from the suprapatellar pouch and then applies pressure to the medial infrapatellar space while feeling for a bulge in the lateral infrapatellar space. Repeat the test on the lateral side (**Fig. 6.54**).
Patellar tap	The clinician places one hand on the proximal aspect of the knee to displace synovial fluid down from the suprapatellar pouch and then pushes the patella downward. If the patella moves, then there is fluid in the knee. If there is no movement appreciated, the patella is against the femur.

FIGURE 6.27. Normal AP x-ray of the knee.

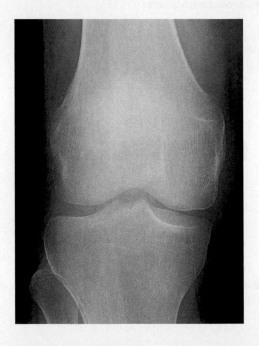

talofibular ligament (ATFL), calcaneofibular ligament (CFL), and posterior talofibular ligament (PTFL) (**Fig. 6.28A**). Muscles that move the ankle and the extrinsic muscles of the foot are summarized in **Table 6.11**.

The foot is composed of 7 tarsal bones, 5 metatarsals, and 14 phalanges. The intertarsal joints, namely, the subtalar and transverse tarsal (talonavicular and calcaneocuboid) joints, facilitate inversion and eversion of the foot (**Fig. 6.28B**). Muscles that move the foot and toes are either extrinsic or intrinsic. Extrinsic muscles include muscles of the anterior, lateral, superficial posterior, and deep posterior compartments of the leg. There are 20 intrinsic muscles, which are innervated by the medial and lateral plantar nerve branches of the tibial nerve.

Physical Examination

Examination of the ankle and foot begins with inspection for masses, deformities, erythema, or effusions (**Table 6.2**). The medial and lateral malleoli, tarsals, and metatarsals (particularly the base of the fifth digit) are palpated for tenderness or deformities.

The ROM of the ankles, intertarsal, and metatarsophalangeal (MTP) joints is assessed with ankle dorsiflexion and plantar flexion, foot eversion and inversion, and toe flexion and extension.

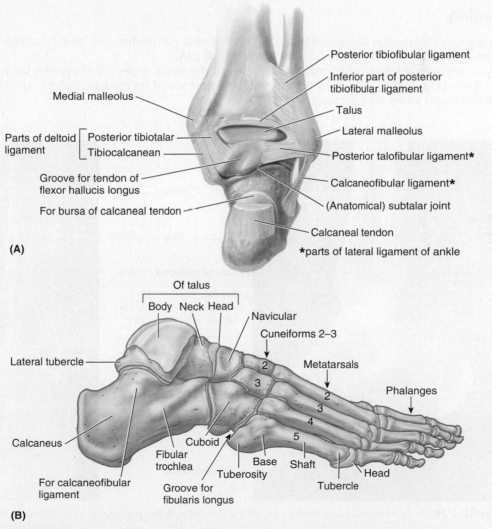

FIGURE 6.28. Bones and ligaments of the foot and ankle. A. Posterior view. B. Lateral view.

TABLE 6.11. Compartments and nerve supply of the lower extremity

Anterior Compartment	Lateral Compartment	Superficial Posterior Compartment	Deep Posterior Compartment
Muscles and Actions			
Tibialis anterior (ankle dorsiflexion) Extensor digitorum longus (toe extension) Extensor hallucis longus (great toe extension) Peroneus tertius (weak ankle dorsiflexion and foot eversion)	Peroneus longus Peroneus brevis (resist inadvertent inversion, limited foot eversion)	Gastrocnemius Soleus (ankle plantar flexion)	Tibialis posterior (foot inversion) Flexor digitorum longus (toe flexion) Flexor hallucis longus (great toe flexion)
Nerves			
Deep peroneal nerve	Superficial peroneal nerve	Tibial nerve	Tibial nerve

Imaging

In a normal ankle x-ray, the articulation of the talus with the medial and lateral malleoli is preserved with a visible and symmetric joint space (**Fig. 6.29A**).

In a normal foot x-ray, the articulations between the tarsal bones are congruent with visible joint space (**Fig. 6.29B**). The bony arch of the foot is preserved on the lateral view. All MTP and interphalangeal joints are congruent.

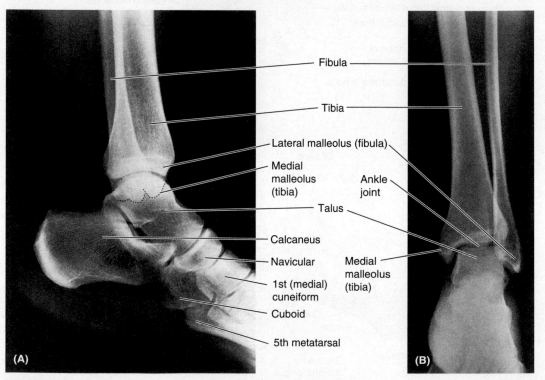

Fibula

Tibia

Lateral malleolus (fibula)

Medial malleolus (tibia)

Ankle joint

Talus

Calcaneus

Navicular

Medial malleolus (tibia)

1st (medial) cuneiform

Cuboid

5th metatarsal

(A)

(B)

FIGURE 6.29. A. Normal oblique/mortise x-ray of the left ankle. **B.** Normal lateral x-ray of the left ankle.

CLINICAL CASES

 ## CRYSTAL INFLAMMATORY ARTHRITIS

Presentation

A 56-year-old male presents to his health care provider with a 2-day history of pain, redness, and swelling in his right big toe. He has a past medical history of hypertension and a previous episode of right toe swelling several years ago.

Definition

Crystal inflammatory arthritis is stimulated by the deposition of uric acid (gout) or calcium pyrophosphate dihydrate (CPPD) crystal in joints.

What are common causes?

Gout occurs with uric acid crystals deposition in the joint. Risk factors for gout include male sex, past medical history of gout, and cardiovascular disease. Pseudogout occurs with CPPD crystal deposition in the joint.

What is the differential diagnosis?

Monoarthritis: The differential diagnosis includes septic arthritis, crystal arthritis, seropositive and seronegative inflammatory arthritis, trauma, hemarthrosis, and osteoarthritis (OA).

What symptoms might be observed?

Symptoms of gout and pseudogout include joint pain and decreased ROM. Gout usually has a more insidious onset compared to pseudogout, which is often more acute in onset. Gout is more likely to involve the first MTP.

What are the possible findings on examination?

Vital signs: Tachycardia and fever may be present.
Inspection: Inspect involved joint(s) for erythema and swelling. Also inspect the pinna of the ears, feet, and fingers for tophi, which are uric acid crystal deposits in soft tissue and joints (**Fig. 6.30**).
Palpation: Affected joint(s) will feel warm and tender with an effusion.
ROM: Reduced in acute gout and pseudogout secondary to inflammation of the joint.

What tests should be ordered?

Laboratory tests: CBC, metabolic panel (elevated creatinine [Cr], serum uric acid, hypercalcemia, hypomagnesemia, phosphate, low parathyroid hormone [PTH], high thyroid-stimulating hormone [TSH], and ALP [**Table 6.12**]; note that elevated uric acid is not diagnostic of gout and may be normal during a gout attack). Other serology (elevated ESR and CRP).
Imaging: In gout, x-ray findings are initially normal, with possible evidence of soft tissue swelling. Late findings include bony, round erosions and "punched-out" lesions with overhanging edges; tophi may be visible as soft tissues calcify (**Fig. 6.31A**). In CPPD, x-rays may reveal calcium deposits in fibrocartilage of the menisci in the knee and triangular fibrocartilage of the wrist and the symphysis pubis (**Fig. 6.31B**).

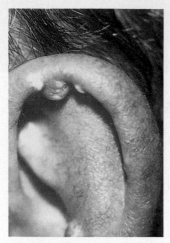

FIGURE 6.30. Tophi, which are deposits of uric acid crystals in tissue, in the ear.

TABLE 6.12. Differences in crystals on synovial fluid analysis	
Uric Acid Crystals	**CPPD Crystals**
Needle shaped	Rhomboid shaped
Negatively birefringent	Positively birefringent

Special Tests

Synovial fluid: Fluid from arthrocentesis may exhibit an inflammatory pattern with more than 2,000 white blood cells (WBCs)/mm³ and differential of >50% neutrophils. In addition, it may reveal intracellular birefringent crystals on microscopy (**Fig. 6.32**).

Crystal and bacterial arthritis cannot always be distinguished by presentation and peripheral blood tests. Joint fluid aspiration and culture is needed to reliably rule out septic arthritis. A negative Gram stain does not exclude infection. Similarly, the presence of crystals does not rule out infection, as crystals may occur concomitantly with infection.

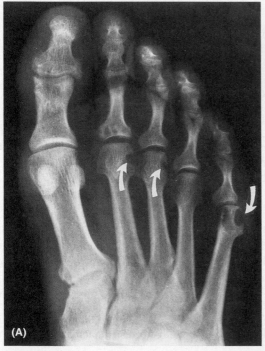 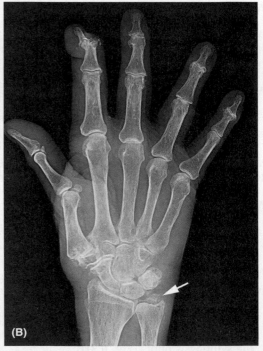

FIGURE 6.31. A. X-ray of a foot affected by gout demonstrating para-articular punched-out lesions in the distal metatarsal bones (*arrows*). **B.** X-ray of the hand and wrist with pseudogout (calcium pyrophosphate deposition disease [CPPD]). Note the narrowing of the joint spaces and the chondrocalcinosis of the triangular fibrocartilage (*arrow*).

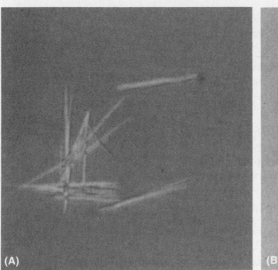
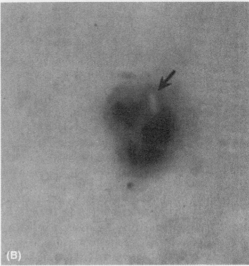

FIGURE 6.32. A. Needle-shaped urate crystals in synovial fluid. **B.** CPPD crystals phagocytized by white blood cells in synovial fluid (*arrow*).

 MYOPATHY

Presentation

A 67-year-old female presents to her health care provider with fatigue and weakness, particularly when climbing stairs or standing from a sitting position, as well as a low-grade fever and rash on the dorsum of her hand.

Definition

Myopathy is a condition that affects the muscle fibers and often presents as weakness despite an intact nerve supply and functioning neuromuscular junction (NMJ).

What are common causes?

Common etiologies of myopathy include

Type of Myopathy	Etiologies
Inflammatory	Immune system–related myopathies, including polymyositis, dermatomyositis, rheumatoid arthritis (RA), systematic lupus erythematosus (SLE), and inclusion body myositis
Metabolic/congenital	Myopathy related to metabolic abnormalities, primarily genetic deficits in lipid and glycogen breakdown as well as mitochondrial diseases. Other congenital causes include Duchenne muscular dystrophy
Endocrine	Addison disease, Cushing disease, hypo/hyperthyroid conditions, and hyperparathyroidism
Malabsorption	Inadequate absorption of electrolytes or nutrients such as osteomalacia-related myopathy, hypo/hyperkalemic myopathy, and complications of celiac disease

continued

Drug/toxin	Myopathy resulting from toxins or pharmaceutical substances such as alcohol (acute and chronic use) steroids, colchicine, statins, cytochrome P450 (CYP3A4) inhibitors in conjunction with simvastatin, cocaine, and heroin
Infection	Common sources of infectious myopathies include trichinosis, coxsackievirus A/B, cysticercosis, Lyme disease, influenza, *Staphylococcus aureus*, and human immunodeficiency virus (HIV)

The timing of onset of muscle weakness helps differentiate the cause of myopathy. An acute presentation is more likely related to toxins. Rhabdomyolysis, a syndrome caused by a rapid breakdown of skeletal muscle, often presents over days. Polymyositis and steroid-induced or endocrine causes are likely to present over weeks. It is also helpful to identify the pattern of muscle weakness as predominantly proximal muscle weakness, predominantly distal muscles weakness, or both. The clinician should determine if the weakness is symmetric.

What is the differential diagnosis?

Muscle weakness: Based on an anatomic approach, the differential diagnosis can include central nervous system (CNS) pathology (e.g., stroke or subdural hematoma), demyelinating conditions (e.g., multiple sclerosis [MS] or Guillain-Barré syndrome), myelopathy, ventral horn pathology (e.g., amyotrophic lateral sclerosis [ALS]), motor root pathology, peripheral neuropathy, NMJ pathology (e.g., myasthenia gravis or botulism), myopathy, and chronic medical conditions (e.g., diabetes, heart disease, and depression).

What symptoms might be observed?

Symptoms of myopathies include symmetric proximal muscle weakness, which often presents as difficulty climbing stairs or standing up from a chair. Distal muscle weakness is less common and may present with difficulty writing or with a weak handgrip. Generalized malaise, fatigue, and dark urine may also be present.

What are the possible findings on examination?

Vital signs: Fever may be present.
Inspection: Examine the weak muscle groups for any asymmetry in muscle size or evidence of inflammation or swelling. The skin should be inspected for rashes such as Gottron papules (on the dorsum of the fingers), heliotrope rash (over the eyebrows), or shawl sign (rash on the back, shoulders, and upper chest).
Palpation: Palpate for asymmetry in muscle size, pain, or tenderness.
Neurologic examination: Assess for weakness in the affected muscles. The muscle strength is graded using the Medical Research Council (MRC) scale (Chapter 7). Test deep tendon reflexes to rule out neurologic causes of weakness. Sensation is typically normal.

What tests should be ordered?

Laboratory tests: CBC; metabolic panel (CK, lactate dehydrogenase [LDH], serum myoglobin, and aminotransferases may be elevated due to muscle breakdown, elevated Cr and BUN if renal injury, electrolytes, and TSH); urine dipstick may be positive for blood (suggestive of myoglobinuria); toxicology screen (alcohol, cocaine); other serology (if inflammatory etiologies are suspected, ESR, CRP, ANA, anti–Sjögren syndrome-related antigen A [Anti-Ro/SSA], La/SSB, anti-Sm, anti-ribonucleoprotein [RNP], and anti-Jo-1 [myositis specific] as suggested by history and physical examination).
Imaging: MRI can visualize muscle tissue well and is useful in diagnosing inflammatory myopathy; MRI can also help determine appropriate sites for muscle biopsy.

Special Tests

Electrophysiologic (EMG) testing: Assess the peripheral nervous system and NMJ function. EMG may also help determine the optimal site for muscle biopsy.

Muscle biopsy: Assess microscopic level changes in the physical structure of muscle and measure the accumulation of lipids or glycogen in muscle.
Genetic testing: If applicable, test for inheritable myopathies and muscular dystrophy.

 # OSTEOARTHRITIS

Presentation

A 76-year-old obese female presents with a 1-year history of progressive right hip pain that radiates to her groin. The pain is aggravated with weight-bearing and physical activity. The pain improves with rest.

Definition

Idiopathic OA is a progressive degenerative joint disease resulting in a loss of articular cartilage and chronic reactive bone changes resulting in bone destruction and the formation of new bone at the margins called *osteophytes*. Secondary OA is a loss of articular cartilage and chronic reactive bone changes as a result of an injury or pathology affecting the joint(s).

What are common causes?

OA may be caused by trauma, congenital or developmental joint disorders, avascular necrosis (AVN), endocrine disorders (e.g., acromegaly, hyperparathyroidism, hypothyroidism), metabolic disorders (e.g., gout, pseudogout, Wilson disease, hemochromatosis), neuropathic disorders (e.g., Charcot joint from diabetes, syphilis), or Paget disease. Risk factors for OA include age, obesity, gender (female), and genetic predisposition.

What is the differential diagnosis?

Joint pain: The differential diagnosis includes trauma (e.g., fracture, dislocation), infection (e.g., septic arthritis, OM, cellulitis), inflammatory processes (e.g., gout, pseudogout, RA, bursitis), musculoskeletal injuries (e.g., muscle strain, tendinopathy, ligament/meniscal injury), and neuropathy or referred pain (e.g., meralgia paresthetica, back pain).

What symptoms might be observed?

Symptoms of OA include joint pain and stiffness that is worse with activity and at the end of the day. The most commonly affected joints are the DIP, PIP and first CMC in the hands, and the knees and hips. Patients may notice weakness and knee locking or instability.

What are the possible findings on examination?

Vital signs: Typically normal.
Inspection: Assess the gait pattern (e.g., antalgic or Trendelenburg). Inspect the joints for swelling, joint alignment, flexion contractures, bony deformity, and muscle atrophy. Inspect the hands for bony enlargements at the DIP joints (Heberden nodes) and PIP joints (Bouchard nodes) and squaring of the CMC joint (**Fig. 6.33**).
Palpation: Palpate the affected area, noting any joint line tenderness, joint effusion, or bursa inflammation. Crepitus may be felt with joint movement.
ROM: Motion may be reduced, and pain may occur with movement.

FIGURE 6.33. Heberden nodes at the DIP joint indicative of OA.

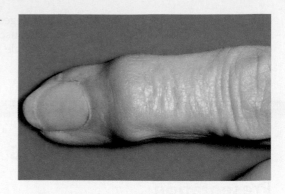

Special Tests

Trendelenburg sign: See section overview.

Patellar grind test: With the patient supine, apply downward pressure on the superior pole of the patella. While maintaining pressure on the patella, the patient should flex the quadriceps muscles, pulling the patella proximally against resistance. Pain during this maneuver is suggestive of patellofemoral joint disorder.

What tests should be ordered?

Laboratory tests: CBC (leukocytosis) and other serology (inflammatory work-up to rule out other etiologies and diagnoses including RF and ANA, which should be normal in primary OA).

Imaging: X-rays of the affected joints can help diagnose OA. For the lower extremity joints, weight-bearing x-rays are useful (**Fig. 6.34**). Common radiologic features of OA include

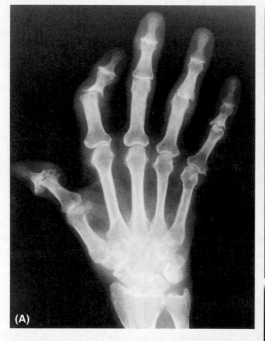

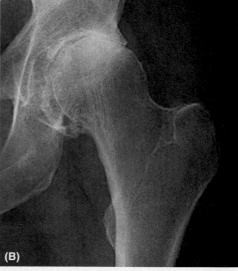

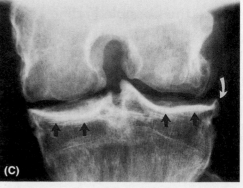

FIGURE 6.34. Osteoarthritis. **A.** Erosive osteoarthritis demonstrating "gull winging" of the cartilage of the DIP joints of the first three digits. **B.** Hip joint demonstrating marked joint space narrowing and osteophyte formation. **C.** Knee joint demonstrating subchondral sclerosis (*straight arrows*) and an osteophyte (*curved arrow*).

- Asymmetric joint space narrowing
- Osteophyte formation
- Subchondral sclerosis
- Subchondral cysts

A special 3-foot standing x-ray can be used to assess the alignment of the knee and the amount of genu valgus or varus deformities based on the Q angle. CT scan may be used to rule out secondary causes of hip or knee pain, such as an occult or stress fracture. MRI may be used to directly visualize the articular cartilage and to rule out soft tissue pathology to the meniscus, tendons, or ligaments.

Special Tests

Synovial fluid: Clear, viscous fluid with WBCs <2,000 cells/mm^3.

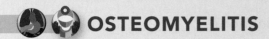

OSTEOMYELITIS

Presentation

A 55-year-old male with diabetes presents to his health care provider. Two weeks prior, he had sustained a cut on his left fifth toe, which is now painful and red.

Definition

Osteomyelitis (OM) is an infection of the bone characterized by inflammation and bony destruction.

What are common causes?

In general, OM is caused by the following mechanisms:

Mechanism	Description
Hematogenous	Source of infection originates in the blood (e.g., intravenous [IV] drug use); vertebrae are the most common bones infected
Contiguous focus	Direct inoculation of the bone such as following surgery, trauma, penetrating injury, and arterial insufficiency; causative agents include bacteria, mycobacteria, and fungi
Chronic	Fractures, diabetic ulcers, and poor wound repair (such as medications or poor nutrition)

The most common pathogens causing OM in adults are *S. aureus* (including methicillin-resistant *S. aureus* [MRSA]), *Enterobacter*, and *Streptococcus* species. *Escherichia coli* and fungal infections are less common causes of OM.

Risk factors for OM include immunocompromised states, indwelling chronic venous access lines (e.g., dialysis lines), sickle cell disease, diabetes, and neuropathies causing repetitive trauma (Charcot foot). Patients with diabetes may not present with the typical symptoms of OM because of associated neuropathies. Given the significant consequences of diabetes-associated foot infections, the clinician and the patient should closely inspect the feet, toes, and open wounds.

> • CLINICAL PEARL
>
> In patients with joint replacements, blood-borne infections can seed and grow on the prosthesis. Infection must be considered in the setting of new-onset pain or loosening of hardware in those with orthopedic implants.

What is the differential diagnosis?

Monoarthritis: The differential diagnosis includes septic arthritis, crystal arthritis, seropositive and seronegative inflammatory arthritis, trauma, hemarthrosis, and OA.

Unilateral extremity erythema and swelling: The differential diagnosis includes cellulitis/erysipelas, ischemia, deep vein thrombosis (DVT)/phlebitis, and lymphatic drainage obstruction.

What symptoms might be observed?

Symptoms of OM include pain around the region of infection, a new or worsening ulcer, discharge from the ulcer, and slow-healing (>2 weeks) ulcers.

What are the possible findings on examination?

Vital signs: Fever, tachycardia, or hypotension may be present, although vital signs may also remain normal.

General examination: Primary assessment should be performed, looking for portals of entry including injection sites, trauma, decubitus ulcers, or open wounds. Also check for any indwelling lines, which should be inspected for erythema or discharge. Assess for sources of bacteremia, including possible infective endocarditis (Chapter 2).

Inspection: Inspect the affected area for open wounds or injuries, discharge, erythema, and swelling. Likelihood of OM is based on ulcer characteristics including ulcer size >2 × 2 cm (likelihood ratio [LR]+ 7.2) and the ability to probe to bone or visualize bone at the ulcer site (LR+ 6.4). The presence of surrounding pale or blue tissue may indicate vascular compromise.

Palpation: Palpate the affected area, noting any swelling, induration, pain, or warmth. The clinician or wound care specialist should probe open wounds to determine the depth of the wound and possible bone involvement.

ROM: Assess the ROM of the joint above and below the affected area.

Special Tests

Neurologic examination: Assess the power and sensation in the affected extremity and compare it to the opposite side.

Vascular examination: Palpate peripheral pulses, check capillary refill, and assess for signs of vascular compromise such as pallor, shiny skin, and hair loss.

What tests should be ordered?

Laboratory tests: CBC (leukocytosis in acute cases); microbiology (blood cultures to check for bacteremia). A bone biopsy is the most accurate method of determining the causative pathogen. Cultures from skin swabs generally have little utility given the high rate of contamination with normal skin flora; other serology (ESR) may be elevated in acute and chronic OM and helpful for monitoring response to treatment. An ESR >70 mm/h is associated with an LR+ 11. CRP may be elevated in OM and decreases faster than does ESR in successful treatment regimens.

Imaging: Orthogonal plain x-rays of the affected area should be performed to rule out infection, sclerotic bone, edema, or a gas bubble associated with OM (**Fig. 6.35A**). CT scan can further characterize the severity of bone destruction and may help to identify more complex areas of involvement not visualized on x-rays. MRI can accurately detect OM (**Fig. 6.35B**). Additionally, it is useful for investigating soft tissue injuries for abscesses such as an epidural abscesses related to vertebral OM.

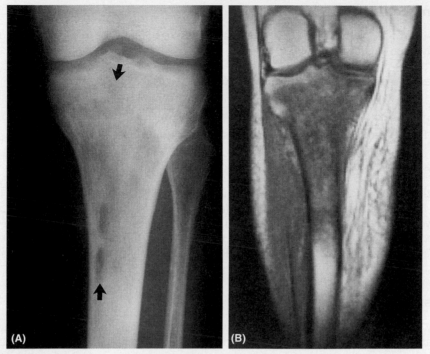

FIGURE 6.35. A. X-ray of the proximal tibia demonstrating osteomyelitis (*arrows*). **B.** Coronal T1-weighted MRI demonstrates osteomyelitis of the proximal tibia. The infection extends to the joint line.

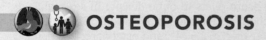

OSTEOPOROSIS

Presentation

An 80-year-old female was admitted to the hospital with a hip fracture caused by a fall from standing height. Her health care provider considers whether she has osteoporosis.

Definition

Osteoporosis is a skeletal disease characterized by low bone mass and abnormal bone microarchitecture leading to an increased risk of fracture (**Fig. 6.36**).

What are common causes?

Risk factors for osteoporosis include age (>65 years), previous osteopenia on imaging, prolonged glucocorticoid use (at least 3 months in the last year at a dose of at least 7.5 mg/d), low body weight (<60 kg), family history of osteoporotic fracture, smoking, and excess alcohol intake. Medical comorbidities associated with osteoporosis include early menopause, intestinal malabsorption, chronic disease, hyperparathyroidism, and eating disorders.

What is the differential diagnosis?

Fragility fracture: The differential diagnosis includes hematologic malignancy (e.g., leukemia, lymphoma, and multiple myeloma), metastatic disease (e.g., kidney, prostate, breast, thyroid, and lung cancer), and renal osteodystrophy.

What symptoms might be observed?

Osteoporosis is often asymptomatic. Patients may notice loss of height due to vertebral compression fractures or other fragility fractures.

What are the possible findings on examination?

Vital signs: Typically normal.
Inspection: Evidence of kyphosis (Chapter 5).
Palpation: Palpate along the spine for tenderness or deformities.

Special Tests

Serial height: A loss of 2 cm (0.8 in.) in an office-measured height or 4 cm (1.6 in.) based on a recalled height is concerning for a vertebral fracture.
Lateral lower rib to iliac crest distance: Measure the distance from the lowest rib to the iliac crest. A distance <3 cm (1.2 in.) is suggestive of a vertebral fracture.
Gait and balance: Assess gait and perform the Romberg test (Chapter 7) to assess the risk of falling and fractures.

What tests should be ordered?

Laboratory tests: CBC (anemia), metabolic panel (hyper- or hypocalcemia, hypomagnesemia, phosphate, albumin, PTH, liver enzymes and function, Cr [metabolic bone disease may be associated with chronic kidney disease such as renal osteodystrophies], ALP [elevated in fracture or lytic bone lesion], urine and serum protein electrophoresis to rule out multiple myeloma, TSH, and low 25-OH vitamin D. Vitamin D levels should be reassessed 3–4 months after supplementation. Luteinizing hormone [LH], follicle-stimulating hormone [FSH], and testosterone may be considered), and urine studies (24-hour urine collection for calcium and Cr excretion).
Imaging: Perform thoracolumbar x-rays to assess for vertebral compression fractures (**Fig. 6.37**). Dual energy x-ray absorptiometry (DEXA) is performed to quantify bone mass, which correlates with the risk of fragility fracture (**Fig. 6.37**). The T-score refers to bone density in sex-matched, young, healthy adults. A normal T-score is greater than -1.0 standard deviations (SD). Osteopenia is defined as a T-score less than -1.0 and greater than -2.5 SD, and osteoporosis is defined as a T-score below -2.5 SD. Z-scores compare bone density to age-matched controls.

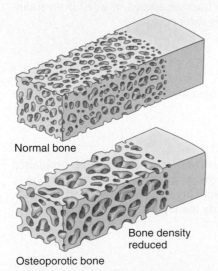

Normal bone

Bone density reduced

Osteoporotic bone

FIGURE 6.36. Normal and osteoporotic bone.

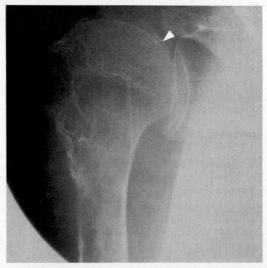

FIGURE 6.37. AP x-ray demonstrating osteoporosis in the proximal humerus. Chondrocalcinosis is present too (*arrowhead*).

Diagnostic Scores

The World Health Organization (WHO) Fracture Risk Assessment (FRAX) score calculates a 10-year probability of a hip fracture or other major osteoporotic fracture (spine, proximal humerus, or forearm) in untreated patients between ages 40 and 90 years. The calculator is based on clinical risk factors for fracture and femoral neck bone mineral density (BMD) and on the risk of an osteoporotic fracture. The calculator is available online.

RHEUMATOID ARTHRITIS

Presentation

A 36-year-old female presents with bilateral hand pain, swelling, and stiffness. She is experiencing difficulty with fastening her buttons, opening jars, and typing at work. She often experiences fatigue. The clinician suspects she has an inflammatory arthritis such as RA.

Definition

RA is a seropositive inflammatory arthritis. Other seropositive inflammatory arthritides include SLE and systemic sclerosis. RA is a chronic inflammatory condition predominantly targeting the synovial membranes of joints resulting in erosion of adjacent cartilage and bone and damage to surrounding ligaments and tendons. RA can lead to various extra-articular manifestations.

What are common causes?

The etiology of RA is not fully understood but may be attributed to genetics, autoimmunity, and environmental or infectious triggers. The peak onset of RA is 30–50 years of age, and there is a female predominance.

What is the differential diagnosis?

Polyarthritis: The differential diagnosis includes infection (e.g., viruses such as cytomegalovirus [CMV], parvovirus B19, and Epstein-Barr virus [EBV]; Lyme disease; tuberculosis [TB]; and septic arthritis secondary to bacteremia), crystal arthritis, seropositive or seronegative arthritis, vasculitis, and OA.

What symptoms might be observed?

Symptoms of RA include pain and swelling particularly of small joints, morning joint stiffness lasting more than 1 hour, constitutional symptoms such as fatigue and anorexia, and joint deformities.

What are the possible findings on examination?

Vital signs: Tachycardia, tachypnea, and fever may be present.
General examination: Perform a complete physical examination, focusing on joints and extra-articular manifestations of RA. Extra-articular manifestations of seropositive inflammatory arthritides include:
Skin: Rheumatoid nodules on extensor surfaces, sicca of the eyes and mouth, and white or red changes in the fingers and toes are suggestive of Raynaud phenomenon.
Eye: Ocular redness associated with scleritis/episcleritis and corneal ulcers (corneal melt).
Neurologic: C-spine instability, peripheral neuropathy, and mononeuritis multiplex.
Cardiac: Pericardial rub or effusion and valvular nodules causing murmur.
Respiratory: Crackles associated with pulmonary fibrosis and pleural friction rub.
Gastrointestinal: Splenomegaly may be seen in Felty syndrome, which is a triad of RA, neutropenia, and splenomegaly.

FIGURE 6.38. Joint deformities secondary to RA. Note the swan neck (left third and fourth digits), boutonniere deformities (fifth digits), and Z-deformity of the thumbs.

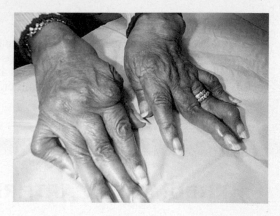

Inspection: Inspect joints for erythema, swelling, and deformities (**Fig. 6.38**) including the following:

- PIP and DIP joints may have swan neck and/or boutonniere deformities.
- Thumbs may have a Z-deformity.
- MCP joints may have ulnar drift and subluxation.
- Wrist joints may have radial deviation and volar subluxation.
- Feet may have hind foot valgus deformity.
- MTP joints may have subluxation.

Palpation: Palpate joint lines for tenderness and effusions. The flexor tendons should be palpated for thickening and nodules. The ulnar styloid of the wrist should be pressed; RA can cause laxity of the ulnar styloid ("piano key" laxity).

ROM: Active joints may have reduced ROM.

What tests should be ordered?

Laboratory tests: CBC (anemia of chronic disease, neutropenia), metabolic panel (Cr, electrolytes, and liver enzymes for a baseline before starting treatment), and other serology (RF is positive

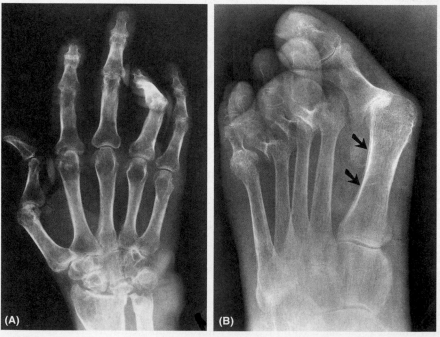

FIGURE 6.39. A. X-ray of the hand and wrist demonstrating erosive changes in the metacarpophalangeal, proximal interphalangeal, and wrist joints. **B.** X-ray of the foot demonstrating erosive changes and subluxation of the MTP joints.

in 30%–50% of patients early in the disease course, but in 70%–85% with established disease, anti–cyclic citrullinated peptide [CCP; Sp 95%], elevated ESR, and CRP).

Imaging: Obtain x-rays of affected joints to assess for symmetrical joint space narrowing, erosive changes, periarticular osteopenia, periarticular swelling and joint effusions, and deformities (**Fig. 6.39**).

Special Tests

Synovial fluid analysis: Clear, yellow-white color with >2,000 WBCs/mm³.

> ● CLINICAL PEARL
>
> The cornerstone of treatment for RA and seropositive arthritides includes disease-modifying antirheumatic drugs (DMARDs) and, when appropriate, anti–tumor necrosis factor (TNF) therapy.

SEPTIC ARTHRITIS

Presentation

A 55-year-old male with diabetes develops a fever and symptoms suggestive of a urinary tract infection. Shortly after, he develops rapidly progressing pain, swelling, and redness in his knee and is unable to bear weight. In the Emergency Department, the health care provider suspects septic arthritis.

Definition

Septic arthritis is an inflammatory arthritis secondary to bacterial invasion of a joint.

What are common causes?

Bacteria can seed the joint through the bloodstream, contiguous infections from cellulitis or osteomyelitis, or inoculation of the joint from a penetrating trauma. Risk factors for septic arthritis include older individuals, underlying joint disease such as RA or prosthetic joints, comorbidities or immunosuppressants such as diabetes or corticosteroids, and sexually transmitted infections. The most common organisms for septic arthritis include

Type of Organism	Species
Gram-positive cocci (80%)	*S. aureus* (60%), *S. epidermidis* (especially in prosthetic joints), *Streptococcus* species (20%), and *Enterococcus*
Gram negative (15%)	Seen in immunocompromised patients and includes *H. influenza*, *E. coli*, *P. aeruginosa*, and *Serratia marcescens*
Anaerobes	Less common but may be seen in immunocompromised patients and include *Clostridium perfringens* and *Bacteroides fragilis*
Other	Disseminated gonococcal disease

What is the differential diagnosis?

Polyarthritis: The differential diagnosis includes infections (e.g., viruses such as CMV, parvovirus B19, and EBV; Lyme disease; TB; and septic arthritis secondary to bacteremia), crystal arthritis, seropositive or seronegative arthritis, vasculitis, and OA.

What symptoms might be observed?

Symptoms of septic arthritis include joint pain and swelling, chills, fatigue, anorexia, and purulent skin lesions.

What are the possible findings on examination?

Vital signs: May present with fever, hypotension, tachycardia, and tachypnea, suggesting acute infection or sepsis.
Inspection: Joint erythema and effusion may be seen along with surrounding cellulitis.
Palpation: Joint may be warm, tender, and effused.
ROM: Active joints may have reduced ROM.

What tests should be ordered?

Laboratory test: CBC (leukocytosis predominantly neutrophils), microbiology (blood cultures are positive in ~50% of confirmed cases of septic arthritis; synovial fluid cultures; urine cultures including for gonorrhea and chlamydia), and other serology (elevated ESR and CRP).
Imaging: Presence of x-ray findings depends on duration of the infection (**Fig. 6.40**). Early x-ray findings are usually normal with only soft tissue swelling. These x-rays can help rule out contiguous OM. Later x-ray findings include aggressive and rapid joint destruction. If a lesion involves or crosses a joint space, it most likely has an inflammatory or infectious origin. Tumors typically do not extend across a joint space.

Special Tests

Synovial fluid analysis: Cloudy or purulent appearance with a WBC > 20,000 cells/mm³, predominantly neutrophils (>75% polymorphonuclear neutrophils [PMNs]). The higher the WBC, the greater the likelihood of an underlying infection. Crystals may be concomitantly present; Gram stain and culture may be positive.

● **CLINICAL PEARL**

Empiric treatment with broad-spectrum antibiotics should be initiated early to avoid rapid joint destruction and overwhelming sepsis. Ideally, blood, urine, and synovial fluid cultures are obtained prior to initiating therapy.

FIGURE 6.40. X-ray of the great toe demonstrating osteomyelitis and joint space infection of the interphalangeal joint in a patient with diabetes.

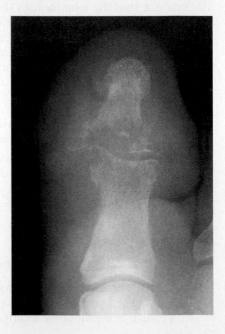

CLAVICLE FRACTURE

Presentation

A 28-year-old male ran over a pothole while cycling and was thrown over the handlebars of his bicycle. He presents to the Emergency Department with pain over his right collarbone and difficulty moving his right arm.

Definition

A clavicle fracture is the presence of one or more breaks in the clavicle and is classified based on the fracture location. For this classification, the bone is divided into thirds, and fractures are described as either medial, midshaft, or distal/lateral. Further description is provided by the amount and direction of displacement of the fracture.

• CLINICAL PEARL

In high-energy trauma, the clavicle fracture may be part of a more significant injury. Scapulothoracic dissociation occurs when the entire shoulder girdle is dislocated from the axial skeleton and should be considered in widely displaced clavicle fractures with asymmetry in the distance of the scapula from the vertebral spine compared to the uninjured side (**Fig. 6.41**). Scapulothoracic dissociation can be associated with significant neurovascular injury.

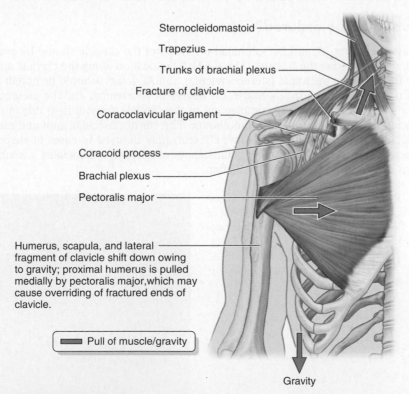

Sternocleidomastoid

Trapezius

Trunks of brachial plexus

Fracture of clavicle

Coracoclavicular ligament

Coracoid process

Brachial plexus

Pectoralis major

Humerus, scapula, and lateral fragment of clavicle shift down owing to gravity; proximal humerus is pulled medially by pectoralis major, which may cause overriding of fractured ends of clavicle.

▬ Pull of muscle/gravity

Gravity

FIGURE 6.41. Clavicle fracture.

What are common causes?

Fractures of the clavicle are usually caused by acute trauma, most commonly by direct impact to the shoulder or clavicle, as seen in contact sports or high-speed activities.

What is the differential diagnosis?

Clavicle pain: The differential diagnosis includes AC joint injury, rotator cuff pathology, rib fracture (especially the first three ribs), sternoclavicular joint pathology (especially septic or crystal), and shoulder dislocation.

What symptoms might be observed?

Symptoms of clavicle fracture include pain that is worse with movement of the shoulder.

What are the possible findings on examination?

Vital signs: Typically normal.

Inspection: Inspect for asymmetry or deformity of the affected side. Inspect for stretching of the skin caused by underlying bony deformity (tenting) and whitening of the skin without return of capillary refill at the site of tenting (blanching). Also inspect for bone protruding through the skin. This is called an *open fracture* and requires immediate orthopedic evaluation.

Palpation: Palpate along the entire clavicle and surrounding tissue for tenderness.

ROM: Pain will limit active and passive movements of the shoulder girdle, although movement distal to the elbow distal should be normal.

Special Tests

Neurovascular examination: Distal neurologic examination should be performed to assess motor function and sensation of the axillary, radial, median, and ulnar nerves. Distal pulses including radial and ulnar pulses should be palpated, and capillary refill should be assessed.

What tests should be ordered?

Imaging: X-rays including AP and 30° cephalad tilt views of the clavicle should be ordered to help diagnose and characterize the fracture (**Fig. 6.42**). The location along the clavicle and any extension of the fracture into the joints (sternoclavicular and AC joints) should be noted; further, note the direction and amount of displacement, the degree of shortening, and the presence of comminution. The chest x-ray is a useful complement to the clavicle x-ray to help rule out scapulothoracic dissociation or an associated pneumothorax. The sternoclavicular joint and medial clavicle can be difficult to visualize on plain x-ray; CT scan may be used in cases of suspected medial clavicle fracture or dislocation. In rare circumstances of suspected associated vascular injury, CT angiography can be used for further evaluation.

FIGURE 6.42. X-ray demonstrating a fracture of the left clavicle. (Courtesy of Joel Vilensky, Department of Anatomy and Cell Biology, Indiana University School of Medicine.)

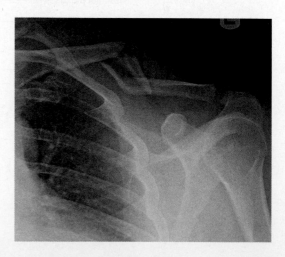

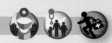 **ROTATOR CUFF TEAR**

Presentation

A 56-year-old male painter presents to his health care provider with a 1-month history of pain in his shoulder. The pain is worse with movement, especially when the arm is raised above his head.

Definition

Rotator cuff tear is an interruption in the physical continuity of any rotator cuff tendon (**Fig. 6.14**).

What are common causes?

The etiologies of rotator cuff tear are classified as acute or chronic. Acute tears occur following a sudden, forceful tension that exceeds the elastic capacity of the tendon. As a result, the tendon ruptures or is avulsed from its bony insertion. Chronic tears are multifactorial and include repetitive movements and bony changes (e.g., spurring of the acromion) to the shoulder (**Fig. 6.43**).

What is the differential diagnosis?

Shoulder pain: The differential diagnosis includes trauma (clavicle fracture or shoulder dislocation), C-spine pathology (strains, disc injuries, radiculopathy), rotator cuff pathology, referred pain (diaphragmatic irritation), biceps tendinitis, inflammatory arthritis (especially seronegative disease), crystal arthritis (hydroxyapatite crystals), and OA.

What symptoms might be observed?

Symptoms of a rotator cuff injury include pain located over the lateral aspect of the arm (specifically, in the area of the deltoid muscle). It is common to have pain that is worse when lifting the

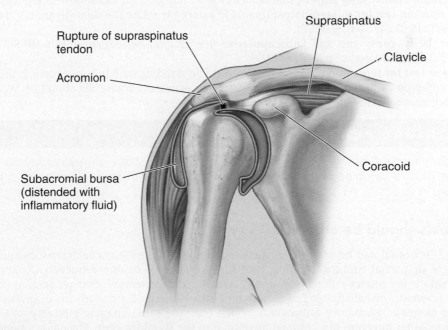

FIGURE 6.43. Rupture of the supraspinatus tendon and inflammation of the subacromial bursa secondary to a rotator cuff injury.

TABLE 6.13. Differences in etiology rotator cuff tears	
Acute Rotator Cuff Tear	**Chronic Rotator Cuff Tear**
Occurs as a result of acute trauma to the shoulder girdle such as a fall on an outstretched hand Pain is sharp, intense, and instantaneous with inability to perform various movements at the shoulder joint. May be accompanied by other orthopedic injuries, such as a clavicle fracture or shoulder dislocation	Occurs due to gradual attrition of the tendon over time Typically found in occupations requiring repetitive overhead activities Also found in athletes who perform repetitive movements (e.g., throwing) Pain will be limited initially but will gradually worsen over time.

hand over the head and when sleeping on the side of the affected shoulder. Acute and chronic rotator cuff pathology may have different presentations (**Table 6.13**).

What are the possible findings on examination?

Vital signs: Typically normal.
Inspection: Inspect for asymmetric muscle atrophy related to decreased use of the affected side.
Palpation: Palpate the affected area for tenderness at the site of the rotator cuff insertion on the greater tuberosity. Frequently, there is concomitant AC joint arthritis with tenderness to palpation of the joint.
ROM: Reduced, secondary to pain.

Special Tests

Muscle strength: Patients usually demonstrate motor weakness, pain with resistance, or inability to perform specific motions.
Neer test for acromial impingement: See chapter introduction (Sn 0.50–0.92, Sp 0.27–0.69).
Jobe or "empty can" test for supraspinatus: See chapter introduction (Sn 0.32–0.99, Sp 0.40–0.91).
External rotation test for infraspinatus: Unable to externally rotate the shoulder that is at 0° abduction (Sn 0.19–0.84, Sp 0.53–0.90).
Lift-off or belly press test for subscapularis: See chapter introduction (lift-off Sn 0.0–0.79, Sp 0.59–1.00; belly press Sn 0.40, Sp 0.98).
Hornblower test for teres minor: The patient should be standing with his or her arm in the scapular plane and elbows flexed to 90°. Ask the patient to externally rotate the shoulder. Weakness or pain indicates a positive test (Sn 1.00, Sp 0.93).

● CLINICAL PEARL

No single physical examination test is best for diagnosing rotator cuff pathology, and a constellation of tests combined with a detailed history should be utilized to develop a differential diagnosis.

What tests should be ordered?

Imaging: Ultrasound can be used to visualize tendons and assess tear characteristics such as size, complete or partial rupture, location, and the presence of tendon retraction. X-rays will not demonstrate any rotator cuff tears; however, associated degenerative changes such as bone spurs at the acromion or calcific tendinitis may be visible. The gold standard for diagnosing tendon tears is magnetic resonance arthrogram, which uses the same imaging modality as MRI but is performed after injection of a contrast medium into the shoulder joint. This allows more detailed imaging of the shoulder anatomy that can reveal subtle tendon tears that may not be detected on ultrasound (**Fig. 6.44**).

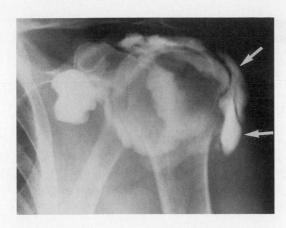

FIGURE 6.44. Complete rotator cuff tear. This shoulder arthrogram shows contrast injected into the glenohumeral joint extravasating into the subacromial/subdeltoid bursa (*arrows*).

 DISTAL RADIUS FRACTURE

Presentation

A 78-year-old female presents with pain and the inability to move her left wrist after she slipped on ice. She fell forward onto her outstretched hands.

Definition

A distal radius fracture involves the epiphysis and/or metaphysis of the distal radius.

What are common causes?

The most common etiology is a "fall onto outstretched hand" or FOOSH (**Fig. 6.45**). These fractures are more common in elderly patients and those with osteoporosis.

What is the differential diagnosis?

Wrist deformity: The differential diagnosis includes trauma or inflammation secondary to conditions such as RA that damage the joint alignment. Particular fractures of the wrist are summarized in **Table 6.14**.

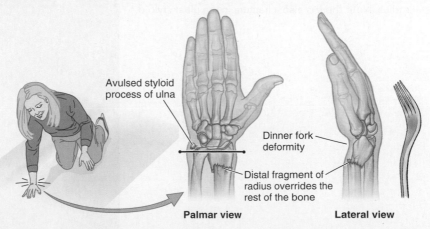

Avulsed styloid process of ulna

Dinner fork deformity

Distal fragment of radius overrides the rest of the bone

Palmar view

Lateral view

FIGURE 6.45. Distal radius fracture.

TABLE 6.14. Classification of distal radius fractures

Fracture Type	Characteristics
Colles fracture	The distal fracture fragment is displaced dorsally, creating a characteristic "dinner fork" deformity.
Smith fracture	Also known as a *reverse Colles* in which the distal fracture fragment is displaced volarly
Barton fracture	An intra-articular fracture of the distal radius with associated radiocarpal dislocation: also referred to as a *volar shear fracture* or *dorsal shear fracture*, depending on orientation of the fracture
Chauffeur fracture	A fracture of the radial styloid process, caused by compression of the scaphoid against the styloid: sustained by chauffeurs when the crank handle in old cars backfired

What symptoms might be observed?

Symptoms of a distal radius fracture include wrist pain and tenderness, with difficulty moving the wrist.

What are the possible findings on examination?

Vital signs: Typically normal.

Inspection: Inspect the forearm, wrist, and hand for asymmetry, ecchymosis, and deformities. Deformities depend on the fracture pattern, but the most common distal radius fracture pattern is a Colles fracture that presents with a "dinner-fork" deformity. Significant swelling of the wrist tracking into the hand and fingers may also occur.

Palpation: Palpate the forearm, wrist, and hand. Tenderness may be appreciated at the fracture site. Tenderness in the anatomical snuffbox or in the radial side of the wrist may be present in a scaphoid fracture.

ROM: Flexion–extension of the wrist may be limited or absent due to pain, although elbow and finger movements will be preserved. If elbow or finger ROM is reduced, suspect involvement of additional joints.

What tests should be ordered?

Imaging: The fracture type and pattern can be assessed from x-rays of the wrist and forearm (**Fig. 6.46**). Typically, four views (AP, lateral, and two oblique views) are obtained to visualize the fracture. CT scans of the wrist are helpful when intra-articular fractures are suspected and are required for preoperative planning.

FIGURE 6.46. A comminuted, intra-articular compression fracture of the distal radius. Note there is also a fracture in the ulnar styloid.

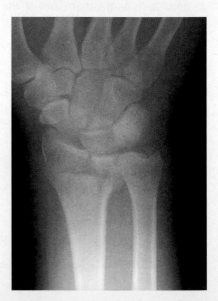

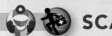

SCAPHOID FRACTURE

Presentation

A 19-year-old female presents to the Emergency Department with persistent pain at the base of her right thumb after being tackled in a soccer game and falling onto her outstretched hand.

Definition

A scaphoid fracture is a fracture of the scaphoid bone (**Fig. 6.47**). The scaphoid is the most commonly fractured carpal bone.

It is important to determine the location of the fracture within the scaphoid bone. The scaphoid bone has a retrograde blood supply where the flow of blood runs distal to proximal and not proximal to distal as seen in most bones. This has significant implications for the risk of avascular necrosis (AVN).

What are common causes?

Scaphoid fractures occur after FOOSH with the wrist in hyperextension. In general, scaphoid fractures occur in younger individuals engaged in high-energy sports.

What is the differential diagnosis?

Thumb pain: The differential diagnosis includes trauma (distal radius fracture, dislocation, or scaphoid fracture), De Quervain tendinitis, tenosynovitis, and OA.

What symptoms might be observed?

Symptoms of a scaphoid fracture include pain that is worse with gripping. The location of pain depends on the fracture site: volar prominence of the distal wrist for distal pole fractures, anatomical snuffbox for waist or midbody fractures, and distal to the Lister tubercle for distal pole fractures.

What are the possible findings on examination?

Vital signs: Typically normal.
Inspection: Inspect the hand and wrist for swelling at the thumb base. Typically, scaphoid fractures are not associated with obvious asymmetry.
Palpation: Palpate the hand, wrist, and anatomic snuffbox for tenderness and deformities.
ROM: Movements involving the thumb may be normal, although opposition of the thumb may reproduce the pain.

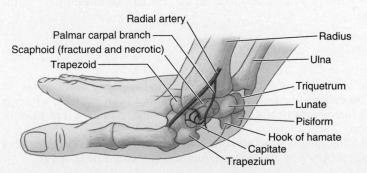

FIGURE 6.47. Scaphoid fracture.

FIGURE 6.48. X-ray of the scaphoid demonstrating a fracture. (Courtesy of Joel Vilensky, Department of Anatomy and Cell Biology, Indiana University School of Medicine.)

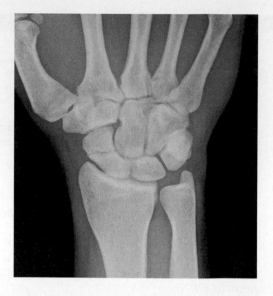

Special Tests

Grip strength: May be reduced.

What tests should be ordered?

Imaging: Plain film radiography with dedicated scaphoid views is the first-line diagnostic tool for scaphoid fractures (**Fig. 6.48**). However, scaphoid fractures may not be visible on initial injury. In this instance, a thumb spica cast is placed and the thumb is immobilized for 7–10 days, at which time x-rays are repeated to assess for fractures. In patients with persistent pain and repeat negative x-rays, MRI remains the gold standard imaging modality to diagnose scaphoid fractures. Subtle changes in the tissue such as bone edema or callus formation around the fracture site will be detected with MRI. If an MRI is not available, a CT scan may be performed to evaluate for fracture.

 # FEMUR HEAD AND NECK FRACTURES

Presentation

A 26-year-old male is involved in a motor vehicle accident (MVA). He has significant pain in his right hip on arrival to the hospital.

Definition

Fractures of the femoral head are less common and may be associated with hip dislocations. In fact, 5%–15% of posterior hip dislocations are associated with a femoral head fracture, which is caused by the femoral head being forced against the posterior rim of the acetabulum. Fractures of the femoral neck are more common.

The femoral head and neck are intracapsular structures that lack a periosteal layer, affecting callus formation and overall healing. Blood supply may also be compromised in fractures (**Fig. 6.49**).

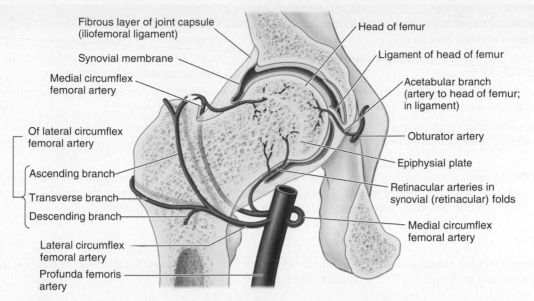

FIGURE 6.49. Anterior view of the coronal section demonstrating blood supply to the hip.

What are common causes?

In athletes, stress and repetitive motion can lead to fractures. Other common causes include:

Type of Fracture	Etiologies
Femoral head fractures	Impaction injuries, avulsion, or shear forces including MVA (e.g., when an unrestrained passenger hits the knee against the dashboard), fall from height, or injuries sustained during contact sports
Femoral neck fractures	Low-energy falls in older patients with low bone density or high-energy trauma in younger patients

What is the differential diagnosis?

Unilateral hip pain: The differential diagnosis includes trauma, bursitis, arthritis (inflammatory, septic, and OA), AVN of the hip, labral tear, piriformis syndrome, or hamstring syndrome, and neurologic causes such as sciatica should be considered especially if pain originates in the back and radiates down the leg.

● CLINICAL PEARL

True hip pain typically localizes to the groin.

What symptoms might be observed?

Symptoms of hip fracture include pain localized to the groin or proximal thigh and difficulty with ambulation.

What are the possible findings on examination?

Vital signs: Typically normal.
Inspection: Inspect for signs of trauma including ecchymosis, swelling, wounds, or abrasions. Also, assess the resting position of the leg (**Table 6.15**).
Palpation: Palpate the pelvis and femur, especially the greater trochanter, for tenderness.

TABLE 6.15. Deformities in hip fractures

Femoral Head Fracture	Femoral Neck Fracture
Limb may appear shortened if there is an associated acetabular fracture.	Displaced neck fractures often result in an external rotated and shortened leg.
In cases of associated posterior hip dislocation, the leg may be flexed, adducted, and internally rotated.	No deformities are present with impaction or stress fractures.
Associated anterior dislocations present with the hip extended, abducted, and externally rotated.	

ROM: In displaced fractures, even a gentle log roll (internal and external rotation) of the leg will produce pain and muscle spasm. In undisplaced or valgus impacted fractures, more extensive ROM may be possible; however, it will often be accompanied by groin pain.

Special Tests

Neurovascular examination: Assess sciatic nerve function, palpate peripheral pulses, and assess for capillary refill and circulation distal to the fracture.

● **CLINICAL PEARL**

In femoral head and neck fractures, the knee should be examined for associated trauma.

What tests should be ordered?

Laboratory tests: See Osteoporosis section, as hip fractures are common fragility fractures. Because operative management is highly beneficial to these patients, ordering a CBC, metabolic panel (electrolytes, Cr), and coagulation studies is helpful to prepare for surgery.

Imaging: For a femoral head fracture, AP pelvis and AP and cross-table lateral (taken supine with unaffected hip and knee flexed to 90°) hip x-rays should be obtained. For femoral neck fractures, AP pelvis and AP and lateral radiographic views of the hip should be obtained. CT or MRI scan is obtained if an occult hip fracture is suspected (**Fig. 6.50**). If the hip is dislocated, a CT scan should also be obtained after reduction of the hip to identify loose bone fragments in the joint, to assess the position and pattern of the femoral head fracture, and to assess for acetabular or pelvic fractures.

FIGURE 6.50. X-ray of the left hip demonstrating a stress fracture of the femoral neck. Note the linear lucency with surrounding sclerosis in the femoral neck.

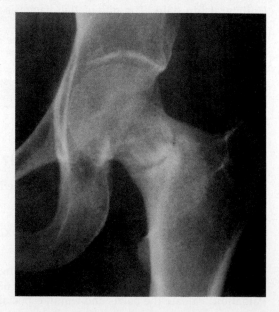

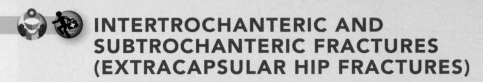

INTERTROCHANTERIC AND SUBTROCHANTERIC FRACTURES (EXTRACAPSULAR HIP FRACTURES)

Presentation

A 76-year-old female fell from a standing height and landed on her right side. She is experiencing right hip pain and is unable to ambulate.

Definition

Extracapsular fractures are a break in the proximal segment of the femur outside of the joint capsule. There are two types of extracapsular fractures. The first type is an intertrochanteric fracture, which occurs between the neck of the femur and the lesser trochanter. The second type is a subtrochanteric fracture, which occurs between the lesser trochanter and 5 cm distal to the lesser trochanter. Subtrochanteric fractures may have an accompanying intertrochanteric fracture (**Fig. 6.51**).

What are common causes?

Extracapsular hip fractures are often caused by low-energy falls in elderly patients with osteoporosis or cancer (primary or metastatic) affecting the hip. In younger patients, fractures may be caused by high-energy trauma.

What is the differential diagnosis?

Unilateral hip pain: The differential diagnosis includes trauma, bursitis, arthritis (inflammatory, septic, and OA), AVN of the hip, labral tear, piriformis syndrome or hamstring syndrome, and neurologic causes such as sciatica particularly if the pain originates in the back and radiates down the leg.

What symptoms might be observed?

Symptoms of extracapsular hip fractures include pain in the hip, thigh, or groin, particularly in the acute phase of the injury, and difficulty with ambulation.

What are the possible findings on examination?

Vital signs: Typically normal.
Inspection: Inspect the hip for signs of trauma and deformities such as a short, externally rotated leg.
Palpation: Palpate the pelvis, hip, and femur for tenderness, especially at the greater trochanter and the trochanteric bursa.
ROM: Decreased movement of the hip joint may be seen due to the fracture and associated pain.

Special Tests

Neurovascular examination: Perform a screening examination to assess the sensation and motor function of the distal leg. Also, palpate peripheral pulses and assess capillary refill of the distal leg.

What tests should be ordered?

Laboratory tests: See Osteoporosis section, as hip fractures are common fragility fractures. Since operative management is highly beneficial, ordering a CBC, metabolic panel (electrolytes, Cr), and coagulation studies is helpful in preparation for surgery.

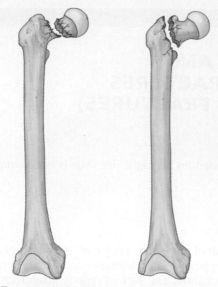

(A) Transcervical fracture **(B) Intertrochanteric**
of femoral neck **fracture**

FIGURE 6.51. Schematic of transcervical **(A)**
and intertrochanteric fracture **(B)**.

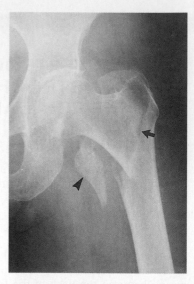

FIGURE 6.52. X-ray of a comminuted intertrochanteric fracture
(*arrows*) of the left proximal femur.

Imaging: For intertrochanteric fractures, AP pelvis, AP hip, and cross-table lateral (horizontal projection) x-rays of the hip should be obtained (**Fig. 6.52**). CT or MRI scan is indicated if x-rays are negative and if there remains a high clinical suspicion for fracture.

For subtrochanteric fractures, AP and lateral hip, AP pelvis, and x-rays of the ipsilateral femur should be obtained. CT or MRI scan may be indicated if x-rays are negative.

● **CLINICAL PEARL**

Hip fractures have a 20%–30% mortality risk in the first year following fracture. Expedient time to surgery has been demonstrated to decrease mortality risk.

 MENISCUS INJURIES

Presentation

A 29-year-old male presents with persistent right knee pain after slipping down the stairs several weeks ago. The patient reports that his knee "seizes" when he descends stairs.

Definition

A meniscal injury is a disruption of the knee menisci that results in painful and/or mechanical symptoms. Meniscal injuries are typically described anatomically. Medial meniscus tears are more common than lateral meniscus tears (with the exception being acute ACL injuries, in which lateral tears are more common; **Fig. 6.53**). Degenerative tears in older patients are typically found in the posterior horn of the medial meniscus, but acute/subacute tears may be found anywhere on the meniscus.

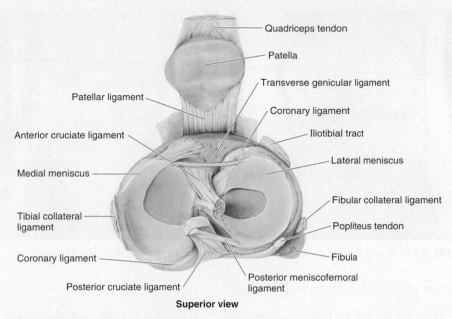

Quadriceps tendon

Patella

Transverse genicular ligament

Patellar ligament

Coronary ligament

Iliotibial tract

Anterior cruciate ligament

Lateral meniscus

Medial meniscus

Fibular collateral ligament

Tibial collateral ligament

Popliteus tendon

Coronary ligament

Fibula

Posterior cruciate ligament

Posterior meniscofemoral ligament

Superior view

FIGURE 6.53. Ligaments and menisci of the knee.

What are common causes?

Meniscal pathology commonly presents in the form of tears that may be described based on radiologic features. Acute, traumatic tears cause mechanical symptoms. Degenerative tears are often seen in association with OA and usually do not cause mechanical symptoms of locking or catching.

What is the differential diagnosis?

Knee pain: The differential diagnosis includes septic arthritis, crystal arthritis, inflammatory arthritis (both seropositive and seronegative), OA, trauma (dislocation or juxta-articular fracture), hemarthrosis, prepatellar bursitis (especially after prolonged kneeling), and ruptured Baker cyst.

What symptoms might be observed?

Symptoms of meniscal injury include persistent knee pain that localize to the medial or lateral side. Typically, pain worsens with weight-bearing or activities such as stair-climbing, pivoting, and squatting. Patients may experience locking or "seizing" of the knee joint. True locking is the inability to fully extend the knee. Patients often describe the locking as occurring when walking up or down stairs or inclines or on uneven ground. Intermittent swelling may also be reported.

What are the possible findings on examination?

Vital signs: Typically normal.
Inspection: Inspect for swelling and deformities.
Palpation: Palpate around the knee joint line for tenderness, particularly in the area of the tear.
ROM: Pain may rarely be reproducible when weight bearing or flexing–extending the knee.

Special Tests

McMurray test: With the patient supine, the clinician flexes the patient's knee and externally rotates the foot. Next, the clinician applies valgus stress to the knee and extends the knee, which tests the medial meniscus. A positive test is the reproduction of pain and locking. The lateral meniscus is tested similarly, except the foot is rotated internally and a varus force is applied while extending the knee.

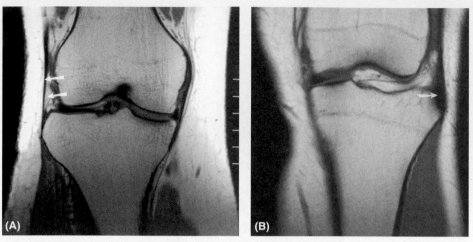

FIGURE 6.54. A and B. MR images of the knee demonstrating a medial meniscus tear (*arrows*).

What tests should be ordered?

Imaging: Plain films have no role in diagnosing meniscal tears, but chondrocalcinosis or calcium deposits on the menisci may be visualized (**Fig. 6.54**). MRI is the gold standard for diagnosing meniscal tears, although it is known to have a high false-positive rate. MRI also provides information on surrounding soft tissues including cartilage and the cruciate and collateral ligaments.

 # ANTERIOR CRUCIATE LIGAMENT TEAR

Presentation

A 26-year-old soccer player presents to the Emergency Department after feeling a sudden "pop" in his knee. He experienced acute-onset knee pain and swelling and was unable to complete the match.

Definition

An ACL tear involves disruption of the ACL anywhere along its length, including its origin and insertion at the femur and tibia.

What are common causes?

An ACL injury is often associated with sporting activity but can occur during any activity in which the anterior tibial translational stress force exceeds the elastic potential of the ACL. ACL injuries are 4.5 times more likely to occur in women due to differences in biomechanics and collagen production. ACL tears may also present with a concomitant meniscal injury (lateral meniscus is most commonly affected).

What is the differential diagnosis?

Knee pain: The differential diagnosis includes septic arthritis, crystal arthritis, inflammatory arthritis (both seropositive and seronegative), OA, trauma (dislocation or juxta-articular fracture), hemarthrosis, prepatellar bursitis (especially after prolonged kneeling), ruptured Baker cyst, and pes anserine bursitis.

What symptoms might be observed?

Symptoms of ACL tears include pain immediately following the injury, difficulty with ambulation, and decreased movement. Patients may hear or feel a "pop" sensation at the time of the injury, which is suggestive of an ACL tear.

What are the possible findings on examination?

Vital signs: Typically normal.
Inspection: Inspect the knee for swelling.
Palpation: Palpate the affected knee for tenderness and signs of an effusion (see chapter Introduction).
ROM: The patient may be unable to extend the knee. During extension, the tibia may show excessive anterior translation. This is also demonstrated as a quadriceps avoidance gait, whereby the patient minimizes extension of the quadriceps during ambulation.

Special Tests

Pivot shift: The patient is supine with the hip flexed to 30° and the knee extended. The clinician applies internal rotatory force to the tibia and valgus pressure to the knee and slowly flex the knee. A reduction of the tibia may be felt as a "clunk."
Anterior drawer test for ACL testing: The patient is supine with knees flexed to 90°. The clinician pulls the proximal tibia anteriorly. Laxity or excess anterior displacement of the tibia when it is pulled forward indicates a positive test (**Fig. 6.55**).

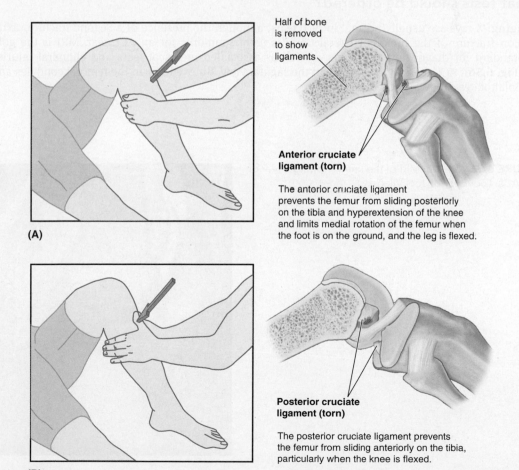

Half of bone is removed to show ligaments

Anterior cruciate ligament (torn)

The anterior cruciate ligament prevents the femur from sliding posteriorly on the tibia and hyperextension of the knee and limits medial rotation of the femur when the foot is on the ground, and the leg is flexed.

(A)

Posterior cruciate ligament (torn)

The posterior cruciate ligament prevents the femur from sliding anteriorly on the tibia, particularly when the knee is flexed.

(B)

FIGURE 6.55. **A.** Anterior drawer sign to examine for torn ACL. **B.** Posterior drawer sign to examine for torn PCL.

Lachman test for ACL testing: The patient is supine with knees flexed to 30°. The clinician stabilizes the distal femur with one hand and pulls the proximal tibia anteriorly with the other hand. Increased anterior translation of the tibia is a positive test. The extent of translation of the tibia is graded as:

- Grade I: <5 mm of translation
- Grade II: 5–10 mm of translation
- Grade III: >10 mm of translation

Posterior drawer test for PCL testing: The patient is supine with knees flexed to 90°. The clinician pushes the proximal tibia posteriorly. Laxity or excess posterior displacement of the tibia when it is pushed posterior indicates a positive test.

MCL testing: The patient is supine with knees flexed to 30°. The clinician applies valgus stress to the knee. Excess movement of the knee indicates a positive test for MCL injury.

LCL testing: The patient is supine with knees flexed to 30°. The clinician applies varus stress to the knee. Excess movement of the knee indicates a positive test for LCL injury.

● CLINICAL PEARL

In ACL injuries, all ligaments and menisci should be assessed, as it is common for multiple injuries to coexist.

What tests should be ordered?

Imaging: X-rays are usually normal in ACL tears, although the presence of a Segond fracture (avulsion fracture of the proximal lateral tibia) is pathognomonic for an ACL tear. MRI is the gold standard for diagnosing ACL tears as well as associated meniscal tears and chondral injuries (**Fig. 6.56**). ACL tears are best seen on the sagittal view. Bony edema in the femoral condyles and tibial plateau may also be seen.

FIGURE 6.56. Sagittal MRI of the knee showing a tear of the ACL. (Courtesy of Joel Vilensky.)

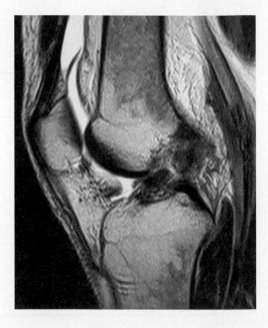

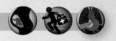 # DEEP VEIN THROMBOSIS

Presentation

A 72-year-old obese male presents with new-onset left leg pain. He had a hip replacement 4 weeks ago and has had limited mobility due to ongoing pain. In addition to the pain, his leg is swollen, red, and warm.

Definition

A DVT is a blood clot in a deep venous system. DVTs can be classified as provoked or unprovoked. Provoked venous thrombosis refers to the development of a clot in the setting of a known risk factor. Unprovoked (idiopathic) venous thrombosis refers to the development of a clot without an identifiable risk factor.

What are common causes?

DVTs are caused by a number of conditions. A clot can be provoked by immobility (e.g., long flight or postsurgery), damage to the vein (e.g., previous clot or surgery), and hypercoagulability. These three factors are referred to as *Virchow triad*. Hypercoagulability includes inherited factors (factor V Leiden, prothrombin mutation, antithrombin deficiency, and protein C and S deficiency), active cancer, pregnancy or postpartum (up to 6 weeks), hormone replacement therapy (including the oral contraceptive and testosterone therapy), obesity, nephrotic syndrome, inflammatory conditions (e.g., inflammatory bowel disease), myelodysplastic syndromes (e.g., polycythemia vera and essential thrombocythemia), and antiphospholipid antibody syndrome.

What is the differential diagnosis?

Leg swelling, redness, and pain: The differential diagnosis includes infection (cellulitis), musculoskeletal injury (muscle trauma, strain or tear, tendonitis, bone fracture), venous insufficiency, previous DVT with postthrombotic syndrome, ruptured popliteal/Baker cyst, postsurgical pain, and lymphedema.

What symptoms might be observed?

Symptoms of a DVT include leg pain and swelling along with calf tenderness. Patients may also have shortness of breath if pulmonary embolism (PE) is present as a complication.

Physical Examination

Vital signs: Patients may develop tachycardia, tachypnea, decreased oxygen saturation, and hypotension in the case of a PE.
Inspection: Inspect for unilateral leg swelling, erythema, and prominent superficial veins.
Palpation: Palpate for unilateral leg tenderness, swelling, and palpable venous cords. Check the temperature of the extremity for warmth.

Special Tests

Calf circumference: Measure the calf circumference 10 cm below the tibial tuberosity on both legs. A calf circumference discrepancy of >3 cm is considered significant.

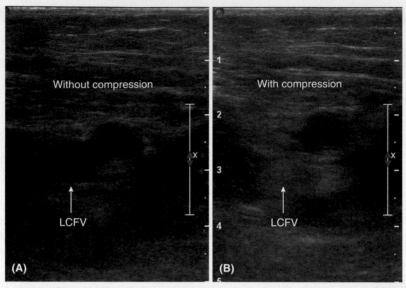

FIGURE 6.57. Ultrasound images of the left common femoral vein (*LCFV*): **(A)** without compression and **(B)** with normal compression. A lack of or incomplete compressibility may indicate a thrombus.

What tests should be ordered?

Laboratory tests: CBC (anemia, thrombocytopenia); metabolic panel (serum albumin, liver enzymes, Cr, and brain natriuretic peptide [BNP]). Urine studies include urinalysis for proteinuria and Cr to rule out secondary causes of swelling; other serology (D-dimer has high sensitivity but low specificity and can rule out DVT when the pretest probability is low).

Imaging: Compression ultrasonography tests for full compressibility of proximal vein to rule out proximal DVT (**Fig. 6.57**). Ultrasonography is used for direct visualization of the thrombus and for assessing competence of deep vein valves. Contrast venography is the gold standard of imaging modalities due to its high sensitivity and specificity. However, one limitation of this test is the potential of adverse reactions with the use of contrast, and it is not frequently performed.

Diagnostic Scores

A Wells score ≥ 2 suggests that DVT is likely, whereas a score < 2 suggests that DVT is not likely (**Table 6.16**).

TABLE 6.16. Pretest probability of deep vein thrombosis	
Clinical Feature	**Score**
Active cancer	1
Immobilization of the lower extremities (e.g., paralysis, paresis, or recent plaster)	1
Bedridden for more than 3 days or major surgery within 4 weeks	1
Localized tenderness along the distribution of the deep venous system in the lower leg	1
Entire leg swollen	1
Asymmetric calf swelling with affected leg >3 cm in diameter compared to unaffected leg	1
Pitting edema	1
Collateral superficial veins	1
DVT is not the leading diagnosis in the differential.	−2

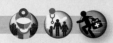 # PERIPHERAL ARTERY DISEASE

Presentation

A 50-year-old male, with a history of diabetes and smoking, presents with calf pain that is precipitated by walking. His pain is relieved with rest.

Definition

PAD is narrowing of arteries outside of the brain and heart that results in decreased perfusion. PAD is categorized based on the extent of arterial occlusion by the Fontaine stages:

Stage I: Asymptomatic with incomplete arterial obstruction
Stage II: Mild claudication
Stage IIA: Claudication with walking a distance >200 m
Stage IIB: Claudication with walking a distance <200 m
Stage III: Rest pain, primarily in the feet
Stage IV: Necrosis and/or gangrene of the limb

Stages II and III are referred to as *intermittent claudication*, which classically presents with leg pain, discomfort, and/or fatigue associated with walking and activity. Symptoms are typically relieved with rest.

What are common causes?

The most common cause of PAD is atherosclerosis due to age, hypertension, dyslipidemia, smoking, diabetes, and genetic factors. Other causes of PAD include aneurysmal disease (acquired or hereditary), thromboembolic disease, inflammatory (e.g., vasculitis), trauma, adventitial cysts, entrapment syndromes (e.g., popliteal artery entrapment syndrome), and congenital vascular malformations.

What is the differential diagnosis?

Calf pain: The differential diagnosis includes venous causes (e.g., DVT and venous insufficiency), infections (e.g., septic arthritis or cellulitis), arthritis (e.g., OA and inflammatory arthritis), chronic compartment syndrome, symptomatic Baker cysts, and trauma (Achilles tendon rupture or proximal tibia fracture).

What symptoms might be observed?

Symptoms of PAD include leg pain, especially with activity (claudication) that relieves with rest. Critical ischemia manifests with persistent and severe pain.

What are the possible findings on examination?

Vital signs: Hypertension may be present. In critical leg ischemia, hypotension, tachycardia, tachypnea, and fever may be present.
Inspection: Inspect for skin changes, pallor, erythema, wounds, and signs of necrosis or gangrene. Nonhealing wounds typically develop over distal bony prominences, such as ankles, heels, and toes. Also note any hair loss, trophic skin changes, and nail thickening.
Palpation: Palpate the skin for coolness, and palpate distal pulses (which may be reduced or difficult to palpate). Check for delayed capillary refill in the digits.
Auscultation: Abdominal and femoral bruits are suggestive of turbulent blood flow.

Special Tests

Pallor on elevation and rubor on dependency: With the patient supine, the clinician elevates the patient's legs above the level of the heart for 15–30 seconds. Marked skin pallor in the leg during this maneuver suggests poor arterial supply. Next, the clinician lowers the legs and instructs the patient to sit up and allow the legs to dangle over the edge of the examination table. If the legs turn red (rubor on dependency), arterial insufficiency should be suspected.

● CLINICAL PEARL

A thick layer of inelastic connective tissue called *fascia* surrounds muscle compartments. Extremity trauma (e.g., fractures, burns, and crush injuries), vascular compromise, and tight casts can substantially increase the pressure within a compartment. Consequently, the intracompartment pressure may surpass the arterial pressure, causing hypoperfusion. This is termed *compartment syndrome* and is considered a surgical emergency. Patients experience symptoms of ischemia including pain, paresthesia, paralysis, pulselessness, cool skin temperature (polar), and skin pallor. In an awake and alert patient, compartment syndrome is diagnosed clinically, but compartment pressure measurements may be used to confirm the diagnosis.

What tests should be ordered?

Laboratory tests: CBC (leukocytosis), metabolic panel (Cr, electrolytes, and risk-factor stratification with fasting lipids and hemoglobin A1c), and microbiology (blood cultures especially if signs of gangrene or necrosis are present).

Imaging: X-rays may be performed to assess for other orthopedic causes of leg pain and may reveal signs of calcified arteries. Ultrasound arterial Doppler studies can detect abnormalities in arterial blood flow waveforms that are associated with PAD. MR angiogram using gadolinium enhancement and CT angiogram can determine the location and severity of PAD for consideration of endovascular intervention.

Special Tests

ABI: ABI is the most cost-effective way to assess PAD (see chapter introduction).

Treadmill testing with pre- and post-ABI: May be useful to assess for lower extremity PAD when resting ABI is within normal limits.

ANKLE SPRAINS

Presentation

A 19-year-old female presents to the Emergency Department with pain and swelling in his right ankle. Earlier that afternoon, he was playing basketball. He had jumped up for the ball and landed on another player's foot, rolling his ankle with his foot turned inward. He experienced immediate pain and swelling and is ambulating with significant discomfort.

Definition

Ankle sprain is a stretching or tearing of a ligament of the ankle (**Fig. 6.58**). Low lateral ankle sprain is an injury to one or more of the lateral ligaments of the ankle (ATFL, CFL, and PTFL). Low medial ankle sprain is an injury to one or more parts of the medial (deltoid) ligament of the ankle (tibionavicular, tibiocalcaneal, and posterior tibiotalar parts of medial ligament). High ankle sprain (syndesmotic injury) is an injury to one or more parts of the distal tibiofibular syndesmotic ankle ligaments.

Ankle sprains are graded as:

Grade I: Mild sprain with microscopic tearing of ligaments; the ankle joint remains stable.

Grade II: Moderate sprain with partial tear of some ligaments; the ankle joint may be normally aligned but is unstable.

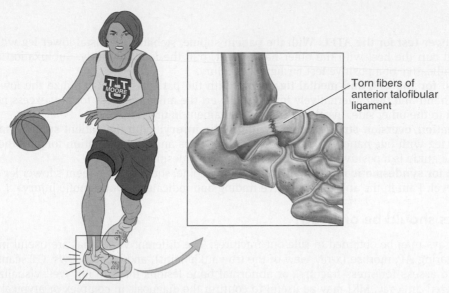

Torn fibers of
anterior talofibular
ligament

FIGURE 6.58. Anterior talofibular ligament tear.

Grade III: Severe sprain with complete tear of ligaments; the ankle joint is highly unstable.

What are common causes?

Lateral ankle sprains are the most common type of ankle sprain and usually occur from excessive inversion and plantar flexion of the ankle beyond the normal ROM. Medial ankle sprains typically involve eversion of ankle beyond the normal ROM. High ankle sprains result from excessive external rotation and dorsiflexion of the foot, with internal rotation of the tibia during active movement. These injuries are typically seen in high-energy sports including ice hockey and football.

What is the differential diagnosis?

Ankle pain and swelling: The differential diagnosis includes trauma (e.g., a fracture), infection (e.g., septic arthritis, OM, or cellulitis), crystal arthritis (e.g., gout), degenerative changes (e.g., OA and impingement syndromes), hematologic causes (e.g., hemophilic arthropathy), PAD, and neuropathy (e.g., tarsal tunnel syndrome).

What symptoms might be observed?

Symptoms of a lateral ankle sprain include pain at the anterolateral side of the ankle, ankle swelling, and instability when walking on uneven ground. Symptoms of a medial ankle sprain are similar except that the instability is worse when walking downhill or down stairs. A high ankle sprain may present with pain at the anterior ankle, especially when the toe pushes off the ground or pivots, ankle swelling, and difficulty bearing weight.

What are the possible findings on examination?

Vital signs: Typically normal.

Inspection: Inspect for signs of ankle swelling, ecchymosis, and deformities. Valgus alignment may be present with a medial ankle sprain, whereas a varus alignment may be present in a lateral ankle sprain.

Palpation: Tenderness along the ankle joint line or over bony landmarks, including the distal tibia, fibula, and foot, suggests underlying fracture. Tenderness of the anterior and lateral malleolus as well as the lateral ankle joint line may be present in lateral ankle sprain. Tenderness of the anterior and medial malleolus may be present in medial ankle sprain, and tenderness of the anterior ankle joint line and posterior to malleoli may be present in a high ankle sprain.

ROM: Reduced ankle movements due to pain and swelling.

Special Tests

Anterior drawer test for the ATFL: With the patient supine, stabilize the distal lower leg with one hand, and cup the heel with the other hand. Next, pull the foot anteriorly. Subluxation of the ankle is indicative of a positive test for ligament injury.

Talar tilt test for the CFL and medial ligament: With the patient supine, stabilize the lower leg with one hand and then alternatively invert and evert the ankle to assess for any excess motion compared to the other side. Instability indicates ligament injury (**Fig. 6.59**).

External rotation/eversion stress test for syndesmotic injury: With the patient supine, stabilize the lower leg with one hand while the other hand applies an external rotation force to the foot. Pain in the ankle is a positive finding and indicates a syndesmotic injury.

Squeeze test for syndesmotic injury: With the patient supine, squeeze the patient's lower leg at the midcalf level. Pain in the ankle is a positive finding and indicates a syndesmotic injury.

What tests should be ordered?

Imaging: X-rays may be obtained to rule out fractures. The different views that are useful include weight-bearing AP, mortise (x-ray view of the true ankle joint), and lateral views. CT scans may be used to assess for stress fractures or abnormal bone lesions that are not well visualized or characterized on x-ray. MRI may be useful to confirm the diagnosis in complex or atypical cases and exclude other pathology involving soft tissue.

Diagnostic Scores

The Ottawa ankle rules are clinical guidelines to determine if x-rays of the ankle are warranted by quantifying the probability of an ankle or foot fracture. In patients aged 18 years or older, obtain an ankle x-ray series (AP, lateral, and mortise) if there is pain in the malleolar region and any of the following:

- Bony tenderness at the posterior edge or tip of the lateral malleolus (examine the distal 6 cm of the fibula)
- Bony tenderness at the posterior edge or tip of the medial malleolus (examine the distal 6 cm of the tibia)
- Inability to bear weight both immediately following injury and in the Emergency Department

In patients aged 18 years or older, obtain a foot x-ray series (AP, lateral, and oblique) if there is any pain in the midfoot region and any of the following:

- Bony tenderness at the base of the fifth metatarsal
- Bony tenderness at the navicular
- Inability to bear weight both immediately after injury and in the Emergency Department

In cases of intoxicated or uncooperative patients or patients with other distracting injuries and obvious deformity or swelling, clinical judgment should supersede these rules.

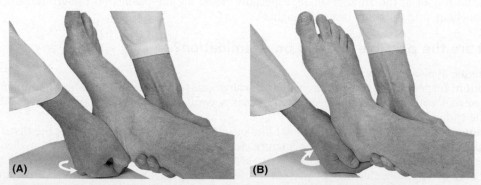

FIGURE 6.59. Talar tilt test demonstrating ankle inversion (**A**) and eversion (**B**).

Head and Neck

KRISTEN M. KRYSKO • GAVIN J. LE NOBEL •
JEFFREY E. ALFONSI • AARON IZENBERG • MOLLY ZIRKLE

7

The head and neck consists of the cranium, brain, cranial nerves (CNs), cervical spinal cord, sensory organs (eyes, ears, mouth, and nose), sinuses, and major blood vessels. This region is responsible for cognition, movement, sensation, and interaction with surroundings.

■ INITIAL EVALUATION AND ASSESSMENT

Head and neck pathology can manifest in a wide array of symptoms. **Table 7.1** summarizes the most common neurologic and otolaryngeal presentations.

General Head and Neck Examination

Depending on the extent of the examination, the patient may be draped in a gown, exposing the back and extremities as needed. In many cases, the patient can be sitting upright with the neck exposed. A systematic head and neck examination follows the sequence: inspection, palpation, percussion, auscultation, and special maneuvers. In many cases, percussion and auscultation are not applicable. For the neurological examination, the level of consciousness (LOC) should be evaluated using a scale such as the Glasgow Coma Scale (GCS), as shown in **Table 7.2**. The neurological examination also involves an assessment of the mental status, cranial nerves, motor system, sensory system, coordination, gait, and stance.

Laboratory Tests

Laboratory investigations are used to help diagnose systemic causes of neurologic and otolaryngeal symptoms. A complete blood count (CBC) is ordered to investigate possible infection or thrombocytopenia that may predispose to bleeding. Measuring electrolytes, calcium, magnesium, creatinine (Cr), liver enzymes/function, fasting glucose, and hemoglobin (Hb) A1c and obtaining a urine and serum toxicology screen are important as abnormalities in these investigations can cause seizures, confusion, or neuropathy. Vitamin B_{12} may also be ordered to investigate cognitive impairment, myelopathy, or neuropathy. When thyroid disease is suspected, thyroid-stimulating hormone (TSH) and a free thyroxine (T_4) level should be ordered. Other neurologic investigations include tests for systemic rheumatologic conditions and other infections (syphilis, HIV, lyme). Other investigations relevant to otolaryngology include Epstein-Barr virus (EBV) testing, oropharyngeal swab for streptococcal infection, and skin prick testing or serum immunoglobulins (IgEs) to diagnose allergens.

Head and Neck Imaging

The major imaging modalities for the brain and spinal cord are computed tomography (CT) and magnetic resonance imaging (MRI) scans. CT scans are quick, are readily available, and provide information on bony structures and sinuses. CT scans can identify acute bleeds, cranial fractures, and cancers. However, CT scans are not as effective at imaging the brain parenchyma, especially in the posterior fossa.

> ● **CLINICAL PEARL**
>
> When reading a plain CT scan of the head, the ABBBCS mnemonic provides a framework:
>
> **A**ir-filled spaces (sinuses, mastoid air cells)
> **B**ones
> **B**lood (epidural, subdural, subarachnoid, intraparenchymal)
> **B**rain (stroke, edema, masses, midline shift)
> **C**erebral spinal fluid (CSF)
> **S**paces (sulci, ventricles, cisterns)

TABLE 7.1. Common presenting symptoms

Structure	Symptoms
Ears	Hearing loss, tinnitus, vertigo, fullness, pain, discharge
Eyes	Diplopia, visual field loss (unilateral, bilateral, or quadrants), visual acuity changes, eye pain, redness, sicca, or discharge
Nose	Rhinorrhea, congestion, loss of smell (anosmia), postnasal drip (with cough), pain, epistaxis
Throat and neck	Pain, globus, dysphagia, odynophagia, tooth pain, oral ulcers, voice hoarseness, lumps or masses, swollen glands
Sinuses	Pain and tenderness, headache, nasal discharge or congestion, anosmia, loss of taste (dysgeusia)
Cortex	Level of alertness, disruption of cognitive domains (e.g., memory, executive function, language, or visuospatial), neglect, alexia, agraphia, and personality changes
Brainstem	Level of alertness, respiratory drive, diplopia, dysarthria (slurred speech), dysphagia (difficulty swallowing), drop attacks
Sensory	Numbness, paresthesia, burning pain, loss of proprioception or balance, glove and stocking sensation loss
Motor (motor nerves, Neuromuscular junction [NMJ], myopathy)	Weakness (unilateral, bilateral, proximal, or distal), fatigability, fasciculations, and myalgia
Cerebellum	Ataxia (wide-based gait), poor balance, poor coordination, scanning dysarthria (jerky, slurred, or loud speech)
Bowel and bladder	Urinary symptoms including retention, urgency or incontinence, fecal incontinence or constipation, and saddle anesthesia

TABLE 7.2. Glasgow coma scale

Score	Eye	Verbal[a]	Motor[b]
1	No eye opening	No sounds	No movements
2	Opens eyes to pain	Incomprehensible sounds	Extension to pain
3	Opens eyes to voice	Inappropriate words	Flexion to pain
4	Spontaneous eye opening	Confused, disoriented	Withdraws from pain
5		Oriented	Localizes to pain
6			Follows commands

[a]An intubated patient is assigned a score of "1T" on the verbal component.
[b]Central pain can be elicited through rubbing the sternum or pressing against the superior orbital bone.

TABLE 7.3. Common magnetic resonance imaging sequences and uses		
Sequence	**Identifying the Sequence**	**Use**
T1	Gray matter dark White matter bright CSF dark	Demonstrates anatomy Pathology often dark
T2	Gray matter bright White matter dark CSF bright	Demonstrates pathology, which is often bright
FLAIR	Gray matter bright White matter dark CSF dark	Demonstrates pathology, which is bright and easier to identify as CSF dark
DWI/ADC	Cytotoxic edema bright on DWI, dark on ADC (diffusion restriction) Vasogenic edema bright on DWI and ADC (T2 shine through)	Demonstrates cytotoxic edema (helpful in acute stroke)

FLAIR, fluid-attenuated inversion recovery; DWI, diffusion weighted imaging; ADC, apparent diffusion coefficient.

MRI scans are excellent at imaging the brain parenchyma, spinal cord, and inner ear. However, MRI scans are expensive and less readily available than CT scans. When an MRI scan is obtained, a number of pulse sequences may be used to highlight specific pathology or anatomical regions (**Table 7.3**). Contrast dye can be given with both CT and MRI scans to image blood vessels and to highlight breakdown of the blood brain barrier, as indicated by abnormal enhancement, which may occur in some masses and inflammatory lesions. For neck imaging, ultrasound can be used to visualize the great vessels, thyroid gland, and lymph nodes.

> ● **CLINICAL PEARL**
>
> Neurons have cell bodies that are located in the gray matter of the central nervous system (CNS) and myelinated axons that are located in the white matter. In the brain, gray matter is located in the external aspect of the cerebral cortex, whereas in the spine, it is in the internal aspect.

Special Tests

Electrophysiologic tests including electroencephalogram (EEG), nerve conduction studies/electromyography (NCS/EMG), and evoked potentials (EPs) are useful in assessing brain activity and nerve function. Audiology studies may also be obtained to assess hearing. CSF obtained by lumbar puncture (LP) is helpful in assessing inflammatory, infectious, and neoplastic conditions. Biopsy of the brain, lymph nodes, thyroid nodules, nerves, and muscles may also be helpful in confirming certain diagnoses.

SYSTEMS OVERVIEW

■ CRANIUM, SCALP, AND MENINGES

Overview

The brain is contained within the bones of the cranium (skull) as shown in **Figure 7.1.** Superficial to the cranium is the scalp, which includes the skin and subcutaneous tissue. Deep to the cranium are the meninges, which are membranous coverings of the brain that provide protection to the brain and support blood vessels. The meninges include the dura mater (tough thick external fibrous layer), the arachnoid mater (thin intermediate layer), and the pia mater (delicate internal vascular layer), as shown in **Figure 7.2**.

Physical Examination

The scalp and face are inspected for asymmetries and signs of trauma and then palpated for tenderness, deformities, and soft tissue swelling.

Imaging

The cranium can be imaged using x-ray (**Fig. 7.3**), CT or MRI scans. The meninges are best visualized using MRI.

■ CEREBRUM

Overview

The brain is divided into the cerebrum, diencephalon, brainstem, and cerebellum (**Fig. 7.4A and B**).

The cerebrum includes two hemispheres, and each consists of four lobes: frontal, parietal, temporal, and occipital lobes (**Fig. 7.4A**). The frontal lobe is involved in planning, reasoning, problem solving, and movement (primary motor area within the precentral gyrus) as well as in the motor component of speech (Broca area). The parietal lobe is important in sensation (primary somatosensory area within the postcentral postcentral gyrus), orientation, recognition, and visuospatial skills. It is also involved in carrying out complex movements. The occipital lobe is important in visual processing and contains the primary visual cortex. The temporal lobe is important in perceiving auditory stimuli, understanding speech (Wernicke area) and memory (hippocampus).

Physical Examination

The cerebrum examination includes an assessment of cognition, language, vision, and the motor and sensory pathways. A detailed assessment of cortical function begins during the patient interview. The Mini Mental State Examination (MMSE) and the Montreal Cognitive Assessment (MoCA) are widely used screening tools to assess cognitive function. If any cognitive deficits are identified, formal cognitive testing may be warranted.

> ● CLINICAL PEARL
>
> *Dysarthria* is a disorder of articulation and typically localizes to the brainstem or CNs. *Aphasia* is a disorder of language function (expression or understanding) and typically localizes to the dominant cerebral hemisphere.

The cortex is also involved with language and expression. The language examination consists of six components (**Table 7.4**). The type of aphasia is classified by the pattern of deficits, and each

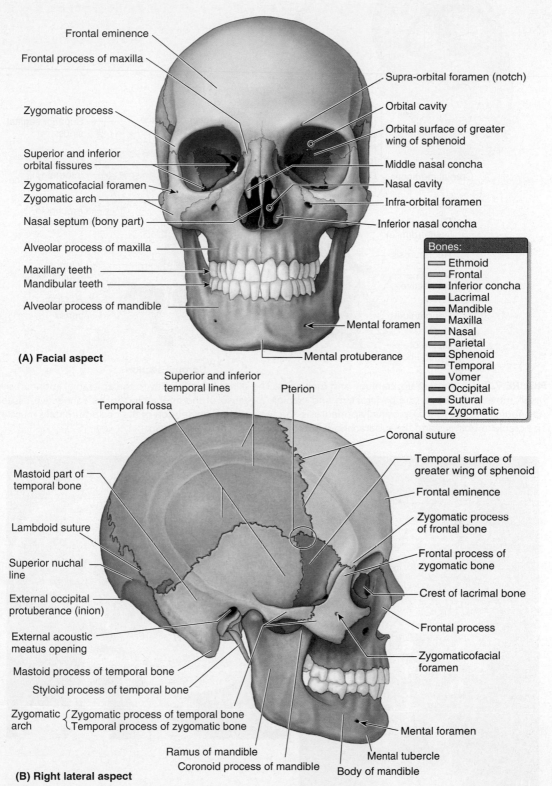

Frontal eminence

Frontal process of maxilla

Zygomatic process

Superior and inferior orbital fissures

Zygomaticofacial foramen

Zygomatic arch

Nasal septum (bony part)

Alveolar process of maxilla

Maxillary teeth

Mandibular teeth

Alveolar process of mandible

Supra-orbital foramen (notch)

Orbital cavity

Orbital surface of greater wing of sphenoid

Middle nasal concha

Nasal cavity

Infra-orbital foramen

Inferior nasal concha

Mental foramen

Mental protuberance

(A) Facial aspect

Bones:
Ethmoid
Frontal
Inferior concha
Lacrimal
Mandible
Maxilla
Nasal
Parietal
Sphenoid
Temporal
Vomer
Occipital
Sutural
Zygomatic

Superior and inferior temporal lines

Temporal fossa

Pterion

Coronal suture

Mastoid part of temporal bone

Lambdoid suture

Superior nuchal line

External occipital protuberance (inion)

External acoustic meatus opening

Mastoid process of temporal bone

Styloid process of temporal bone

Zygomatic arch { Zygomatic process of temporal bone
Temporal process of zygomatic bone

Temporal surface of greater wing of sphenoid

Frontal eminence

Zygomatic process of frontal bone

Frontal process of zygomatic bone

Crest of lacrimal bone

Frontal process

Zygomaticofacial foramen

Mental foramen

Ramus of mandible

Coronoid process of mandible

Mental tubercle

Body of mandible

(B) Right lateral aspect

FIGURE 7.1. Adult cranium. **A.** Anterior view of the bones of the skull, which are color coded. **B.** Lateral view of the bones of the skull.

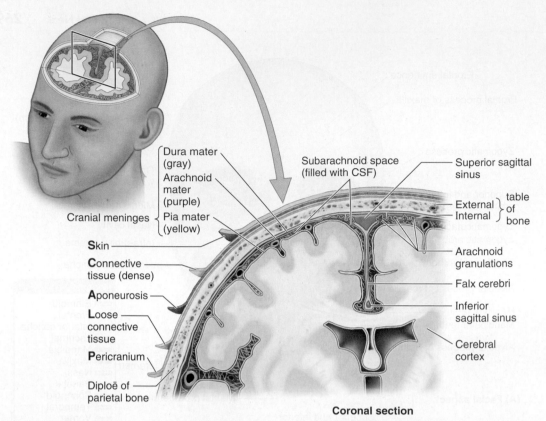

FIGURE 7.2. Layers of scalp, cranium, and meninges. The skin is bound tightly to the epicranial aponeurosis, which moves freely over the pericranium and cranium because of the intervening loose connective tissue. *Aponeurosis* refers to the epicranial aponeurosis, the flat intermediate tendon of the occipitofrontalis muscle. The cranial meninges and the subarachnoid (leptomeningeal) space are shown.

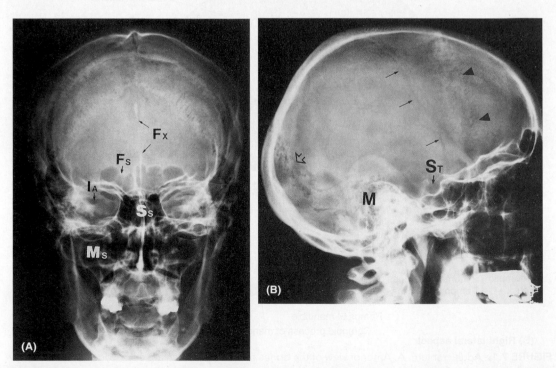

FIGURE 7.3. X-rays of the skull. **A.** PA x-ray of the skull. Note the following structures: falx cerebri (*Fx*), frontal sinus (*Fs*), internal auditory canal (*Ia*), sphenoid sinus (*Ss*), and maxillary sinus (*Ms*). **B.** Lateral x-ray of the skull. Note the following structures: coronal suture (*arrowheads*), occipital suture (*open arrow*), middle meningeal vascular grooves (*straight arrows*), sella turcica (*St*), and mastoid air cells (*M*).

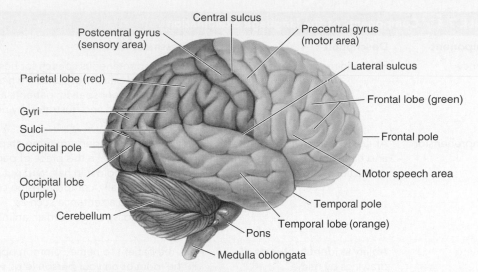

(A) Right lateral view of right brain and lobes of cerebrum

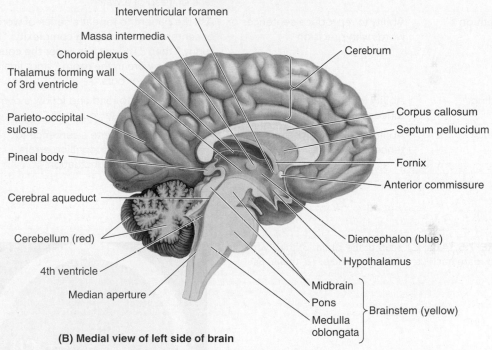

(B) Medial view of left side of brain

FIGURE 7.4. Structure of the brain. **A.** The cerebral surface features the gyri (folds) and sulci (grooves) of the cerebral cortex. **B.** The medial surface of the cerebrum and deeper parts of the brain (diencephalon and brainstem) are shown after bisection of the brain. The parieto-occipital sulcus demarcating the parietal and occipital lobes is seen on the medial aspect of the cerebrum. The lobes of the cerebrum and parts of the brainstem are color coded.

type of aphasia has a particular neurologic localization within the dominant hemisphere, which is usually the left side.

Imaging

MRI and CT scans are used for imaging the cerebrum (**Fig. 7.5**).

TABLE 7.4. Components of the language examination

Component	Description	Assessment Method
Fluency	Flow and magnitude of speech	Observe spontaneous speech for hesitancy, faltering, and paucity of speech, which indicate nonfluent speech; patients are typically aware of and frustrated by nonfluent speech.
Comprehension	Ability to perceive, interpret, and understand language and instructions	Ask the patient to perform three-step commands such as "take this piece of paper in your left hand, fold it in half, and put it on the floor." Verbally, comprehension can be assessed using a sentence such as: "The lion was killed by a tiger. Which animal is dead?"
Naming	Ability to identify objects or drawings by name	Ask the patient to name common objects in the room or on your person (e.g., watch or pen) and less common objects (e.g., the face or clasp of a watch).
Repetition	Ability to reproduce sentences or words with precision	Ask the patient to repeat a series of words or sentences of increasing complexity: "It is sunny," then "The cat hid under the couch when dogs were in the room," and, finally, "No ifs, ands, or buts."
Reading	Ability to read words and sentences correctly	Ask the patient to read and follow a command such as "close your eyes."
Writing	Ability to write words or sentences correctly	Ask the patient to write a sentence to examine for grammar, spelling errors, phrase length, and punctuation.

FIGURE 7.5. Axial CT scan of the brain. *3*, third ventricle; *CN*, caudate nucleus; *L*, lateral ventricle; *Th*, thalamus.

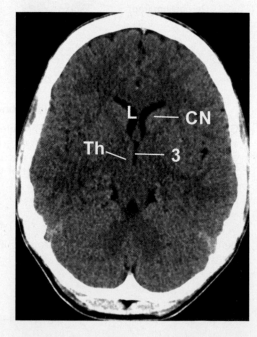

CRANIAL NERVES AND BRAINSTEM

Overview

The brainstem is at the base of the brain and contains the midbrain, pons, and medulla. The medulla includes the cardiac and respiratory regulatory centers of the brain (**Fig. 7.4A**). Below the brainstem lies the spinal cord, which extends down the vertebral column.

The 12 pairs of CNs include bundles of sensory, motor, and/or autonomic fibers carrying impulses to and from the brainstem. CNs exit the brain through cranial foramina and fissures to ultimately synapse with their targets (**Fig. 7.6**).

Physical Examination

The maneuvers to examine the cranial nerves are summarized below:

Olfactory Nerve (I)

- Test sense of smell by placing objects with strong scents (e.g., cloves or coffee) under one nostril while the other nostril is occluded.

Optic Nerve (II)

- Determine best corrected visual acuity using an eye chart.
- Test visual fields by asking the patient to cover one eye and perform finger counting in each quadrant. **Figure 7.7** depicts possible deformities in the visual fields.
- Assess pupillary response to light by shining a light into each eye and watching for direct (the eye the light is shone into) and consensual (the opposite eye) pupillary constriction. The swinging flashlight test involves swinging the light between the two eyes at 1 Hz and can be used to detect a relative afferent pupillary defect (RAPD).
- Funduscopy with ophthalmoscope to examine the retina (**Fig. 7.18**).

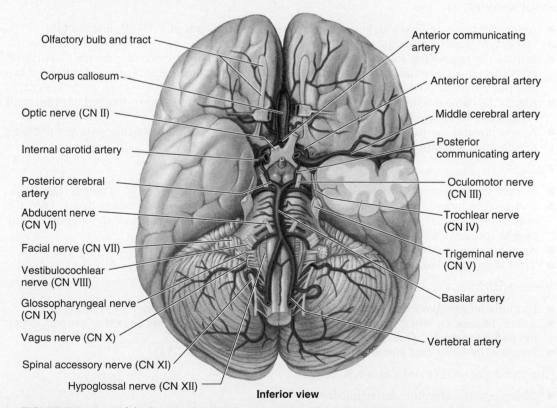

Inferior view

FIGURE 7.6. Base of the brain with cranial nerves and cerebral arterial circle.

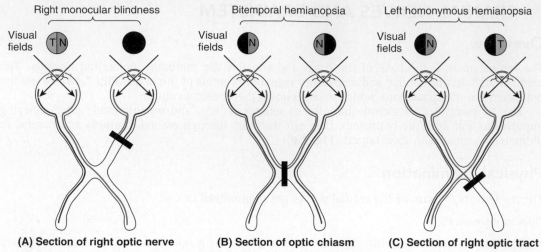

FIGURE 7.7. Visual field pathway from eyes to the optic tracts. **A.** Visual field defect causing right monocular blindness from pathology of the right optic nerve. **B.** Visual field defect causing bitemporal hemianopsia from pathology of the optic chiasm. **C.** Visual field defect of a left homonymous hemianopsia from pathology of the right optic tract.

Oculomotor (III), Trochlear (IV), and Abducens Nerves (VI)

- Inspect the position of the eye, pupil size, and for the presence of ptosis.
- Assess smooth pursuit of the eyes in nine gaze positions (**Fig. 7.8**) and look for nystagmus.
- Examine saccades by asking the patient to shift the gaze quickly between two targets.
- Assess pupillary light reflex as in CN II.

Facial Nerve (V)

- Assess sensation to light touch, pin, and cold sensation in each of $V_1/V_2/V_3$ distributions.
- Inspect for wasting of temporalis muscle.
- Palpate the temporalis and masseter muscle while the patient is clenching the jaw; test lateral pterygoids by asking the patient to hold the mouth open against resistance; test medial and lateral pterygoids by pushing the jaw laterally against resistance.
- Assess the corneal reflex by asking the patient to look up and away; next, touch the cornea with cotton, and observe for a direct and consensual blink response.
- Assess jaw jerk by placing the clinician's index finger on the patient's chin with the patient's mouth open and tapping the finger with a reflex hammer.

Facial Nerve (VII)

- Inspect for facial asymmetry such as a flattened nasolabial fold or a drooping mouth (**Fig. 7.9**).
- Test muscle power by asking the patient to close the eyes tight (orbicularis oculi), raise the eyebrows (frontalis), show the teeth, close the mouth tightly (orbicularis oris), and puff out the cheeks (orbicularis oris and buccinators).
- Assess corneal reflex as in CN V.
- Taste is rarely tested, but should be done unilaterally if tested.

Vestibulocochlear Nerve (VIII)

- Examine for nystagmus secondary to abnormalities in the vestibular system as in CN III.
- Assess hearing by whispering into one ear while rubbing fingers over the other ear and asking the patient to repeat what was said.
- Perform the Rinne and Weber tests (**Figs. 7.20 and 7.21**; **Table 7.13**).

Glossopharyngeal (IX) and Vagus Nerves (X)

- Observe palate elevation for symmetry.
- Assess articulation by asking the patient to enunciate the sounds—"ka," "ga," "pa," "la," and "puthkuh."

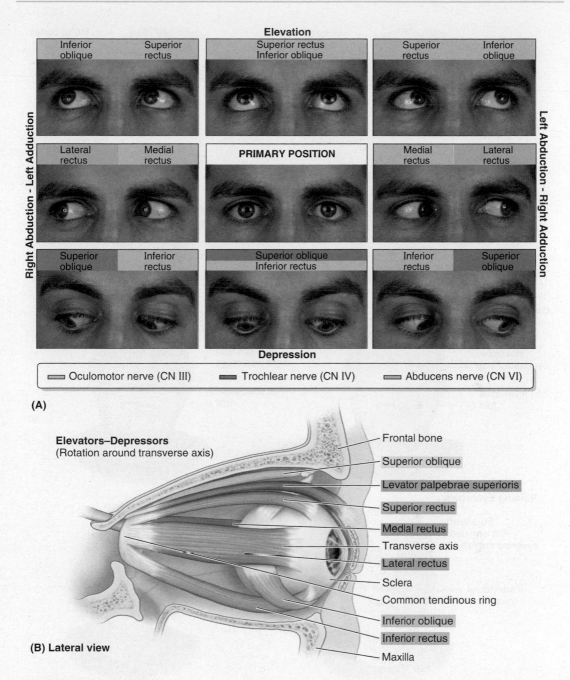

FIGURE 7.8. A. Binocular movements. B. Associated muscles.

- Observe the patient swallowing water.
- Assess the gag reflex by stroking the soft palate with a tongue depressor on each side.

Spinal Accessory Nerve (XI)

- Inspect for atrophy of the trapezius and sternocleidomastoid (SCM) muscles.
- Test the power of the trapezius muscle by asking the patient to shrug the shoulders against resistance; test the power of the SCM by asking the patient to turn the head against resistance (**Fig. 7.10**).

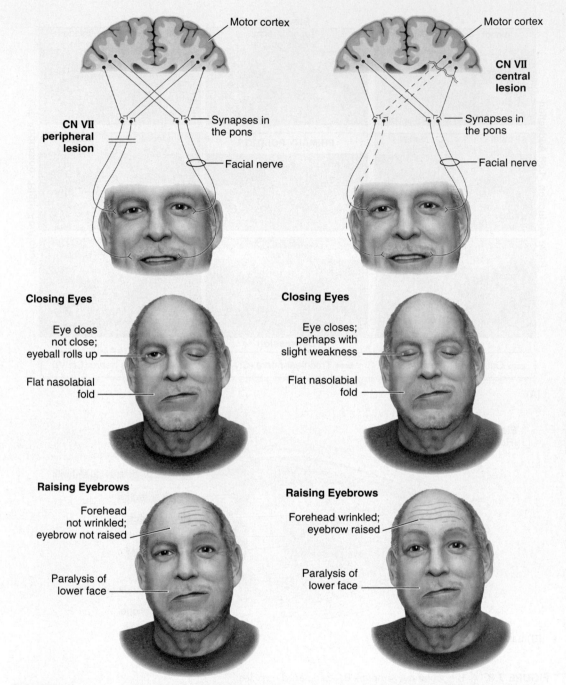

FIGURE 7.9. Lower motor neuron (LMN) versus upper motor neuron (UMN) lesions and facial weakness. In a peripheral lesion of CN VII, there is complete weakness of the ipsilateral facial expression muscles. In a central lesion, bilateral innervation to the frontalis results in sparing of the frontalis, while there is paralysis of the lower face due to unilateral innervation.

Hypoglossal Nerve (XII)

■ Inspect the tongue for atrophy and fasciculations.
■ Test power by asking the patient to stick out the tongue and look for deviation to one side; power can also be tested by asking the patient to push the tongue into each cheek while the clinician applies pressure externally to the cheek.

Common abnormalities in cranial nerve function are summarized in **Table 7.5**.

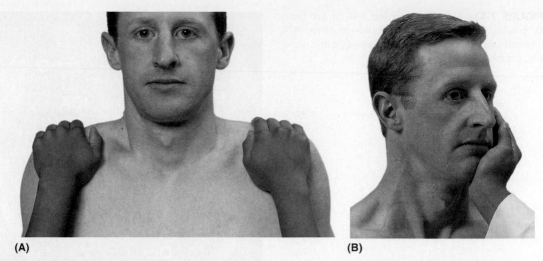

(A)   **(B)**

FIGURE 7.10. Motor examination of the spinal accessory nerve. **A.** Examination of the trapezius muscles. **B.** Examination of the right SCM muscle.

Imaging

MRI is the best modality for imaging CNs and the brainstem (**Fig. 7.11**).

■ MOTOR SYSTEM

Overview

Motor function is a complicated process that involves the central and peripheral nervous systems. The basal ganglia located deep within the brain contain a network of subcortical gray nuclei

TABLE 7.5. Abnormal findings on examination of the cranial nerves	
CN	**Findings in Dysfunction**
I	Unilateral or bilateral anosmia
II	Decreased visual acuity, visual field defect (**Fig. 7.7**), decreased pupil response to light, RAPD (constriction with light shone in normal eye, but when light swings to abnormal eye, both pupils paradoxically dilate), abnormal optic disc (change in color, margins, vessels)
III	Anisocoria (mydriatic), ptosis, dysconjugate gaze/eye deviation ("down and out"), impaired adduction and elevation
IV	Hypertropia, difficulty with combined adduction/infraduction
V	Decreased sensation, temporalis wasting or weakness, jaw deviation to the side of the lesion, absent/asymmetric corneal reflex, brisk jaw jerk
VI	Medial deviated eye, difficulty with eye abduction
VII	Unilateral facial weakness/droop, pattern of facial weakness can determine if the lesion is UMN or LMN; UMN lesion spares the frontalis due to bilateral cortical innervation of frontalis, whereas LMN leads to weakness throughout (**Fig. 7.9**), absent corneal reflex.
VIII	Nystagmus/vertigo, decreased hearing, abnormal Rinne and Weber tests (**Table 7.13**)
IX/X	Palate/uvula may deviate away from the side of the CN X lesion; dysarthria (difficulty articulating) and/or dysphagia (difficulty swallowing), absent gag reflex.
XI	Atrophy and weakness of trapezius and SCM (weakness on turning head left indicates weakness of the right SCM)
XII	Tongue deviates to the side of a CN XII lesion and unable to resist pressure on the cheek contralateral to the lesion, atrophy, and fasciculations in LMN lesion.

FIGURE 7.11. Axial T2-weighted MRI of the brain. *B,* basilar artery; *EOM,* extraocular muscles; *ICA,* internal carotid arteries; *M,* midbrain; *O,* optic nerve; *Oc,* occipital lobe; *V,* vermis.

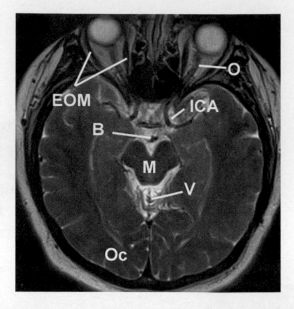

(striatum [caudate and putamen], globus pallidus, substantia nigra, nucleus accumbens, and subthalamic nucleus) that are responsible for initiation of movement through a complex network of connections. The motor pathway begins in the primary motor cortex (precentral gyrus), which is arranged somatotopically with the face represented most laterally and the leg represented most medially (**Fig. 7.12**). This information travels via the corticospinal tract and through the white matter region to reach the brainstem and spinal cord. This upper motor neuron (UMN) synapses on the lower motor neuron (LMN) in the spinal cord, then exits the spinal cord and becomes the peripheral nerve. The peripheral nerve synapses on the muscle at the NMJ.

Physical Examination

The motor examination includes inspection and an evaluation of tone, power, and reflexes. On inspection, muscle bulk (e.g., atrophy or hypertrophy), involuntary movements (e.g., fasciculations and tremor), and posturing are noted.

Elevated muscle tone may be due to rigidity or spasticity. Tone is best assessed with the patient supine. *Rigidity* is a velocity-independent increase in tone throughout the range of motion with a "lead pipe" type of stiffness. To assess for rigidity, the patient's arm is slowly flexed and extended at the elbow and the wrist is slowly rotated. For the lower extremity, the leg is rolled on the examination table, and then the knee is slowly flexed and extended. *Spasticity* is a velocity- and direction-dependent increase in tone. To assess spasticity, the elbow is rapidly extended then the forearm is rapidly supinated. For the lower extremity, the knee is rapidly flexed. If spasticity is present, the entire foot will lift off of the examination table.

In the upper and lower extremities, muscle power is evaluated proximally and distally (Chapter 6). Each muscle group is tested in the neutral position by applying force with a similar muscle group. For example, when testing power in the fingers, the clinician uses his or her fingers to test the patient's power. It is also important to compare muscle groups from the patient's left and right side. Subtle UMN weakness can be elicited by looking for a pronator drift in which the patient holds the arms fully extended at the shoulder level with the palms up. Patients are instructed to hold this position for at least 10 seconds with their eyes closed. If the patient has UMN weakness, the weak arm will drift down and pronate. The power of each muscle tested is scored with the Medical Research Council (MRC) grading scale (**Table 7.6**).

Functioning deep tendon reflexes require intact muscles and nerves. They can be assessed with the patient supine or seated (**Table 7.7**). Using a reflex hammer, the tendon is struck to elicit a reflex. Each reflex is graded on a 0 to 4 + scale: absent (0), present only with reinforcement maneuvers (1 +), normal (2 +), hyperactive without clonus (3 +), and hyperactive with clonus (4 +).

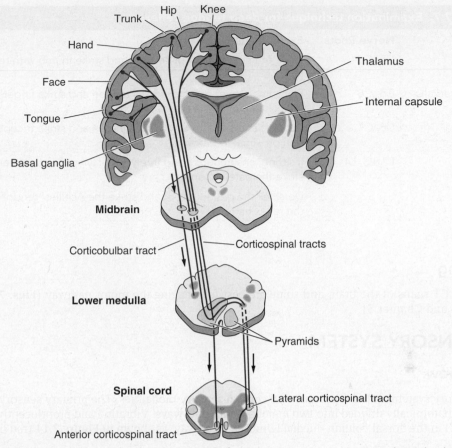

FIGURE 7.12. Corticospinal tract. The UMN travels from the primary motor cortex through white matter tracts to the pyramids where it crosses the midline and then synapses with the LMN in the anterior horn of the spinal cord.

Clonus is tested at the ankle by slightly flexing the knee, rapidly dorsiflexing the foot, and then holding the foot in a flexed position to observe and feel for rhythmic movements. Lastly, the plantar response (Babinski) is tested by stroking the lateral aspect of the sole of the foot upwards and across the ball of the foot medially using a sharp object, such as a tongue depressor. Normally, the toes will flex (**Fig. 7.13A**). An abnormal response is extension and fanning of the toes (**Fig. 7.13B**).

Overall, the findings from the motor examination help determine if a patient's weakness is caused by a UMN or LMN abnormality (**Table 7.8**).

TABLE 7.6. **Medical research council grading scale**	
Grade	Characteristics
5	Active movement against full resistance (normal)
4	Active movement against gravity and some resistance (4– and 4+ can be used)
3	Active movement against gravity but not resistance
2	Active movement with gravity eliminated
1	Flicker or trace of contraction
0	No muscular contraction

TABLE 7.7. Examination technique for deep tendon reflexes

Reflex	Nerve Roots	Exam Technique
Biceps	C5, C6	Place thumb over biceps tendon and strike thumb with reflex hammer
Brachioradialis	C5, C6	Place finger over brachioradialis tendon and strike finger with reflex hammer
Triceps	C6, C7	Support anterior arm on arm of clinician and strike triceps tendon proximal to elbow
Knee	L2, L3, L4	If sitting, ensure legs hang freely and if lying, flex the knee then strike the patellar tendon
Ankle	S1, S2	Dorsiflex the patient's foot and strike the Achilles' tendon with the reflex hammer

Imaging

MRI and CT scans of the brain and spine are best for imaging the motor pathway (**Figs. 7.5, 7.11, and 7.15** and Chapter 5).

■ SENSORY SYSTEM

Overview

The sensory system includes primary and cortical sensory modalities. The primary sensory modalities are anatomically divided into two major sensory pathways. Vibration and proprioceptive sensation travel in the dorsal column–medial lemniscus pathway, as shown in **Figure 7.14** (red line), and

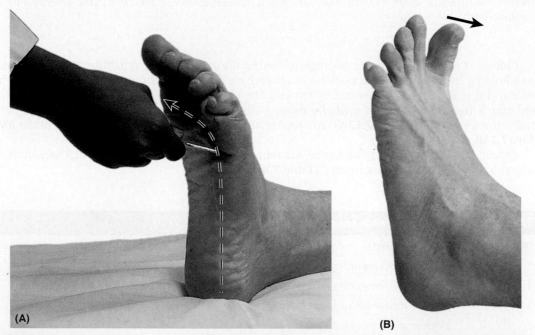

(A)

(B)

FIGURE 7.13. Examination of the plantar response. **A.** Normally, the toes curl downward when the lateral sole is stroked, which is termed "flexor" or "downgoing." **B.** An abnormal response involves "extensor" or "upgoing" toes as shown here.

TABLE 7.8. Clinical findings on the neurologic examination for upper and lower motor neuron lesions

Feature	UMN Lesion	LMN Lesion
Bulk	Usually normal	Atrophy
Involuntary movements	May have spasms	May have fasciculations, cramps
Tone	Increased with spasticity	Decreased (flaccid) or normal

Pattern of weakness	Pronator drift
	Pyramidal pattern:
	  Upper extremities—extensors weaker than flexors
	  Lower extremities—flexors weaker than extensors
	Contralateral to brain lesion
		Depends on process:
		  Nerve root—weakness in associated myotome
		  Nerve—weakness in muscles innervated by involved nerve(s)
		  NMJ—fatigable weakness
		  Muscle—bilateral proximal upper and lower extremity weakness

Reflexes	Hyperreflexia ± clonus	Hyporeflexia or areflexia
Plantar response	Extensor (upgoing)	Flexor (downgoing)

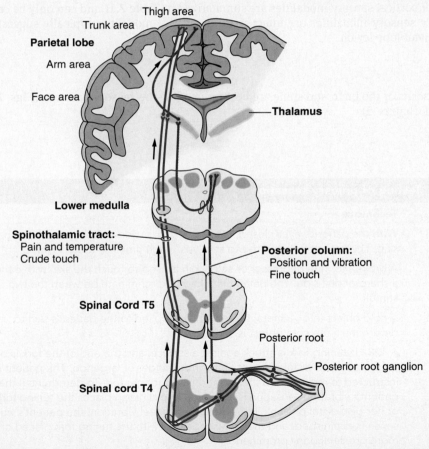

FIGURE 7.14. Dorsal column medial lemniscus (DCML, *red*) and spinothalamic tract (STT, *blue*). The DCML primary order neuron travels up the spinal cord in the ipsilateral posterior columns and then synapses in the medulla. The second-order neuron crosses the midline and travels to the thalamus where it synapses on the third-order neuron that travels to the sensory cortex. The STT primary order neuron synapses in the dorsal horn. The second-order neuron crosses the midline within a few levels and travels to the thalamus where it synapses on the third-order neuron that travels to the sensory cortex.

pain and temperature travel in the spinothalamic tract (blue line). The cortical sensory modalities are two-point discrimination, graphesthesia, stereognosis, and neglect, which are located in the contralateral parietal lobe.

> ● CLINICAL PEARL
>
> The diencephalon lies deep within the brain and contains the thalamus and hypothalamus. The thalamus relays sensory information to the cortex. The hypothalamus is involved in homeostasis, including regulation of temperature, heart rate, and blood pressure. The hypothalamus also produces hormones that impact the pituitary gland, which is important in producing hormones.

Physical Examination

The sensory examination starts with an assessment of each primary sensory modality in the distal aspect of the upper and lower extremities. If there are sensory complaints or abnormal findings, a more detailed examination of the area of impaired sensation is performed to map the location of sensory loss. For each sensory modality, side-by-side comparison should be performed (**Table 7.9**).

By mapping the pattern of sensory loss, it is possible to localize the lesion causing the patient's symptoms (**Table 7.10**).

Testing for cortical sensory modalities are summarized in **Table 7.11** and can only be conducted if the primary sensory modalities are intact. Loss of cortical modalities typically suggests a contralateral parietal lobe lesion.

Imaging

MRI and CT scans of the brain and spine are best for imaging the sensory pathway (**Figs. 7.5, 7.11, and 7.15** and Chapter 5).

TABLE 7.9. Testing of primary sensation	
Sensation	**Technique**
Light touch	With the patient's eyes closed, a cotton swab is used to lightly touch the patient's skin. The patient is instructed to say "yes" each time the touch is felt.
Pain	A broken tongue depressor or safety pin is used to touch the skin with either a sharp or dull side. The patient is asked to discriminate between the two stimuli.
Temperature	A cold object (e.g., a metal tuning fork) is applied to the patient's skin to determine if the cold object is sensed.
Vibration	A 128-Hz tuning fork is struck against a surface, and the end of the fork is placed on the patient's distal phalanx of the index finger or large toe. The patient is instructed to report when the vibration is no longer felt. To determine if the patient's vibration sensation is abnormal, the clinician places the tuning fork on his or her own distal phalanx. If the clinician can feel vibration, the patient's vibration sense is diminished, and the test is repeated with the tuning fork placed on a more proximal bony prominence.
Proprioception	The patient's index finger or large toe is stabilized at the distal interphalangeal joint on the medial and lateral sides. The tip of the digit is moved up or down, and the patient is instructed to detect the direction of movement. If movements are not detected, repeat the test on more proximal joints (similar to vibration testing).

TABLE 7.10. Clinical abnormalities on sensory examination and the most likely location of the lesion

Pattern of Sensory Loss	Localization
Unilateral face/arm/leg	Contralateral brain
Crossed sensory findings (one side of face, opposite side of arm and leg)	Brainstem
Sensory level (loss of all dermatomes below a given level)	Spinal cord
Dermatomal pattern	Nerve root
Specific nerve territory	Nerve

■ COORDINATION

Overview

The cerebellum is involved in the coordination of movement and motor learning. Impairment in motor or sensory functions also impact coordination testing. Cerebellar lesions typically cause impaired ipsilateral coordination. In general, slightly greater coordination may be seen in the dominant hand relative to the nondominant hand.

Physical Examination

Coordination is generally tested with three maneuvers: finger-to-nose, rapid alternating movements, and heel-to-shin. In the finger-to-nose test, the patient is asked to touch the nose with the index finger and then fully extend the arm to touch the clinician's index finger. The patient should repeat these back-and-forth movements quickly and accurately, while the clinician notes the smoothness and accuracy of the movements. In cerebellar disease, dysmetria and intention tremor may be observed.

Rapid alternating movements are tested by having the patient rapidly pronate and supinate the forearm to pat their thigh, alternating between the dorsal and palmar surfaces of the hand. The rate, rhythm, accuracy, and smoothness of the alternating movements should be noted. In cerebellar disease, these movements may be slow and lack rhythmicity and are often characterized by hesitation and pauses. In the heel-to-shin test, instruct the patient to place the heel of one foot on the opposite knee and slide it up and down along the tibia several times. In cerebellar disease, the patient may overshoot or undershoot the knee and demonstrate jerky or unsteady movements.

TABLE 7.11. Testing cortical sensory function

Sensation	Technique
Two-point discrimination	Using an open paperclip or calipers, one or two points of stimulus are applied to the index finger. The patient is asked whether the one or two points of contact are detected. Normally, patients can detect points that are 4–5 mm apart.
Graphesthesia	A number is drawn on the palm of the patient's hand (with patient's eyes closed), and the patient must identify the number.
Stereognosis	An object (e.g., coins or keys) is placed in the patient's hand, and the patient is instructed to identify it with the patient's eyes closed.
Neglect	Neglect can be tested using touch, sound, or visual stimuli. To assess sensory extinction, the patient closes the eyes, and the clinician touches one or both of the patient's hands. The patient is asked to identify which hand was touched (e.g., touched the right, left, or both hands). In the case of neglect, the patient will be able to distinguish right and left, but will not be able to detect when both hands are simultaneously stimulated. The test can also be done with finger wiggling or finger rubbing near one or both ears.

FIGURE 7.15. Axial T2-weighted MRI of the cerebellum. *4*, fourth ventricle; *Cb*, cerebellum; *ICA*, internal carotid artery.

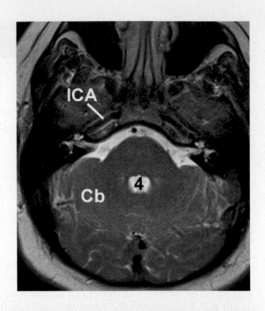

● **CLINICAL PEARL**

Abnormal coordination testing (ataxia) may be secondary to cerebellar dysfunction (cerebellar ataxia) or loss of proprioceptive sensation (sensory ataxia). In an intention tremor, oscillations become more coarse and irregular as the finger approaches a target. Dysmetria is impaired coordination leading to overshooting or undershooting the target. Dysdiadochokinesis is the inability to smoothly perform rapid alternating movements.

Maintaining a stable stance and normal gait requires intact sensation (e.g., vision, proprioception, vestibular systems) and motor function. Sensorimotor integration occurs in the cerebellum. If the cerebellar system is impaired, balance will be impaired even if the eyes are open. If proprioception is impaired, then balance is maintained when the eyes are open and imbalance is seen when the eyes are closed.

The examination of stance begins with inspection of the patient's natural stance. In the Romberg test, the patient stands with the feet together and, if comfortable, with eyes closed. In cerebellar ataxia, the patient will be unable to stand with the feet together even with the eyes open, and this is not indicative of a positive Romberg test. If the patient is steady with the eyes open and off balance when the eyes are closed, this is considered a positive Romberg test and a sign of sensory ataxia. Postural stability is assessed with the forced pullback test, in which the clinician pulls the patient backwards while the patient attempts to maintain stability. When postural stability is impaired (e.g., parkinsonian disorders), there may be retropulsion (several steps taken backward) or the patient may fall backward, requiring support by the clinician. Upon completing the examination of stance, examine the gait and tandem gait (Chapter 6).

Imaging

MRI scan is best for imaging the cerebellum (**Fig. 7.15**).

■ ARTERIES AND VEINS OF THE BRAIN

Overview

Arterial supply to the brain is provided by a pair of internal carotid and vertebral arteries. These four arteries are connected by one anterior and two posterior communicating arteries to form the

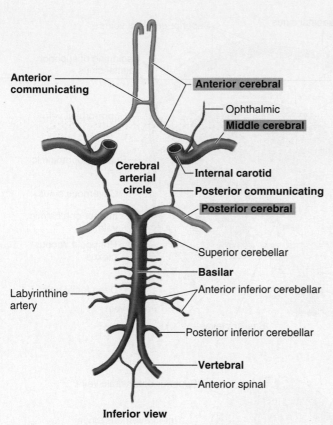

FIGURE 7.16. Schematic representation of the circle of Willis.

circle of Willis (**Fig. 7.16**). The carotid arteries supply the anterior circulation of the brain, and the vertebral arteries supply the posterior circulation of the brain (**Table 7.12**).

A series of cortical veins and venous sinuses drains blood from the brain into the jugular veins (**Fig. 7.17**).

TABLE 7.12. **Major arteries serving the brain**		
Artery	**Origin**	**Distribution Supplied**
Anterior Circulation		
Middle cerebral artery	Internal carotid artery	Lateral cerebral hemispheres and temporal pole
Anterior cerebral artery	Internal carotid artery	Medial cerebral hemispheres and frontal pole
Anterior communicating artery	Connects the anterior cerebral arteries	
Posterior Circulation		
Basilar artery	Formed by joining of the vertebral arteries	Brainstem
Posterior cerebral artery	Basilar artery	Inferior cerebral hemispheres and occipital pole
Posterior communicating artery	Joins internal carotid artery and posterior cerebral artery	
Posterior inferior cerebellar artery	Vertebral artery	Posterior–inferior cerebellum Lateral medulla
Anterior inferior cerebellar artery	Basilar artery	Anterior–inferior cerebellum
Superior cerebellar artery	Basilar artery	Superior cerebellum

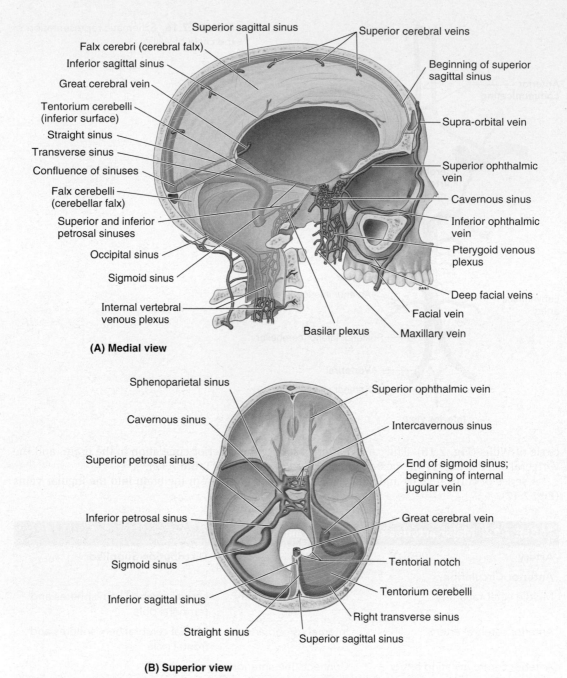

(A) Medial view

(B) Superior view

FIGURE 7.17. Venous sinuses. A. Schematic of left half of cranial cavity and right facial skeleton. B. Venous sinuses of the cranial base.

Physical Examination

As part of the examination of the arteries and veins of the head and neck, a complete neurologic examination is performed. The carotid arteries are palpated to determine the strength and pattern; however, this should be done with caution as pressure can occlude the vessel or dislodge plaques. Next, the carotid arteries are auscultated for bruits. Funduscopy should be performed to inspect for papilledema, loss of venous pulsations, and hemorrhages, which can be seen in elevated intracranial pressure related to venous thrombosis (**Fig. 7.18**).

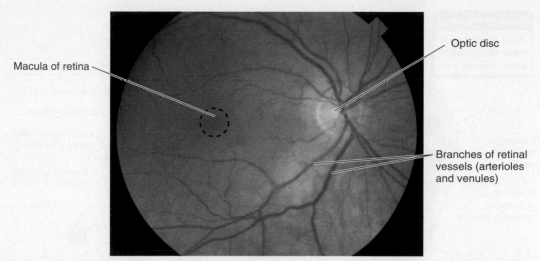

Macula of retina

Optic disc

Branches of retinal vessels (arterioles and venules)

FIGURE 7.18. Fundus of the right eye. Retinal venules (wider) and retinal arterioles (narrower) radiate from the center of the oval optic disc. The dark area lateral to the disc is the macula. Branches of retinal vessels extend toward this area, but do not reach its center, the fovea centralis—the area of most acute vision.

Imaging

The arteries and veins of the head and neck can be assessed using CT or MRI angiogram (for arteries) or venogram (for veins). For extracranial vessels such as the carotid artery, ultrasound can be used.

■ EAR

Overview

The ear is an important sensory organ for hearing and balance through CN VIII. The ear is divided into three parts: external, middle, and internal ear (**Fig. 7.19**). The external ear consists of the auricle and external acoustic meatus. The middle ear is an air space that contains the auditory ossicles. The internal ear contains the membranous labyrinth; its primary divisions are the cochlear labyrinth and the vestibular labyrinth.

Physical Examination

Examination of the ear begins with inspection of the external ear, noting the position, size, symmetry, and any evidence of scars, masses, lesions, or discharge. Next, the pinna and mastoid process are palpated for pain, swelling, or nodules.

The Weber and Rinne tests are bedside screening tests for hearing loss. Sensorineural hearing loss is related to pathology in CN VIII, the inner ear, or the cochlear nucleus in the brainstem. Conductive hearing loss is related to pathology of the outer ear, tympanic membrane, or middle ear such that sound waves are not conducted to the inner ear.

For the Weber test, a 512-Hz tuning fork is struck and placed on the top of the patient's head (**Fig. 7.20**). If the patient reports hearing sound equally in both ears, it is a normal result. If the patient reports that the sound is louder in one ear than the other, this indicates either unilateral conductive hearing loss in the louder ear, or unilateral sensorineural hearing loss in the softer ear. For the Rinne test, a 512-Hz tuning fork is struck and placed on the patient's mastoid process. The patient is instructed to tell the clinician when the sound is no longer heard. At this time, the tuning fork is placed in the front of the patient's ear, and the patient is asked whether the sound was louder when the tuning fork was against the mastoid process or when in front of the ear (**Fig. 7.21**). Normally, the sound should be louder when the tuning fork is held in front of the patient's ear, because

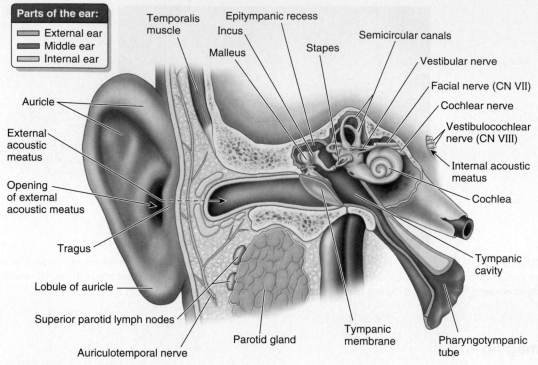

Parts of the ear:
- External ear
- Middle ear
- Internal ear

Temporalis muscle

Epitympanic recess

Incus

Malleus

Stapes

Semicircular canals

Vestibular nerve

Facial nerve (CN VII)

Cochlear nerve

Vestibulocochlear nerve (CN VIII)

Auricle

External acoustic meatus

Internal acoustic meatus

Opening of external acoustic meatus

Cochlea

Tragus

Tympanic cavity

Lobule of auricle

Superior parotid lymph nodes

Auriculotemporal nerve

Parotid gland

Tympanic membrane

Pharyngotympanic tube

FIGURE 7.19. Coronal section of the ear.

air-conducted sound is typically greater than bone-conducted sound. Findings on the Weber and Rinne tests are associated with different patterns of hearing loss (**Table 7.13**).

Otoscopy is an essential aspect of the ear examination to examine the ear canal and tympanic membrane. Holding the otoscope like a pencil or hammer, the pinna is gently pulled posterosuperiorly, and the otoscope is carefully inserted to avoid damage to the external auditory canal and tympanic membrane. The normal tympanic membrane should be intact, ovoid,

FIGURE 7.20. Weber test.

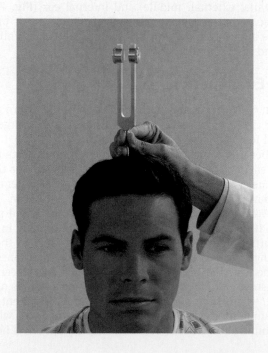

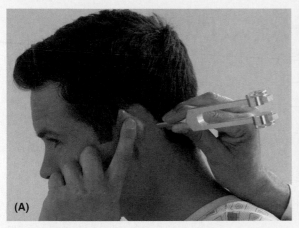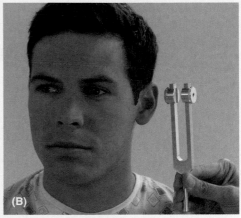

FIGURE 7.21. Rinne test. **A.** Testing bone conduction. **B.** Testing air conduction.

semitransparent, and gray. Examine the external ear canal for erythema, swelling, tenderness, foreign bodies, discharge, and any other abnormalities (**Fig. 7.22**). Next, the tympanic membrane is inspected noting the color, integrity, transparency, and position. Lastly, the pars tensa, pars flaccida, handle of malleus, and light reflex should be identified (**Fig. 7.23**).

Imaging

Imaging of the ear can be achieved with CT scan or MRI (**Fig. 7.24**).

■ NOSE AND SINUSES

Overview

The nose consists of two nostrils separated by the nasal septum. The lateral walls of the nose contain the inferior, middle, and superior turbinates (conchae) that help regulate airflow and moisten and humidify air in conjunction with the sinuses (**Fig. 7.25A**). The four sinuses are the ethmoid, sphenoid, frontal, and maxillary sinuses (**Fig. 7.25B**). The nose also plays a role in olfactory sensation in conjunction with CN I.

Physical Examination

Examination begins with inspecting the size and symmetry of the nose as well as noting any scars, swelling, signs of trauma, or nasal deviation. Next, the patency of the nostrils is assessed by occluding one nostril at a time and assessing ease of air movement through the other nostril. The external nose and frontal and maxillary sinuses are palpated for tenderness that may indicate a sinus infection. The internal nose is inspected using an otoscope or nasal speculum. The septum, vestibule,

TABLE 7.13. Interpretation of tuning fork tests		
Pattern of Hearing Loss	**Weber Test[a]**	**Rinne Test**
Normal or bilateral SNHL	Central	AC > BC bilaterally
Right-sided CHL; normal left ear	Right	Left side AC > BC; right side AC < BC
Right-sided SNHL; normal left ear	Left	Left side AC > BC; right side AC > BC
Right-sided severe SNHL; normal left ear	Left	Left side AC > BC; right side BC > AC

SNHL, sensorineural hearing loss; CHL, conductive hearing loss; AC, air conduction; BC, bone conduction.
[a]Left and right refer to which ear the vibration is louder. Central refers to the vibration being heard equally in both ears.

FIGURE 7.22. Surface anatomy of the external ear.

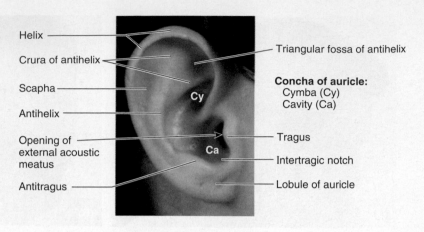

Helix

Crura of antihelix

Scapha

Antihelix

Opening of external acoustic meatus

Antitragus

Triangular fossa of antihelix

Concha of auricle:
Cymba (Cy)
Cavity (Ca)

Tragus

Intertragic notch

Lobule of auricle

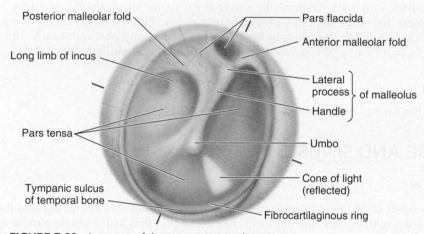

Posterior malleolar fold

Long limb of incus

Pars tensa

Tympanic sulcus of temporal bone

Pars flaccida

Anterior malleolar fold

Lateral process
Handle } of malleolus

Umbo

Cone of light (reflected)

Fibrocartilaginous ring

FIGURE 7.23. Anatomy of the tympanic membrane.

FIGURE 7.24. CT scan at the base of the skull demonstrating the external auditory canals. Note the following structures: *CA*, carotid artery; *E*, opening of the eustachian tube; *EAC*, external auditory canal; *J*, jugular foramen; *M*, mandibular condyle.

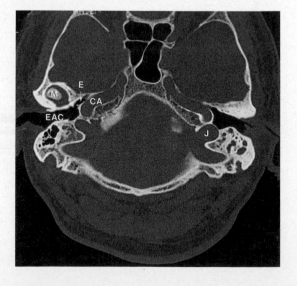

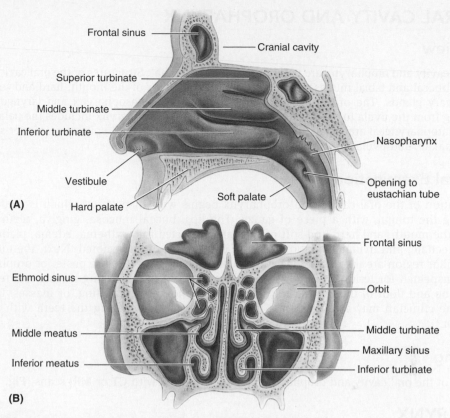

(A)

(B)

FIGURE 7.25. Nasopharynx and paranasal sinuses. **A.** Midsagittal dissection of the posterior part of the lateral wall of the nasal cavity and the palate. **B.** Coronal dissection of the paranasal sinuses and nasal cavity.

mucous membranes, and the middle and inferior turbinates are inspected for signs of inflammation, exudates, bleeding, discharge, trauma, masses, and polyps.

Imaging

Imaging of the nose and sinuses can be obtained using x-rays (**Fig. 7.26**) or CT scan.

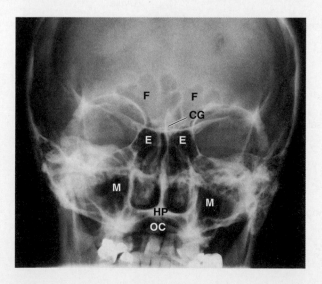

FIGURE 7.26. X-ray of the cranium demonstrating the nasal cavity and paranasal sinuses. *CG*, crista galli; *E*, ethmoidal air cells; *F*, frontal sinus; *HP*, hard palate; *M*, maxillary sinus; *OC*, oral cavity.

ORAL CAVITY AND OROPHARYNX

Overview

The oral cavity and oropharynx are part of the alimentary canal. Structures of the oral cavity include the lips, buccal and labial mucosa, gingiva, teeth, tongue, floor of the mouth, hard and soft palate, and salivary glands. The oropharynx is continuous with the nasopharynx and laryngopharynx, extending from the uvula to the level of the hyoid bone. The oropharynx includes the palatoglossal arch, palatopharyngeal arch, palatine tonsils, base of the tongue and epiglottis, inferior surface of the soft palate, and uvula (**Fig. 7.27**).

Physical Examination

Examination of the oral cavity and oropharynx begins with inspection, which is facilitated by retracting the tongue with a piece of gauze. The lips, buccal mucosa, gingiva, teeth, tongue, floor of the mouth, and hard and soft palates are inspected for erythema, edema, plaques, papules, petechiae, and uvular deviation. Overall dentition should be noted. Next, the tonsils and peritonsillar region are inspected for exudates and swelling. Lastly, the posterior oropharyngeal wall is inspected for lesions, discharge, swelling, and ulceration. Using a bimanual technique, the tongue and floor of the mouth are palpated for tenderness, swelling, or masses. In certain cases, the clinician may examine for a dental abscess by percussing the teeth with a tongue depressor.

Imaging

Imaging of the oral cavity and oropharynx can be performed with CT or MRI scans (**Fig. 7.28**).

LARYNX

Overview

The larynx extends vertically from the tip of the epiglottis to the inferior border of the cricoid cartilage and is divided into three compartments: the vestibule, middle compartment with left and right ventricles, and the infraglottic cavity. The vocal cords are contained within the larynx (**Fig. 7.29**).

FIGURE 7.27. Anatomy of the oral cavity.

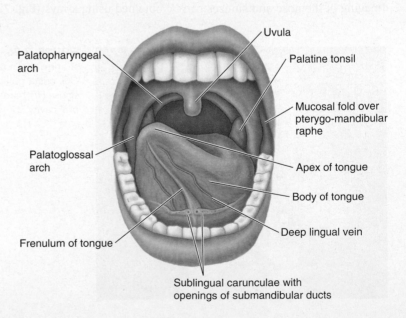

Uvula

Palatopharyngeal arch

Palatine tonsil

Mucosal fold over pterygo-mandibular raphe

Palatoglossal arch

Apex of tongue

Body of tongue

Deep lingual vein

Frenulum of tongue

Sublingual carunculae with openings of submandibular ducts

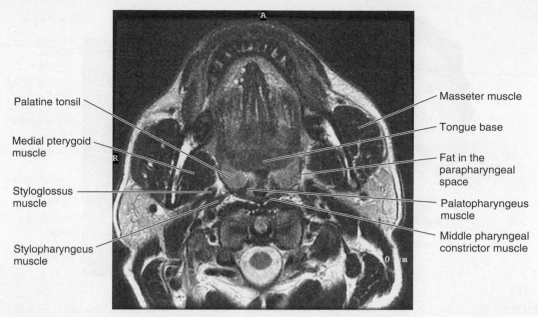

FIGURE 7.28. Axial T2-weighted MRI of the oropharynx.

Labels: Palatine tonsil, Medial pterygoid muscle, Styloglossus muscle, Stylopharyngeus muscle, Masseter muscle, Tongue base, Fat in the parapharyngeal space, Palatopharyngeus muscle, Middle pharyngeal constrictor muscle

Physical Examination

Examination of the larynx is performed via indirect laryngoscopy. The tongue is gently retracted, and a small angled mirror is placed at the back of the oropharynx to visualize the larynx. The epiglottis, vallecula, piriform sinuses, arytenoids, aryepiglottic folds, false vocal folds, true vocal cords, and the subglottic region are examined for nodules, lesions, or ulcerations (**Fig. 7.30**). The dynamic movements of the vocal cords are assessed by instructing the patient to phonate (e.g., ask the patient to say "eeeee") and deeply inspire, looking for asymmetrical movements. These maneuvers cause the vocal cords to adduct and abduct, respectively.

Imaging

The larynx is best imaged with CT or MRI scans.

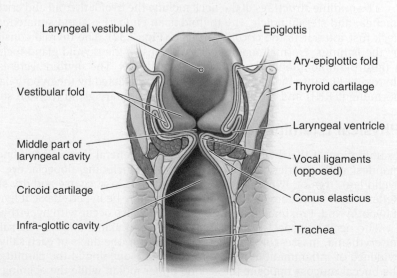

FIGURE 7.29. Posterior view of the coronal section of the larynx.

Labels: Laryngeal vestibule, Vestibular fold, Middle part of laryngeal cavity, Cricoid cartilage, Infra-glottic cavity, Epiglottis, Ary-epiglottic fold, Thyroid cartilage, Laryngeal ventricle, Vocal ligaments (opposed), Conus elasticus, Trachea

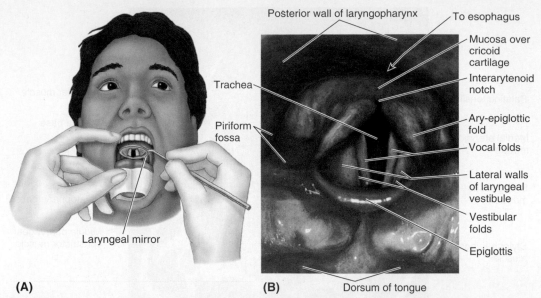

Posterior wall of laryngopharynx

To esophagus

Mucosa over cricoid cartilage

Interarytenoid notch

Trachea

Piriform fossa

Ary-epiglottic fold

Vocal folds

Lateral walls of laryngeal vestibule

Vestibular folds

Epiglottis

Laryngeal mirror

(A)

(B)

Dorsum of tongue

FIGURE 7.30. Examination of the laryngopharynx. **A.** Indirect laryngoscopy. **B.** View of the larynx by indirect laryngoscopy.

◼ NECK

Overview

The neck includes muscles, salivary glands, great vessels, thyroid and parathyroid glands, and lymph nodes.

The muscles of the neck are divided into anterior and posterior triangles by the SCM muscles. The anterior triangle is bound by the mandible superiorly, the SCM muscle laterally, the midline of the neck medially, and the sternum inferiorly.

The three major pairs of salivary glands in the neck are the parotid, submandibular, and sublingual glands. The parotid glands lie inferior and anterior to the acoustic meatus, while the submandibular and sublingual glands lie beneath the mandible and tongue (**Fig. 7.31**).

The great vessels include the carotid artery and the jugular vein, which splits into the internal jugular vein that lies deep to the SCM muscle and the external jugular vein that lies superficial to the SCM.

The midline structures of the neck include the hyoid, thyroid and cricoid cartilage, thyroid gland, trachea, and sternal notch. The thyroid is an endocrine gland situated in the anterior aspect of the neck just inferior to the cricoid cartilage (**Fig. 7.32**). The thyroid consists of two lobes connected by the isthmus. Normal anatomical variations of the thyroid gland include an absent isthmus and a third pyramidal lobe located above the isthmus. The thyroid secretes triiodothyronine (T_3) and thyroxine (T_4) into the bloodstream, which is regulated by the hypothalamus (thyrotropin-releasing hormone [TRH]) and the anterior lobe of the pituitary gland (thyroid stimulating hormone [TSH]).

Physical Examination

Examination of the thyroid gland begins with general inspection. Abnormal thyroid function can manifest with a variety of systemic symptoms including alopecia, eye changes (e.g., proptosis or eyelid lag), tremor, hyperhidrosis, weight gain or loss, coarse and dry skin, and peripheral edema. Reflexes and power are also tested. A patient may be hyperreflexic if hyperthyroid and hyporeflexic if hypothyroid. Proximal muscle weakness may also occur with hyperthyroidism or hypothyroidism.

The neck is inspected for masses, scars, and skin changes. The salivary glands are examined for erythema, masses, or asymmetry. In addition, the ducts of each salivary gland are inspected for evidence of inflammation, pus, or a stone. The opening of the parotid duct (Stensen duct) lies on the buccal mucosa opposite the second upper molar, while the opening of the submandibular duct

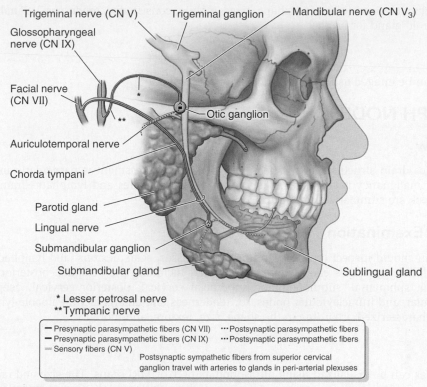

FIGURE 7.31. Innervation of the salivary glands.

(Wharton duct) opens into the floor of the mouth just lateral to the midline at the junction of the tongue and the floor of mouth. The clinician should palpate the salivary glands for masses, tenderness, and regional lymphadenopathy.

The thyroid is palpated by first identifying the cricoid cartilage, located in the lower portion of the neck inferior to the thyroid cartilage and anterior to the C5 vertebrae. Once the cricoid cartilage is identified, the clinician should palpate the isthmus and lobes of the thyroid gland. Asking the patient to swallow helps displace the thyroid gland superiorly to aid in palpation. Any nodules

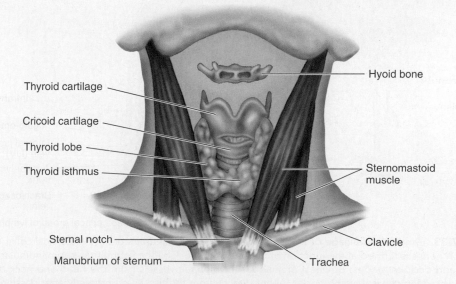

FIGURE 7.32. Location of the thyroid gland and surrounding structures.

should be characterized (e.g., size, shape, fixed/mobile, consistency, tenderness). Finally, auscultate the thyroid gland for bruits.

Imaging

The neck can be imaged using ultrasound, CT or MRI scan.

■ LYMPH NODES

Overview

Lymph nodes drain structures of the head and neck, and assessment is particularly important if infection or malignancy is suspected. The groups of lymph nodes and lymphatic drainage of the head and neck are summarized in **Figure 7.33**.

Physical Examination

The clinician should inspect the head and neck for masses, scars, lesions, and lymphadenopathy. Next, the clinician palpates each lymph node group, including the occipital, posterior auricular, pre-auricular, submental, submandibular, superficial cervical, posterior cervical, deep cervical, supraclavicular, and infraclavicular nodes, for tenderness and enlargement. Palpable lymph nodes should be characterized according to the shape, size, texture, and mobility.

Imaging

Lymph nodes can be visualized using ultrasound and CT or MRI scans. The size and radiographic characteristics of lymph nodes can help determine if they are normal, benign or malignant enlargements. Possible radiographic findings of malignant lymph nodes include calcification, irregular borders, large size, and lymphovascular invasion.

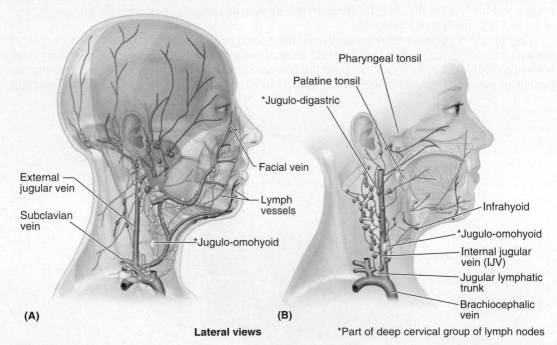

(A)

External jugular vein

Subclavian vein

*Jugulo-omohyoid

Facial vein

Lymph vessels

(B)

Pharyngeal tonsil

Palatine tonsil

*Jugulo-digastric

Infrahyoid

*Jugulo-omohyoid

Internal jugular vein (IJV)

Jugular lymphatic trunk

Brachiocephalic vein

Lateral views

*Part of deep cervical group of lymph nodes

FIGURE 7.33. Lymphatic drainage of face and scalp. **A.** Superficial drainage. A pericervical collar of superficial lymph nodes is formed at the junction of the head and neck by the submental, submandibular, parotid, mastoid, and occipital nodes. **B.** Deep drainage. All lymphatic vessels from the head and neck ultimately drain into the deep cervical lymph nodes, either directly from the tissues or indirectly after passing through an outlying group of nodes.

CLINICAL CASES

 ISCHEMIC STROKE

Presentation

A 72-year-old male with atrial fibrillation, dyslipidemia, hypertension, and type 2 diabetes mellitus (DM) is suddenly unable to speak or understand language. He also has right-sided face and arm weakness.

Definition

Ischemic stroke is a clinical syndrome characterized by a sudden onset of focal neurological deficits, presumed to be due to a perfusion defect in a vascular territory. Transient ischemic attack (TIA) is a sudden and transient episode of neurological dysfunction caused by ischemia without evidence of infarction on imaging. The signs and symptoms depend on the affected vascular territory.

What are common causes?

Common causes include

Etiology	Description
Large artery atherosclerosis	Caused by thromboembolism and includes large artery-to-artery embolism with clot originating from one artery and blocking a distal artery
Cardioembolic	Caused by embolism from the heart and includes atrial fibrillation, left atrial or ventricular thrombi, valvular thrombi (e.g., endocarditis), and paradoxical emboli through a patent foramen ovale or atrial septal defect
Small vessel occlusion (lacunar)	Caused by lipohyalinosis, which involves changes to small blood vessel walls secondary to hypertension
Other determined etiology	Caused by arterial dissection, vasculitis, hypercoaguable states, vasculopathy due to drugs such as cocaine, and rare genetic causes
Undetermined etiology (cryptogenic)	Etiology undetermined after investigations

● CLINICAL PEARL

Stroke risk factors include hypertension, DM, dyslipidemia, family history of stroke and coronary artery disease, and smoking.

What is the differential diagnosis?

Acute-onset focal neurologic deficits: The differential diagnosis includes intracranial hemorrhage, intracranial tumors, seizures, migraine with aura, metabolic disturbances (hypo-/hyperglycemia), brain abscess, hypertensive encephalopathy, and conversion disorder.

TABLE 7.14. Symptoms based on vascular territory

Vascular Territory	Symptom
Middle cerebral artery	Contralateral weakness, contralateral numbness, vision changes, difficulty speaking and/or understanding, and ignoring one side of the body
Anterior cerebral artery	Contralateral weakness and contralateral numbness
Posterior cerebral artery	Visual loss, sensory loss, and memory loss
Basilar artery	Weakness in all extremities and difficulty gazing horizontally
Posterior inferior cerebellar artery	Sensory loss, difficulty speaking and swallowing, dizziness, nausea and vomiting, hiccups, and lack of coordination

What symptoms might be observed?

Signs and symptoms depend on the vascular territory and brain areas affected (**Table 7.14**).

What are the possible findings on examination?

Vital signs: Typically normal, but hypertension may be present.

Neurologic examination: In the acute setting, a screening neurologic examination is performed. In the Emergency Department, clinicians determine the time of onset and may calculate a stroke score such as the National Institutes of Health Stroke Scale (NIHSS). The clinical examination is unable to distinguish between ischemic stroke and intracerebral hemorrhage (ICH). Features that increase the likelihood of intracranial hemorrhage include coma (LR 6.2), neck stiffness (LR 5), seizure (LR 4.7), diastolic blood pressure >110 mm Hg (LR 4.3), vomiting (LR 3), and headache (LR 2.9); however, the clinical exam is not accurate enough to reliably exclude intracerebral hemorrhage (ICH). A summary of signs by vascular territory is presented in **Table 7.15**.

Mental status: Occasionally decreased level of alertness or responsiveness.

Language: Expressive aphasia, receptive aphasia, or both, particularly in dominant-hemisphere strokes. Naming, reading, fluency, comprehension, writing, and/or repetition may be impaired.

TABLE 7.15. Signs based on vascular territory

Vascular Territory	Signs
Middle cerebral artery (MCA)	Contralateral UMN pattern of weakness, arm/face > leg Contralateral loss of primary sensory modalities Contralateral homonymous hemianopsia Gaze deviation toward side of lesion Aphasia (left MCA only) Neglect (more in right MCA stroke, neglect to contralateral side)
Anterior cerebral artery	Contralateral UMN pattern of weakness, leg > face/arm Contralateral loss of primary sensory modalities
Posterior cerebral artery	Contralateral homonymous hemianopsia (if bilateral, cortical blindness) Contralateral sensory loss
Basilar artery	"Locked-in" syndrome with quadriplegia and inability to gaze horizontally
Posterior–inferior cerebellar artery	Crossed sensory findings (loss of pain and temperature sensation of the ipsilateral face and contralateral body) Dysphagia and dysarthria Ipsilateral cerebellar dysfunction

Raising Eyebrows

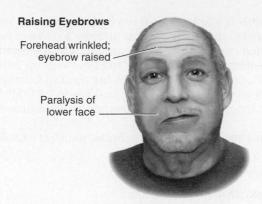

Forehead wrinkled;
eyebrow raised

Paralysis of
lower face

FIGURE 7.34. Upper motor neuron facial paresis.

CNs: Quadrantanopsia or hemianopsia with inability to see part of the visual field. Horizontal eye movements may show a gaze deviation or inability to look in a certain direction. Complete or partial unilateral facial weakness with a UMN pattern may be present (**Fig. 7.34**). The speech may be slurred (dysarthria).

Motor: Weakness of one or more extremities with associated spasticity and hyperreflexia.

Sensory: Loss or decrease in pinprick sensation on one side. If sensation is intact, the clinician can check for neglect or extinction to stimuli on one side of the body.

Coordination: Impaired coordination of the limbs on finger-to-nose or heel-to-shin testing.

What tests should be ordered?

Laboratory tests: CBC, metabolic panel (electrolytes, extended electrolytes, glucose, Cr, liver enzymes), coagulation profile (check for elevated international normalized ration [INR] and partial thromboplastin time [PTT] to determine if anticoagulated), other serology (elevated cholesterol levels in dyslipidemia and elevated HbA1c in DM).

Imaging: MRI scan of the brain is the gold standard to diagnose stroke. Stroke is confirmed by diffusion restriction, which is seen as hyperintense on diffusion-weighted imaging (DWI) and hypointense on apparent diffusion coefficient (ADC) sequences. Given limited availability, plain CT scan of the head is most often used in the acute stroke setting for diagnosis and to rule out ICH (**Fig. 7.35**). Early in ischemic stroke, findings may be subtle with loss of gray-white differentiation and sulcal effacement. Over time, the area of ischemia appears hypodense.

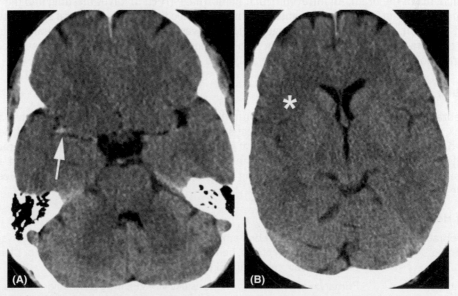

(A)   (B)

FIGURE 7.35. Acute infarct. **A.** Axial CT scan shows a linear density consistent with a "dense MCA" (*arrow*), a sign of thrombosis of the right middle cerebral artery. **B.** At the level of the basal ganglia, there is subtle loss of gray–white differentiation and sulcal effacement (*asterisk*), signs of acute ischemia.

The gold standard for investigating carotid stenosis is a conventional cerebral angiogram. However, this is an invasive procedure with associated risks, so usually patients undergo a noninvasive method of evaluation for carotid stenosis, including carotid Doppler ultrasound, CT angiogram (CTA), or MRI angiogram (MRA). Carotid Doppler ultrasound measures blood flow velocity, with high velocity suggesting high-grade stenosis (Sn 0.91, Sp 0.87). CTA and MRA use contrast to image the carotid arteries; they are effective in detecting high-grade stenosis (CTA Sn 0.85, Sp 0.93; MRA Sn 0.95, Sp 0.92). In those with renal failure who cannot have contrast administered, MRA time of flight can image the carotids (Sn 0.91, Sp 0.88).

Transthoracic or transesophageal echocardiograms are used to rule out a cardiac source of emboli.

Special Tests

A 48-hour Holter monitor is used to assess for paroxysmal atrial fibrillation.

Diagnostic scores: The NIHSS is a rapid neurologic examination performed in acute stroke to determine the severity and distribution. This examination includes components of the neurologic examination and is scored out of 42, with higher scores indicating greater neurologic dysfunction.

INTRACRANIAL HEMORRHAGE

Presentation

A 55-year-old male with a history of hypertension presents with sudden-onset severe headache with associated nausea and vomiting. On arrival at the Emergency Department, he was drowsy and then became unresponsive.

Definition

Intracranial hemorrhage involves bleeding within the cranium. There are multiple areas in which bleeding can occur correspond to different types of intracranial hemorrhages. An ICH involves bleeding within the parenchyma of the brain. An intraventricular hemorrhage (IVH) involves bleeding into the ventricular system of the brain. An epidural hemorrhage involves bleeding into the epidural space between the dura and the skull. A subdural hemorrhage (SDH) involves bleeding into the subdural space, located between the dura mater and arachnoid layer. A subarachnoid hemorrhage (SAH) involves bleeding into the subarachnoid space, located between the arachnoid layer and pia mater (**Fig. 7.36**).

What are common causes?

Intracerebral hemorrhages are caused by ruptured small penetrator arteries, aneurysms, and arteriovenous malformations (AVMs). IVHs are caused by ruptured large arteries or small penetrator arteries, or a large intracranial hemorrhage that ruptures into the ventricles. Epidural hemorrhages are bleeds from the middle meningeal artery, anterior meningeal artery, anterior ethmoid artery, or venous sinuses. SDHs are bleeds from bridging veins in the subdural space. SAHs are bleeds from the Circle of Willis intracranial arteries.

Type of Hemorrhage	Etiologies
Intracerebral hemorrhage	Hypertension, cerebral amyloid angiopathy, trauma, ruptured aneurysm, vascular malformations, hemorrhagic infarction, anticoagulants or bleeding disorder, brain tumor, and drugs (cocaine)
Intraventricular hemorrhages	Primary: vascular malformations (AVM/AVF), intraventricular tumors, intraventricular aneurysms, coagulopathies, drugs (cocaine), pituitary apoplexy, and hypertension Secondary: trauma and ICH/SAH

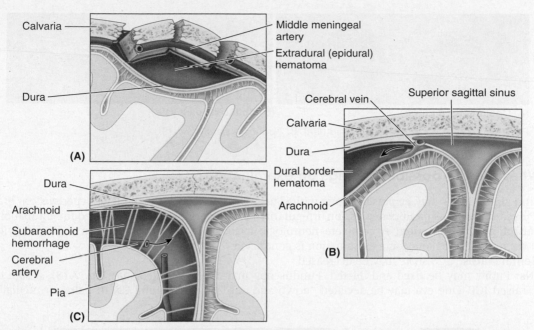

FIGURE 7.36 Intracranial hemorrhages. **A.** Epidural hemorrhage. **B.** Subdural hemorrhage. **C.** Subarachnoid hemorrhage.

Epidural hemorrhage	Trauma (most common), coagulopathy, and dural vascular malformations
Subdural hemorrhages	Trauma (can be minor, especially in elderly) and anticoagulants/coagulopathy; rarely, AVM and meningioma
Subarachnoid hemorrhage	Aneurysmal rupture, AVM, intracranial arterial dissection, trauma, and anticoagulants/coagulopathy

What is the differential diagnosis?

Elevated intracranial pressure (ICP) and focal neurologic symptoms: The differential diagnosis includes intracranial hemorrhage, ischemic stroke, sinus venous thrombosis, intracranial tumor, infection (e.g., brain abscess, meningitis, or encephalitis), metabolic disturbance, hypertensive encephalopathy, and seizure.

What symptoms might be observed?

All hemorrhages can present with nausea, vomiting, and severe headache. Patients may also present with drowsiness, seizures, and focal neurologic deficits which depend on the location of the hemorrhage. An IVH may cause visual changes related to CN palsies from increased ICP. A SDH may present with a more chronic headache and cognitive changes. A SAH may also present with neck stiffness.

> ### ● CLINICAL PEARL
>
> Typically, intracranial hemorrhages result in symptoms of raised ICP, such as headache, nausea, vomiting, and decreased LOC. Increased ICP may also result in herniation syndromes, for instance, uncal herniation that leads to compression of the ipsilateral oculomotor cranial nerve (CN III) resulting in an ipsilateral dilated pupil with lateral and downward ("down and out") eye position. Increased ICP can also lead to abducens nerve (CN VI) palsy via downward displacement of the brainstem causing traction on the fascicular component of CN VI. This results in medial deviation of the eye (**Fig. 7.37**).

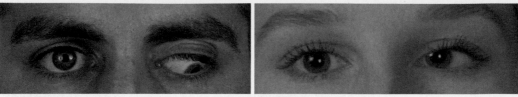

(A) Oculomotor paralysis　　　　　　　　**(B) Abducens paralysis**

FIGURE 7.37. A. Oculomotor paralysis (*left*). B. Abducens paralysis (*left*).

What are the possible findings on examination?

Vital signs: Fever may be present along with signs related to raised ICP, namely, hypertension, bradycardia, and respiratory depression/irregularity (Cushing triad). Patients may require intubation.

Neurologic examination: A complete neurologic exam cannot be completed in a patient with decreased LOC, so a coma examination is conducted.

Mental status: GCS score may be decreased.

CNs: Pupils may be fixed and dilated. Funduscopy may reveal papilledema (**Fig. 7.18**), a sign of raised ICP. One eye may be deviated "down and out," suggestive of a CN III palsy, or medially

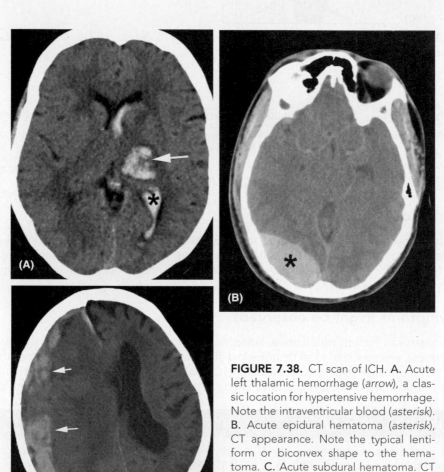

FIGURE 7.38. CT scan of ICH. **A.** Acute left thalamic hemorrhage (*arrow*), a classic location for hypertensive hemorrhage. Note the intraventricular blood (*asterisk*). **B.** Acute epidural hematoma (*asterisk*), CT appearance. Note the typical lentiform or biconvex shape to the hematoma. **C.** Acute subdural hematoma. CT images show a crescentic extra-axial subdural hematoma (*arrows*). There is significant mass effect. This is a neurosurgical emergency.

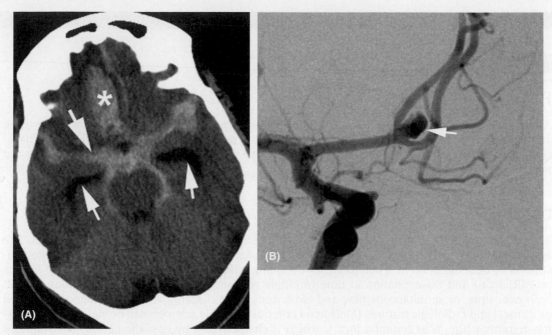

FIGURE 7.39. Subarachnoid hemorrhage with aneurysm of the anterior communicating artery. **A.** Axial CT scan shows acute SAH within the suprasellar cistern (*large arrow*) with extension into the interhemispheric fissure and inferior right frontal lobe (*asterisk*). Note the dilated temporal horns of the lateral ventricles (*small arrows*) consistent with hydrocephalus secondary to intraventricular hemorrhage (not shown). **B.** Cerebral angiogram shows the aneurysm arising from the anterior communicating artery (*arrow*).

deviated in a CN VI palsy. Facial asymmetry may be noted. There may be loss of brainstem reflexes, including the oculocephalic, corneal, and gag reflexes.

Motor: Tone may be spastic and reflexes hyperreflexic.

What tests should be ordered?

Laboratory tests: There are no laboratory abnormalities specific to intracranial hemorrhage, but labs may help evaluate associated conditions (e.g., coagulopathy). Investigations include CBC, metabolic panel (electrolytes, extended electrolytes, glucose, Cr, liver enzymes), and coagulation profile (check for an elevated INR and PTT to determine if the patient is anticoagulated).

Imaging: CT scan is very sensitive in detecting acute hemorrhage and is considered the gold standard for intracerebral hemorrhage. MRI scans of the brain are equally effective in intracerebral hemorrhage and can be done to further characterize the hemorrhage and to determine if there is an underlying lesion such as a tumor or ischemic stroke. Epidural and SDHs are also well detected by CT and MRI scans. For SAH, evidence supports CT scan as being most sensitive within the first 6 hours after symptom onset (Sn 1.0, Sp 1.0), but sensitivity decreases with time (overall Sn 0.93, Sp 1). If a negative CT scan is obtained 6 hours after symptom onset, but clinical suspicion remains high for SAH, an LP is performed to evaluate the CSF for red blood cells and xanthochromia. Refer to **Figure 7.38** for CT scans of the different types of intracranial hemorrhages.

The gold standard for detecting vascular abnormalities, particularly aneurysms in intracranial hemorrhage, and in particular SAH, is conventional cerebral angiography (**Fig. 7.39**). CTA can also be used to detect aneurysms (Sn 0.98, Sp 0.89) and is sensitive for aneurysms >3–5 mm, but may not detect smaller aneurysms.

MULTIPLE SCLEROSIS

Presentation

A 26-year-old Caucasian female presents with 1 week of numbness and paresthesias in the trunk and extremities. She also noticed a shock-like sensation down her spine when she flexes her neck. One year ago, she experienced visual loss in her left eye that fully recovered over several weeks and was diagnosed with optic neuritis.

Definition

Multiple sclerosis (MS) is an autoimmune inflammatory demyelinating condition of the CNS. The age of symptom onset is typically 15–50 years. The diagnosis of multiple sclerosis requires demonstration of dissemination in space (relapses involving different sites in the CNS or multiple lesions on MRI scan) and dissemination in time (multiple relapses, development of new lesions on MRI scan over time, or simultaneous new and old lesions on MRI scan). Therefore, diagnosis is based on clinical and radiologic features (McDonald criteria). Multiple sclerosis can be classified as relapsing–remitting (the most common form), which is characterized by episodic neurologic symptoms with onset over hours to days and improvement over weeks to months, or primary progressive, which is characterized by progressive neurologic disability without relapses. Relapsing remitting MS can transition to secondary progressive MS over time with accumulating disability.

What are common causes?

Multiple sclerosis is multifactorial with several possible etiologies. It is hypothesized that both environmental and genetic factors contribute. Environmental factors associated with multiple sclerosis include viral infections (EBV), low vitamin D levels, geographic factors (higher prevalence further from the equator), and smoking.

What is the differential diagnosis?

Other CNS demyelinating diseases: The differential diagnosis includes acute disseminated encephalomyelitis (ADEM), neuromyelitis optica (NMO), optic neuritis, transverse myelitis, systemic lupus erythematosus (SLE), vasculitis, Behçet disease, sarcoidosis, syphilis, Lyme disease, and vitamin B_{12} deficiency.

What symptoms might be observed?

Symptoms of multiple sclerosis include fatigue, depression, vision loss, double vision, stiffness or weakness, sensory loss and paresthesias, imbalance or incoordination, and bowel and bladder dysfunction with urgency and incontinence. Patients may experience an electrical sensation running down the back with neck flexion (L'hermitte sign). Symptoms may worsen in hot conditions (Uhthoff phenomenon).

What are the possible findings on examination?

Vital signs: Typically normal.
Neurologic examination: A complete neurologic examination should be performed looking for abnormalities.
Mental status: Cognitive testing may show impairments in all domains, but commonly executive function or attention.
CNs: RAPD and decreased color vision may be present in optic neuritis. RAPD is detected using the swinging flashlight test. Normally, both pupils constrict as the light is swung between the eyes. An RAPD is present when both pupils paradoxically dilate when the light is swung from the normal to the abnormal eye. This is generally a sign of dysfunction in the optic nerve or retina of one eye. The affected eye may have optic disc edema on funduscopy acutely, and chronically,

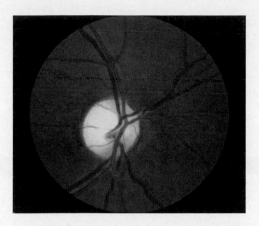

FIGURE 7.40. Pale/white optic disc due to loss of nerve cells after optic neuritis.

the involved optic disc appears pale (**Fig. 7.40**). On examination of extraocular movements, nystagmus (involuntary eye movements) or an internuclear ophthalmoplegia (INO) due to a lesion in the medial longitudinal fasciculus of the brainstem may be present. An INO is observed when testing horizontal eye movements and/or saccades in which the affected eye is unable to fully adduct when looking contralaterally; the contralateral eye demonstrates nystagmus.

Motor: Spasticity, an UMN pattern of weakness, and hyperreflexia/clonus with upgoing plantar responses. Tonic spasms may also be observed.

Sensory: Decreased sensation of pinprick, cold, proprioception, and vibration sensation.

Coordination: Dysmetria.

Gait: Spastic or ataxic gait may be observed.

What tests should be ordered?

Laboratory tests: Other serology (erythrocyte sedimentation rate [ESR], C-reactive protein [CRP], antinuclear antibody [ANA], antineutrophil cytoplasmic antibody [ANCA], rheumatoid factor [RF], anti-dsDNA antibody, complement C3 and C4, antiphospholipid antibodies, vitamin B12, syphilis screen), and CSF (oligoclonal bands [positive in 87.9% of patients] or an elevated IgG index support the diagnosis of MS).

Imaging: There is no gold standard test to diagnose MS. MRI of the brain and spinal cord with gadolinium is the test of choice and is part of the McDonald criteria (Sn 0.35–1.0, Sp 0.36–0.92) (**Fig. 7.41**). Generally, multiple T2 hyperintensities are present in specific locations

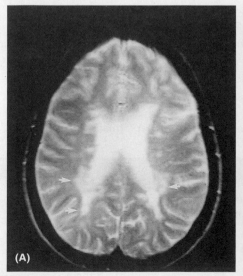
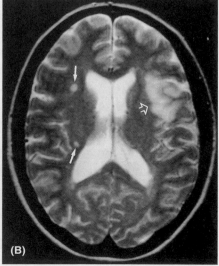

FIGURE 7.41. Multiple sclerosis. **A.** T2-weighted MRI showing areas of ventricular plaques of high signal (*arrows*). **B.** T2-weighted image in another patient shows small periventricular plaques (*solid arrows*) as well as an area of left parietal infarction (*open arrow*).

(periventricular, juxtacortical, infratentorial, spinal cord), and active lesions may show contrast enhancement. CT scan may detect some lesions, but may miss many lesions.

Special Tests

Visual, somatosensory, and auditory brainstem EPs can provide evidence of CNS lesions that are not otherwise clinically apparent.

BRAIN ABSCESS

Presentation

A 55-year-old female on immunosuppressive medications for a heart transplant presents with a 3-day history of increasing headache that worsens with the Valsalva maneuver. She has also had a fever and left arm weakness for 1 day.

Definition

A brain abscess is a collection of infection/pus in the brain parenchyma.

What are common causes?

A brain abscess can develop due to direct spread of infection from a local infection (e.g., otitis media, mastoiditis, sinusitis, dental infection) or following a neurosurgical procedure. Less commonly, a brain abscess can develop from the hematogenous seeding of an infection from a distant site. The microorganism involved depends on the source of infection and is most commonly bacterial.

Source of Infection	Common Microorganisms
Sinuses/dental	*Streptococcus, Haemophilus, Bacteroides, Fusobacterium*, and *Prevotella* species
Ears	Enterobacteriaceae, *Pseudomonas aeruginosa, Streptococcus* and *Bacteroides* species
Head trauma/neurosurgical procedure	*Staphylococcus aureus, P. aeruginosa, Enterobacter, Clostridium*, and *Streptococcus* species
Endocarditis	*Streptococcus viridans* and *S. aureus*
Immunocompromised host	Parasitic: *Toxoplasma gondii* Bacterial: *Listeria, Nocardia* Fungal: *Aspergillus, Cryptococcus neoformans, Coccidioides, Candida*

● CLINICAL PEARL

The most common locations for an abscess are the frontotemporal region followed by the frontoparietal region, parietal, cerebellar, and occipital regions.

What symptoms might be observed?

Symptoms of a brain abscess are variable and include severe headache (75%) that is worse with lying flat, nausea, vomiting, drowsiness, weakness, numbness, and difficulty speaking. Seizures may also occur.

What is the differential diagnosis?

CNS ring-enhancing lesion: The differential diagnosis includes brain abscess, glioblastoma multiforme (GBM), metastatic cancer, CNS lymphoma, multiple sclerosis, infarction (subacute/chronic), hematoma (resolving), and radiation necrosis.

What are the possible findings on examination?

Vital signs: Fever is present in 45%–85% of individuals with a brain abscess. Other vital signs are generally normal, but if there is a systemic infection, hypotension and tachycardia may be present.

Neurologic examination: No specific exam maneuvers exist for a brain abscess, but a complete neurologic examination should be performed to assess for abnormalities.

Mental status: GCS may be altered. Nuchal rigidity/meningismus (neck stiffness) may be present if there is rupture of the brain abscess into the ventricular system and/or coexisting meningitis.

CNs: Papilledema and CN III or VI palsies if ICP is raised.

Motor/sensory/coordination: Any focal neurologic deficit may be present depending on the location of the abscess.

What tests should be ordered?

Laboratory tests: CBC (possible leukocytosis), metabolic panel (electrolytes, extended electrolytes, glucose, Cr, liver enzymes usually normal), other tests (LP is contraindicated in the presence of a mass lesion as herniation may occur; if an LP is performed, findings are similar to bacterial meningitis if the abscess has ruptured into the ventricles).

● CLINICAL PEARL

Brain imaging must be done prior to LP if there are focal neurologic signs or symptoms or papilledema due to the risk of herniation secondary to a CNS mass. Therefore, performing an LP must be carefully considered.

Imaging: There is no gold standard imaging test for diagnosing a brain abscess. Imaging often begins with a CT scan, which may show a hypodense lesion. A contrast-enhanced CT scan will reveal a ring-enhancing mass. MRI scan is more sensitive, and gadolinium can further enhance abscess detection. The mass is typically T1 iso-/hypointense and T2 hyperintense with ring enhancement (**Fig. 7.42**); however, these findings are also seen in tumors. Therefore, hyperintensity on DWI

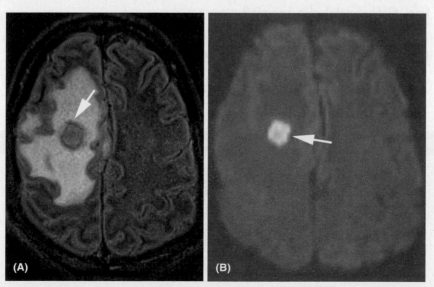

FIGURE 7.42. Pyogenic abscess. **A.** Axial FLAIR images show a round mass with low-signal-intensity rim and a large amount of surrounding edema (*arrow*). **B.** Axial DWI shows a ring-enhancing mass (*arrow*).

and hypointensity on ADC sequences are useful in distinguishing a brain abscess from a tumor (Sn 0.93, Sp 0.91).

Special Tests

When the site of the brain abscess is accessible, a stereotactic CT scan–guided aspiration can be performed for Gram stain, bacterial culture, acid-fast bacilli (AFB) stain, mycobacterial culture, fungal stain, and fungal culture.

 MENINGITIS

Presentation

A 30-year-old male teacher presents with a 1-day history of severe headache, nausea, vomiting, photophobia, fever, and neck stiffness. Neurologic examination was normal.

Definition

Meningitis is inflammation of the leptomeninges, which includes the dura, arachnoid, and pia mater that surround the brain and spinal cord. The brain itself is not involved.

What are common causes?

Meningitis is typically caused by infections and can be classified as bacterial meningitis (**Table 7.16**) or aseptic meningitis. Aseptic meningitis refers to meningitis in which routine bacterial cultures are negative. Aseptic meningitis may be caused by viral, fungal, and mycobacteria infections, as well as malignancy, inflammation, or drugs. Malignancies that seed the CNS include hematologic cancers and metastases from solid tumors. Inflammatory causes include SLE, vasculitis, and sarcoidosis. Drug causes include nonsteroidal anti-inflammatory drugs (NSAIDs), certain antibiotics (sulfa type), and intravenous immunoglobulin (IVIg).

What is the differential diagnosis?

Neck stiffness, headache, and fever: The differential diagnosis includes subdural/epidural empyema, brain abscess, and encephalitis.

Headache, nausea, and vomiting: Mass lesions (e.g., tumors and hemorrhage, particularly SAH), sinus venous thrombosis, arterial dissection, and migraine and other headache disorders.

TABLE 7.16. Common organisms causing meningitis	
Type of Infection	**Microorganism**
Bacterial	*Streptococcus pneumoniae, Neisseria meningitides, Haemophilus influenzae, Listeria monocytogenes* (in neonates and elderly), *S. aureus,* coagulase-negative staphylococci, Gram-negative bacilli
Viral	Enteroviruses (e.g., coxsackie, echovirus), herpes simplex virus (HSV), VZV, West Nile virus, human immunodeficiency syndrome (HIV)
Fungal	*C. neoformans, Coccidioides immitis*
Mycobacteria	Tuberculosis

What symptoms might be observed?

Symptoms of meningitis include headache (Sn 0.5, Sp 0.5), nausea/vomiting (Sn 0.3, Sp 0.6), neck pain (Sn 0.28), and photophobia.

What are the possible findings on examination?

Vital signs: Fever (Sn 0.85, Sp 0.45). Given the systemic infection, individuals may also have hypotension, tachycardia, and tachypnea.
General inspection: Petechia and purpura may be present, particularly in cases of *N. meningitides*.
Mental status: Alteration in mental status ranging from confusion to coma (Sn 0.67).
CNs/motor/sensory/coordination: Focal neurologic deficits of CNs, motor, sensory, or coordination may be present in severe cases of meningitis.

Special Tests

Nuchal rigidity: Neck stiffness is detected with passive neck flexion (Sn 0.3–0.7, Sp 0.68).
Jolt accentuation test: The patient's headache is worsened with rapid horizontal movements of the head (Sn 0.97, Sp 0.6).
Kernig sign: With the patient supine and hip flexed to 90 degrees, the clinician attempts to fully extend the knees. If pain is present the test is positive (Sn 0.05, Sp 0.95) (**Fig. 7.43**).
Brudzinski sign: With the patient supine, the clinician passively flexes the patient's neck. If the knees and hips flex, the test is positive (Sn 0.05, Sp 0.95).

● CLINICAL PEARL

The absence of fever, neck stiffness, and altered mental status rules out meningitis (Sn 0.99–1.0 for at least one of these findings).

What tests should be ordered?

Laboratory tests: CBC (possible leukocytosis, neutrophilia), metabolic panel (possible hyponatremia, elevated Cr, elevated liver enzymes, metabolic acidosis), coagulation profile (elevated INR and PTT, rarely, if disseminated intravascular coagulation develops), microbiology (possible positive blood cultures), and other tests (CSF [findings depend on the type of organism involved]) (**Table 7.17**).

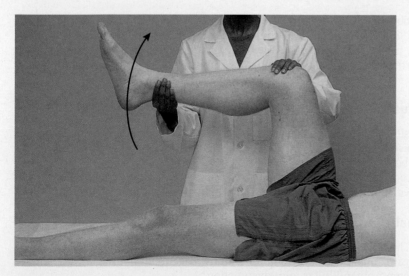

FIGURE 7.43. Kernig sign. The clinician flexes the leg at the hip and knee and then attempts to straighten the knee. The test is positive when there is pain and resistance to extending the knee.

TABLE 7.17. Findings on lumbar puncture based on etiology of meningitis

CSF Test	Bacterial	Viral	Fungal	Tuberculosis
WBC (cells/µL)	Usually >1,000, neutrophilic predominance	Typically <100, lymphocytic predominance	Variable, lymphocytic predominance	Variable, lymphocytic predominance
Protein	Elevated	Normal	Elevated	Elevated
Glucose	Low	Normal	Low	Low
Gram stain and culture	Positive	Negative	Fungal stains and culture positive	Positive AFB and mycobacterial culture
Viral PCR (HSV, VZV)	Negative	Positive	Negative	Negative

WBC, white blood cell count; PCR, polymerase chain reaction.

Imaging: A CT scan of the head is performed prior to a LP to exclude a mass lesion in cases with altered mental status, seizure, papilledema, or focal neurologic deficits or in immunocompromised individuals. CT scan is generally normal in meningitis, but if contrast is given, there may be leptomeningeal enhancement. An MRI scan of the brain is not routinely required in individuals with meningitis, but may show leptomeningeal enhancement when gadolinium is administered.

RHINOSINUSITIS

Presentation

A 50-year-old female presents with a 10-day history of worsening facial pain, purulent nasal discharge, headache, and fever. Prior to the development of these symptoms, her primary care provider had diagnosed her with a viral upper respiratory tract infection.

Definition

Rhinosinusitis is inflammation of the mucosa of the nose and paranasal sinuses. Rhinosinusitis is described by the sinuses involved (maxillary, ethmoid, frontal, or sphenoid sinuses), etiology (viral, bacterial, or fungal), presence of extrasinus involvement (complicated or uncomplicated), and aggravating factors. Furthermore, the clinical course of rhinosinusitis can be divided into five subtypes (**Table 7.18**).

What are common causes?

The majority of acute rhinosinusitis cases are caused by viral infection, specifically rhinovirus. The most common bacterial causes include *S. pneumoniae* and *H. influenzae* followed by *Moraxella catarrhalis,* and oral anaerobes.

Although rhinosinusitis occurs frequently in healthy patients, a number of local, regional, and systemic conditions may predispose a patient to developing rhinosinusitis (**Table 7.19**).

What is the differential diagnosis?

Rhinitis and facial pain: The differential diagnosis includes allergic fungal rhinosinusitis, allergic rhinitis, invasive fungal rhinosinusitis, vasomotor rhinitis, trigeminal neuralgia, migraine or headache disorder, and temporomandibular joint dysfunction.

TABLE 7.18. Subtypes of rhinosinusitis	
Rhinosinusitis Task Force (2007) Clinical Classification Scheme	
Acute rhinosinusitis	Symptoms lasting <4 wk with complete resolution
Recurrent rhinosinusitis	≥4 episodes of acute rhinosinusitis per year with symptom-free intervals
Subacute rhinosinusitis	Symptoms lasting 4–12 wk
Chronic rhinosinusitis	Symptoms lasting ≥12 wk
Acute exacerbation of chronic rhinosinusitis	Sudden worsening of baseline chronic rhinosinusitis with return to baseline

What symptoms might be observed?

Major symptoms of rhinosinusitis include congestion, facial pain/pressure, nasal obstruction, and purulent/colored nasal discharge. Minor symptoms include frontal headache, halitosis, dental pain, otalgia, and cough.

● CLINICAL PEARL

Diagnosis of sinusitis requires either two major symptoms or one major and two minor symptoms.

What are the possible findings on examination?

Vital signs: Fever and/or tachycardia may be present if systemically unwell.
Inspection: The anterior nasal mucosa may demonstrate edema, purulent discharge, and polyps. The oral cavity and oropharynx may demonstrate erythema from postnasal drip or poor dentition. Otoscopy may demonstrate a concomitant middle ear effusion or otitis media.
Palpation: Tender cervical lymphadenopathy may be present with sinusitis.

● CLINICAL PEARL

Rhinosinusitis may result in a number of potential complications (**Table 7.20**), and urgent assessment by an otolaryngologist should be considered.

TABLE 7.19. Predisposing factors for rhinosinusitis		
Local	**Regional**	**Systemic**
Impaired mucociliary transport • Cold/dry air • Medications	Apical dental infection Anatomic derangements • Nasal/midface trauma • Deviated septum • Nasal polyps • Nasal tumors Foreign body • Nasal packing • Nasogastric tubes	General debilitation • Long-term steroid therapy • Uncontrolled DM • Blood dyscrasia • Chemotherapy • Malnutrition • Colonization of upper gastrointestinal and upper respiratory tracts by Gram-negative bacteria Immunodeficiencies • HIV/AIDS • IgG deficiency • Granulomatosis with polyangiitis

TABLE 7.20. **Complications of rhinosinusitis**	
Mucocele/mucopyocele	Collection of sinus secretions trapped due to obstruction of sinus outflow tract May become infected resulting in a mucopyocele
Ophthalmic complications	Preseptal cellulitis Orbital cellulitis Subperiosteal abscess Orbital abscess Cavernous sinus thrombosis
CNS complications	Meningitis Epidural abscess Subdural abscess Parenchymal abscess
Bony complications	Osteomyelitis Pott puffy tumor

What tests should be ordered?

Laboratory tests: CBC (leukocytosis in systemic infection).

Imaging: Medical imaging is not required for acute rhinosinusitis unless systemic toxicity or complications are suspected, in which case CT scan is performed. CT scan offers detailed assessment of the bony anatomy of the paranasal sinuses and may be indicated for assessing for anatomic variants, complications of rhinosinusitis, following medical failure of chronic rhinosinusitis, or with other concerns. Plain film radiography may demonstrate sinus air–fluid levels but has limited specificity and sensitivity. MRI scan can provide excellent soft tissue delineation but poor bony anatomy and is thus limited to assessing for intracranial or intraorbital extension, evaluation of soft tissue masses, and when there is concern regarding possible fungal sinusitis.

RETROPHARYNGEAL ABSCESS

Presentation

An 18-year-old male presents with a 6-day history of throat pain, feeding intolerance, and dysphagia. He developed a fever on the day of presentation. Two weeks earlier, he had an upper respiratory tract infection.

Definition

A retropharyngeal abscess is a suppurative infection in the potential space formed by the fascia located in the retropharynx. Retropharyngeal abscess carries significant risk of morbidity and mortality.

What are common causes?

Retropharyngeal abscess occurs primarily in children, although it can occur in adults. In pediatric patients, retropharyngeal abscess may be caused by direct spread from the nasopharynx, adenoids, and sinuses, whereas in adults, instrumentation of the pharynx, trauma, and foreign bodies are the more common etiologies. The most common pathogens are group A *Streptococcus*, *S. aureus*, and respiratory anaerobes.

What is the differential diagnosis?

Pharyngitis: The differential diagnosis includes viral pharyngitis, bacterial pharyngitis, mononucleosis, Kawasaki disease, and trauma.

What symptoms might be observed?

Symptoms of a retropharyngeal abscess include torticollis, dysphagia/anorexia, cough, trismus, and lethargy.

What are the possible findings on examination?

Vital signs: Fever and/or tachycardia may be present.
Inspection: Posterior pharyngeal swelling and sialorrhea.
Palpation: Tender cervical lymphadenopathy.

> ● **CLINICAL PEARL**
>
> Patients with suspected retropharyngeal abscess should be assessed for any evidence of airway compromise. Other potential complications include septicemia, aspiration pneumonia (abscess rupturing into airway), internal jugular vein thrombosis and thrombophlebitis, carotid artery erosion and rupture, and mediastinitis.

What tests should be ordered?

Laboratory tests: CBC (leukocytosis), metabolic (usually normal Cr, electrolytes), and coagulation profile (INR, PTT if operative management is expected).
Imaging: Lateral neck x-rays are performed to look for widened prevertebral soft tissue (**Fig. 7.44**). In some instances, a contrast-enhanced CT scan may be needed for diagnosis or to diagnose complications.

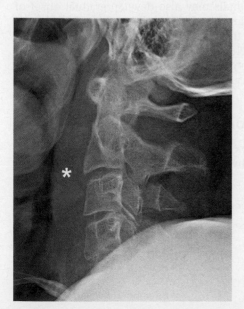

FIGURE 7.44. Lateral neck x-ray. A lateral neck x-ray demonstrating thickened prevertebral tissues (*asterisk*). At the level of C2, the distance from the anterior surface of the vertebrae to the posterior border of the airway should be 7 mm or less. At the level of C6, this distance should be 14 mm or less in children <15 years old and should be <22 mm in an adult. Thickened prevertebral soft tissues may be consistent with a retropharyngeal space infection.

PITUITARY ADENOMA

Presentation

A 20-year-old female presents with a mild headache over the past few months, gradually progressive reduction in peripheral vision, amenorrhea, and galactorrhea.

Definition

A pituitary adenoma is a benign tumor of the anterior pituitary gland. Pituitary adenomas are classified by size, with those <1 cm referred to as *microadenomas*, and those >1 cm referred to as *macroadenomas*. Pituitary adenomas may arise from any of the cell types in the anterior pituitary and can lead to excess of the hormone secreted by the involved cell type or hyposecretion of other pituitary hormones due to compression of the remainder of the gland.

What are common causes?

Pituitary adenomas develop due to clonal expansion of a cell line similar to other neoplasms. This is related to the development of genetic mutations due to genetic and environmental factors. For instance, pituitary adenomas are part of the multiple endocrine neoplasia type 1 syndrome (MEN1), which also includes parathyroid and pancreatic islet tumors.

What is the differential diagnosis?

Sellar region mass: The differential diagnosis includes craniopharyngioma (remnant of Rathke pouch, usually in children), meningioma (benign tumor of the meninges), pituitary gland hyperplasia, germ cell tumors, optic gliomas, aneurysms, and cysts.

What symptoms might be observed?

Symptoms develop due to local mass effect and/or excessive or decreased pituitary function. Classically, individuals develop gradual reduction in peripheral vision, referred to as *bitemporal hemianopsia* (**Fig. 7.45**) because the suprasellar growth of the pituitary adenoma causes compression of the adjacent optic chiasm (**Fig. 7.46**). Individuals may also develop gradual onset of headache due to mass effect. Less commonly, patients develop diplopia due to lateral growth of the adenoma, leading to compression of CN III. Rarely, the pituitary adenoma may hemorrhage (referred to as *pituitary apoplexy*) leading to acute headache, decreased LOC, and diplopia.

Some pituitary adenomas secrete hormones, while others are nonsecreting (**Table 7.21**). All pituitary tumors can cause hypofunctioning of the pituitary gland due to decreased hormone secretion from compression of the remaining pituitary gland.

What are the possible findings on examination?

Vital signs: The vital signs may be affected by hormonal changes, and individuals may be hyper- or hypothermic, tachy- or bradycardic, and hyper- or hypotensive, depending on the hormonal abnormalities.

FIGURE 7.45. Bitemporal hemianopsia. Visual field defect seen in compression of the optic chiasm.

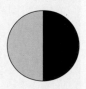

Bitemporal hemianopsia

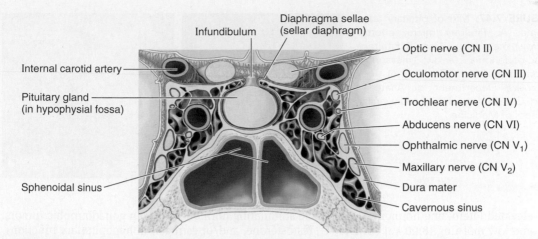

FIGURE 7.46. Pituitary gland and cavernous sinus. Note the close relation of the pituitary gland to the optic nerves superiorly.

CNs: The most classic finding is bitemporal hemianopia. Other abnormalities of pupillary light responses and extraocular movements may be present with CN III compression.

Language/motor/sensory/coordination: Typically normal.

What tests should be ordered?

Laboratory tests: Other serology (elevated prolactin level in a prolactinoma, elevated 24-hour urine cortisol in adrenocorticotropic hormone [ACTH]-secreting tumors, elevated insulin-like growth factor 1 [IGF-1] in growth hormone [GH]-secreting tumors, elevated TSH in TSH-secreting tumors,

TABLE 7.21. Pituitary adenoma cell lines and clinical manifestations		
Cell Line	**Hormone Affected**	**Symptoms and Signs**
Gonadotroph	Generally nonsecreting but could secrete LH/FSH	No hormone-related symptoms usually
Thyrotroph	Elevated TSH or nonsecreting	Goiter, symptoms of hyperthyroidism (fever, tachycardia, heat intolerance, tremor, diarrhea, changes to nails/hair)
Corticotroph	Elevated ACTH	Cushing syndrome (mood changes, hypertension, DM, dorsal fat pad, central obesity, change in fat distribution of the face, striae, thin skin, hirsutism)
Lactotroph	Elevated prolactin	Infertility, amenorrhea, decreased libido, galactorrhea, gynecomastia
Somatotroph	Elevated GH	Acromegaly (excess growth of tissues leading to enlargement of the hands, feet, coarsening of facial features, deepening of the voice)
All types	Hypopituitary (decreased ACTH, TSH, LH/FSH, GH)	Fatigue, lethargy, decreased libido, amenorrhea, hypothyroidism (cold intolerance, bradycardia, changes to skin/nails, constipation)
Compression of pituitary stalk (usually does not occur in adenomas)	Decreased vasopressin release from the posterior pituitary and increased prolactin (decreased dopaminergic inhibition)	Diabetes insipidus (orthostatic hypotension, large urine output, hypernatremia); mildly elevated prolactin may be asymptomatic

FIGURE 7.47. MRI of pituitary adenoma. **A.** Pituitary microadenoma (*arrow*), measuring <1 cm. **B.** Pituitary macroadenoma (*arrow*) measuring more than 1 cm. (Courtesy of Joel Vilensky, Department of Anatomy and Cell Biology, Indiana University School of Medicine.)

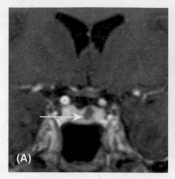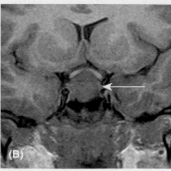

elevated luteinizing hormone [LH]/follicle-stimulating hormone [FSH] in gonadotrophic tumors, and low morning [8:00 AM] cortisol, T_4, testosterone, and/or estrogen in hypopituitary function).

Imaging: No gold standard imaging exists for pituitary adenoma. MRI scan of the brain with sellar views and gadolinium is the best imaging test for suprasellar masses (**Fig. 7.47**). MRI scan is able to depict surrounding structures including the optic chiasm.

Special Tests

Formal Humphrey visual field testing is performed to determine visual field loss.

 # GLIOBLASTOMA MULTIFORME

Presentation

A 56-year-old male presents with a 5-week history of progressively worsening headaches, left-sided upper and lower extremity weakness, and a 3-day history of left focal motor seizures of the upper and lower extremities.

Definition

Glioblastoma multiforme (GBM) is a rapidly progressive brain tumor originating from astrocytic cells with a World Health Organization (WHO) grade IV classification, indicating a high-grade tumor. Histologically, this tumor type is highly cellular and pleomorphic with mitotic activity, microvascular proliferation, and/or necrosis. It has a very poor prognosis.

What are common causes?

GBM originates due to clonal expansion of astrocytic cells in the brain due to both genetic and environmental factors, as in other tumors. In elderly individuals, GBM may arise *de novo* from normal astrocytes. In younger individuals, GBM may evolve from lower-grade gliomas.

What is the differential diagnosis?

CNS mass: The differential diagnosis includes primary CNS tumors such as gliomas, meningiomas, pituitary adenomas, and primary CNS lymphomas, as well as intracranial metastasis, ICH, ischemic infarct, intracranial abscess, and MS.

What symptoms might be observed?

Symptoms of GBM include headache (57%), classically early morning headache, worsened by cough, sneeze, or Valsalva maneuver. Other symptoms include nausea/vomiting (15%), memory loss (39%), personality change (27%), and visual symptoms (21%). Focal or generalized seizures (23%) may occur.

What are the possible findings on examination?

Vital signs: Typically normal, although hypertension, bradycardia, and altered respiratory pattern (Cushing triad) may be present if the ICP is raised.
Neurologic examination: A complete neurologic exam should be performed.
Mental status: GCS may be altered in severe cases (18%). Cognitive impairment (39%) may be present depending on the area of the brain affected by the mass lesion.
CNs: Papilledema and CN III or VI palsies if the ICP is raised.
Language/motor/sensory/coordination: Any focal neurologic deficit, for example, aphasia, weakness, sensory deficit, and dysmetria, may be present.

What tests should be ordered?

Laboratory tests: No lab test exists to diagnose GBM.
Imaging: MRI scan of the brain with gadolinium is the most useful initial test (Sn 0.72, Sp 0.65) to differentiate high-grade gliomas from other grade gliomas. GBM is typically hypointense on T1, hyperintense on T2, and heterogeneously gadolinium enhancing on MRI scan, as shown in **Figure 7.48**. MR perfusion (MRP) scan demonstrates cerebral blood flow, and MR spectroscopy (MRS) scan reveals metabolite ratios in the abnormal tissue, which may aid in distinguishing tumors from other mass lesions and in distinguishing the tumor grade (MRP + MRS Sn 0.93, Sp 0.6 in distinguishing high-grade glioma from other grades). CT scan with contrast is less sensitive but can be used in emergency settings.

Special Tests

Tissue diagnosis is the gold standard in diagnosing GBM. Tissue is obtained during resection or debulking if the tumor is accessible. A stereotactic brain biopsy may also be done if the lesion is too deep for open surgery.

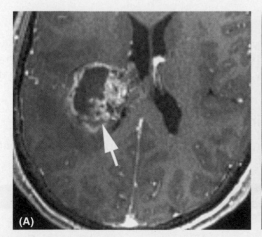 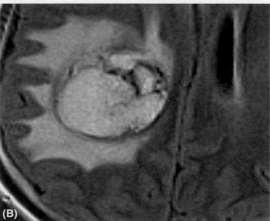

FIGURE 7.48. Glioblastoma multiforme. **A.** MRI T1 with gadolinium. Eccentric nodular enhancement (*arrow*) is suggestive of GBM. **B.** Axial FLAIR shows large amount of increased signal surrounding the mass, representing a combination of edema and infiltrative nonenhancing tumor.

TRAUMATIC BRAIN INJURY

Presentation

A 22-year-old male presents to the hospital after a motor vehicle accident (MVA). He has decreased LOC and a fixed and dilated left pupil that is deviated down and out. He extends his left arm and leg to painful stimuli, but there is no movement on the right side. He is hypertensive and bradycardic.

Definition

Traumatic brain injury (TBI) is trauma to the head resulting in brain injury, and the severity is classified by the GCS (**Table 7.22**).

What are common causes?

The most common causes of head trauma include falls (particularly in the elderly), MVAs, assault, military combat, and sports-related injuries.

Trauma to the head can result in different types of injury to the brain. These include skull fractures, intracranial hemorrhages (epidural, subdural, subarachnoid, intracerebral, and intraventricular hemorrhages), and cerebral contusions as well as focal and diffuse axonal injury (DAI). The primary brain injury occurs at the time of the trauma due to direct impact, acceleration–deceleration, and penetrating and blast injuries. This results in hemorrhage and shearing of white matter tracts (DAI) and cerebral edema. A *coup injury* refers to injury in the brain at the site of impact, while *contrecoup injury* refers to injury on the side of the brain opposite to the impact, likely due to deceleration. Secondary brain injury occurs due to a cascade of molecular injury that continues hours to days after the event due to excitotoxicity, inflammation, cell death, and vasospasm, and this further exacerbates the primary brain injury.

What is the differential diagnosis?

Elevated ICP: The differential diagnosis includes intracranial hemorrhage types, ischemic stroke, venous thrombosis, intracranial tumor, infection (brain abscess, meningitis, encephalitis), metabolic disturbance, hypertensive encephalopathy, and seizure.

What symptoms might be observed?

Symptoms of a TBI include headache, nausea, vomiting, vertigo, amnesia, confusion, slow responses, disorientation, decreased attention, slurring of speech, and incoordination. More severe forms of TBI may cause seizures and coma. Acutely, symptoms related to TBI caused by elevated ICP are summarized in **Table 7.23**.

What are the possible findings on examination?

Vital signs: Hypertension, bradycardia, and respiratory depression/irregularity may be present when the ICP is raised (Cushing triad). Intubation may be required.

TABLE 7.22. Glasgow coma scale in traumatic brain injury	
Severity of TBI	**Initial GCS**
Mild	13–15
Moderate	9–12
Severe	1–8

TABLE 7.23. Symptoms caused by elevated intracranial pressure secondary to a traumatic brain injury

High ICP Syndromes	Signs
Midline shift	Impaired LOC Papilledema Cushing triad
Uncal herniation	Ipsilateral CN III palsy (pupil dilated, down-and-out eye deviation)
Central herniation	Small, dilated, fixed pupils with downward-deviated eyes Fatal
Subfalcine herniation	Abnormal posturing and coma, progresses to central and uncal herniation
Tonsillar herniation ("coning")	Decreased LOC Flaccid quadriplegia Irregular respirations Blood pressure instability Fatal

General inspection: The patient should be examined for other signs of trauma following advanced trauma life support (ATLS) guidelines.

Neurologic examination: A complete neurologic exam should be performed.

Mental status: GCS may be decreased.

CNs: Fixed and dilated pupils may occur. Fundoscopy may reveal papilledema if ICP is high. One eye may be deviated "down and out," suggestive of CN III palsy or deviated medially in CN VI palsy. Facial asymmetry may be noted. Brainstem reflexes, including the pupillary, oculocephalic, corneal, and gag reflexes, may be impaired. Oculocephalic response is only assessed if there is no concern for cervical spine injury. Cold caloric responses can be assessed as an alternative.

Motor: Muscle tone may be spastic, reflexes may be increased, and the plantar response may be upgoing. Observe for spontaneous movements and for response to peripheral stimuli. There may be decreased movements on one side.

Sensory and coordination: Cannot be assessed in a comatose patient.

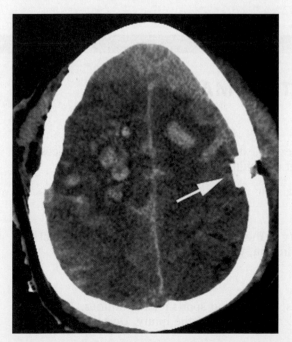

FIGURE 7.49. Depressed skull fracture with ICH. The CT image shows parenchymal and extra-axial hemorrhage (*white areas*) and a depressed fragment (*arrow*).

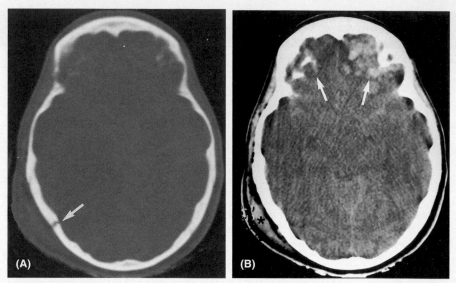

FIGURE 7.50. Contrecoup brain injury. A. CT image in bone windows shows a fracture in the right posterior parietal bone (*arrow*). B. Same image in brain windows shows areas of ICH in the frontal lobes (*arrows*). Note the scalp hematoma (*asterisk*) in the right occipital area.

What tests should be ordered?

Laboratory tests: CBC, metabolic panel (electrolytes, extended electrolytes, glucose, Cr and liver function), and coagulation profile (elevated INR and PTT may indicate a patient is anticoagulated and may need reversal).

Imaging: The imaging in acute head trauma involves a noncontrast CT scan, which is very sensitive in detecting acute hemorrhage, midline shift, brain edema, and signs of herniation. For hemorrhagic lesions, CT and MRI scan have similar sensitivity (CT Sn 0.9; MRI Sn 0.93); however, in nonhemorrhagic lesions (including contusions and DAI), MRI scan has greater sensitivity (CT Sn 0.18; MRI Sn 0.93), with 30% of those with a normal CT head having signs of DAI on MRI scan. **Figure 7.49** shows traumatic ICH, and **Figure 7.50** shows contrecoup injuries.

 # CERVICAL SPINE TRAUMA

Presentation

A 30-year-old male involved in an MVA had a flexion–extension injury with acute-onset neck pain and inability to feel or move his upper and lower extremities.

Definition

Cervical spine trauma involves a traumatic injury to the cervical spine and can lead to spinal cord injury (SCI) due to spinal cord compression, contusion, vascular injury, or transection.

What are common causes?

Cervical spine trauma occurs due to MVAs, falls, assault, and sports-related injuries. The type of injury is classified by the mechanism, stability, and location of the injury. Unstable injuries are more likely to cause SCI (**Table 7.24**).

TABLE 7.24. Types and mechanisms of cervical spine trauma		
Fracture Type	**Mechanism**	**Stability**
Atlanto-occipital or atlantoaxial dislocation	Flexion injury	Unstable
C1 burst fracture	Vertical compression fracture of anterior and posterior arches of C1; transverse ligament may be disrupted.	Very unstable
C1 posterior arch fracture	Compression of posterior elements during neck extension	Unstable
C2 odontoid fracture	Forceful flexion or extension injury Type 1: above transverse ligament Type 2: base of odontoid Type 3: base of odontoid + C2 body	Stable Unstable Unstable
C2 pedicle fracture	Extension injury	Unstable
Anterior wedge fracture	Flexion injury	Usually stable Can be unstable
Spinous process fracture	Lower cervical vertebrae spinous process fracture due to forced flexion	Stable
Burst fracture	Vertical compression fracture due to axial load	Stable, but may impinge cord
Bilateral facet dislocations	Bilateral facet dislocation with flexion injury; disrupts ligaments	Very unstable; often complete SCI
Ligamentous injuries	No bony injury present, but SCI	Unstable

What is the differential diagnosis?

Spinal cord syndromes: The differential diagnosis includes disc herniation, spinal tumor, spinal infarct, infection within the spinal cord, and inflammatory spinal lesion.

What symptoms might be observed?

Symptoms of cervical spine trauma include neck pain, weakness, and sensory loss.

What are the possible findings on examination?

Vital signs: Hypotension and bradycardia may be present in acute SCI due to neurogenic shock. If the level of injury is above C3, there may be respiratory muscle paralysis necessitating urgent intubation.
General inspection: The patient should be examined for other signs of trauma following ATLS guidelines.
Palpation: Spinal tenderness and deformities may be present.
Neurologic examination: A complete neurologic examination should be performed. Findings of specific spinal cord injuries are summarized in **Table 7.25**.
General/mental status: GCS is typically normal unless there is associated brain injury.
CNs: Should be normal in isolated SCI.
Motor: Acutely in spinal shock, muscles will have a flaccid tone, severe bilateral upper and lower extremity weakness, and areflexia below the level of the injury. Days to weeks later, spasticity, hyperreflexia, and upgoing plantar response develop.
Sensory: Loss of the primary sensory modalities below the level of the lesion.
Coordination: Cannot be tested if there is severe weakness as seen in cervical SCI.
Digital rectal examination: Reduced rectal tone.

● CLINICAL PEARL

Distinguishing neurogenic and spinal shock is important. *Neurogenic shock* results in hypotension and bradycardia in acute SCI. *Spinal shock* causes flaccid tone and areflexia in acute SCI.

TABLE 7.25. Signs related to different spinal cord injuries

Extent of Injury	Signs
Complete SCI	Completely absent sensation below the level of the injury Flaccid paralysis below the level of the injury with hyporeflexia acutely and later spasticity and hyperreflexia Urinary retention Decreased rectal tone
Incomplete SCI	Variable loss of sensation below the level of the lesion, partially preserved Weakness below the level of the injury Bowel and bladder dysfunction
Central cord syndrome	Greater motor impairment in the upper than lower extremities Suspended sensory level Bowel and bladder dysfunction
Anterior cord syndrome	Loss of pain and cold sensation below the injury level, but spared vibration and proprioception Weakness below the level of the injury Bowel and bladder dysfunction

What tests should be ordered?

Laboratory tests: There are no specific laboratory investigations.

Imaging: CT scan of the cervical spine is the best imaging modality to assess for cervical spine injuries and should be obtained when there is a high probability of cervical injury (Sn 0.98). Three-view plain radiography (anterior–posterior/lateral/odontoid) can be used in minor trauma without neurologic abnormalities but has lower sensitivity in detecting cervical spine abnormalities compared to CT scan (Sn 0.52). Although excellent for detecting fractures, CT imaging is inadequate in detecting ligamentous injuries, which are much better detected by MRI scans, although fractures may be missed by MRI. Thus, there are pitfalls in all imaging modalities of the cervical spine. **Figures 7.51 and 7.52** display examples of cervical spinal injury imaging including plain x-rays, CT scan, and MRI scan to demonstrate the usefulness of each modality.

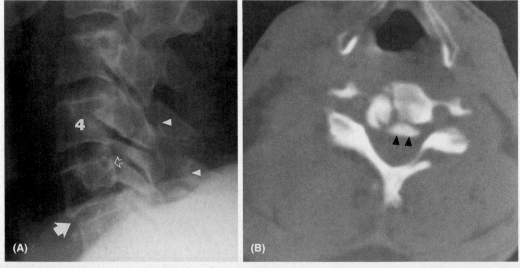

FIGURE 7.51. C5 burst fracture. **A.** Lateral x-ray shows anterolisthesis of C5 on C6 (*large arrow*). There is bowing of the posterior vertebral body line (*open arrow*) and disruption of the spinolaminar line (*arrowheads*). **B.** CT image shows fractures of the body of C5 with retropulsion of a bone fragment into the vertebral canal (*arrowheads*).

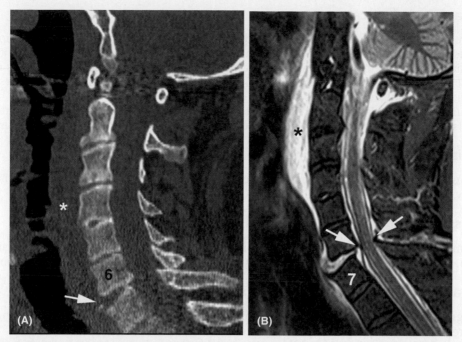

FIGURE 7.52. Wide disc space (*arrows*) in a patient with an extension injury. **A.** Sagittal reconstructed CT image shows that the C6 disc space (*arrow*) is wider than its mates. There is also retrolisthesis of C6 on C7. Note the massive prevertebral hematoma (*asterisk*). **B.** Sagittal T2-weighted MRI shows the wide disc space as well as impingement of the spinal cord by osteophytes anteriorly and posteriorly (*arrows*). The anterior and posterior longitudinal ligaments are ruptured. The patient was quadriplegic.

> ● **CLINICAL PEARL**
>
> Acutely, the cervical spine must be immobilized as soon as possible. Unstable fractures require neurosurgical intervention to decompress the spinal cord or prevent SCI. Steroids are generally given in acute SCI.

FACIAL FRACTURES

Presentation

A 25-year-old male presents to the Emergency Department with a painful jaw, malocclusion, and left-sided lower lip anesthesia the morning after being assaulted.

Definition

A facial fracture is any sudden disruption of the normal bony anatomy of the facial bones. Facial fractures are often coincident and include frontal sinus fractures, orbitozygomatic complex and orbital fractures, midface and nasal fractures, and mandible fractures. Characteristics of the fracture including the location, stability, and comminution of the fracture as well as the displacement and resultant deformity must be considered.

What are common causes?

Facial fractures occur due to trauma sustained during sports, falls, assaults, MVAs, and industrial accidents. Factors influencing the development of and resultant fracture include the point of contact, patient's age, and the amount and direction of force applied to the face. Less force is required for nasal fractures, whereas more force is required for mandible fractures, midface fractures, orbital fractures, and frontal sinus fractures.

A number of complications may result from facial fractures, depending on the nature of the fracture(s) (**Table 7.26**). C-spine injuries may occur in ~10% of patients with facial fractures.

What is the differential diagnosis?

Facial swelling: The differential diagnosis includes contusions, angioedema, anaphylaxis, malignancy, and infections (e.g., parotiditis).

What symptoms might be observed?

Symptoms of facial fractures depend on the bone fractured and include headache, pain, vision loss, diplopia, facial numbness or paresthesias, nasal obstruction, anosmia, hyposmia, and trismus.

What are the possible findings on examination?

Vital signs: Tachycardia, hypotension, tachypnea, and hypoxia may be present, depending on the nature of the facial fractures and other concomitant injuries.

Inspection: Facial deformities, facial lacerations, and ecchymosis may be observed. A broad nasal root, proptosis, enophthalmos, telecanthus, and epiphora may be present, depending on the fracture. Anterior rhinoscopy is used to examine for epistaxis, septal hematoma, and CSF rhinorrhea. The oral cavity and oropharynx may demonstrate postnasal CSF leak as well as lacerations of the gingival and oral mucosa.

Palpation: Deformity, crepitus, and movements of the facial bones may be appreciated.

CNs: Anosmia/hyposmia, vision changes/loss, abnormal extraocular movements, impaired facial sensation, and impaired facial movement may be present, depending on the fracture.

What tests should be ordered?

Laboratory tests: No specific laboratory investigations exist; however, a β-2 transferrin assay can be performed on clear fluid if there is concern for CSF leak.

Imaging: Nasal fractures are diagnosed on clinical grounds. However, for other facial fractures, high-resolution CT scan with reconstructions are essential for diagnosis, preoperative planning, and assessing for complications. An orbital blow-out fracture is depicted in **Figure 7.53**.

TABLE 7.26. Complications of facial fractures

Type	Outcomes
Poor cosmetic outcome	Scar, poor facial contour, soft tissue deformities
Infection	Wound infections, CSF leak, meningitis, osteomyelitis
Hardware related	Hardware infection, plate contours visible through skin, plate exposure, plate or screw failure
Eye, eyelid, orbital complications	Diplopia, lower eyelid injury and malposition, extraocular muscle dysfunction, epiphora
Nasal complications	Epistaxis, septal hematoma, septal abscess, "saddle nose" deformity, septal perforation, synechiae
Malocclusion	Malocclusion, temporomandibular joint dysfunction, trismus, tooth loss, malunion, nonunion
CN injury	Facial paresis/paralysis (especially in temporal bone fracture), facial hypoesthesia/dysesthesia, vision loss
Functional impairment	Nasal airway obstruction, impaired alimentation

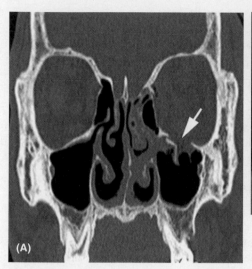
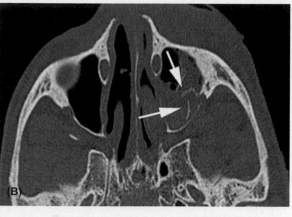

FIGURE 7.53. Blow-out fracture of the left orbital floor. **A.** Coronal reconstructed CT image demonstrating a fracture of the floor of the left orbit (*arrow*) with displacement of bone fragments into the maxillary sinus. **B.** Axial image through the sinus showing bone fragments (*arrows*). Compare with the other side.

 # THYROID NODULES AND MALIGNANCY

Presentation

A 55-year-old male presents with a 2-cm palpable thyroid nodule that was detected during his periodic physical examination.

Definition

A thyroid nodule is an abnormal growth of cells in the thyroid gland. Thyroid nodules are common, occurring in ~5% of the adult population. It is estimated that 5% of these nodules will contain cancerous growth.

What are common causes?

Type	Etiologies
Benign	Colloid nodule, adenoma, focal thyroiditis, thyroid cyst, benign lymph node hypertrophy, parathyroid cyst, cystic hygroma, dermoid, teratoma, laryngocele, and thyroglossal duct cyst
Malignant	Papillary, follicular, medullary, and anaplastic thyroid carcinoma; lymphoma; and metastasis to thyroid

Important risk factors for thyroid malignancy include family history of thyroid malignancy, history of ionizing radiation to the head and neck, male sex, and age (<20 or >60 years old). Other factors that raise concern for malignancy are a large mass, rapidly growing mass, a hard and fixed mass, and lymphadenopathy.

What is the differential diagnosis?

Neck mass: The differential diagnosis includes soft tissue masses (lipomas, sarcomas, and hemangiomas), anatomical fat pad, benign or malignant thyroid nodules, lymphadenopathy, and thyroglossal cyst.

What symptoms might be observed?

Symptoms of thyroid nodules range from asymptomatic to hoarseness, dysphagia, globus sensation, and anterior neck pain. Symptoms of hyperthyroidism may occur if the nodule secretes thyroid hormone.

What are the possible findings on examination?

Vital signs: Typically normal, but tachycardia may be present if hyperthyroid.
Inspection: Visible masses may be present.
Palpation: Thyroid nodules may be present in the right and left thyroid lobes, isthmus, and (if present) pyramidal lobe. The nodule size, shape, firmness, and tenderness should be noted. Cervical lymphadenopathy may be present.

> ● CLINICAL PEARL
>
> Flexible nasopharyngoscopy is performed prior to thyroidectomy to assess vocal cord mobility.

What tests should be ordered?

Laboratory tests: Other serology (TSH, free T_3 and T_4 in patients with nodules >1 cm).
Imaging: A neck ultrasound that includes the thyroid gland and cervical lymph nodes is the best initial investigation for a thyroid nodule or mass. Ultrasonography cannot distinguish between benign and malignant thyroid nodules, but features identified on ultrasound (microcalcifications, hypoechogenicity, irregular margins, absence of hypoechoic halo around the nodule, increased size) can raise suspicion for malignancy. A nuclear scan of the thyroid is performed with radioactive iodine to assess if a nodule is functioning (**Fig. 7.54**).

Special Tests

Ultrasound-guided fine needle aspiration (FNA) biopsy: Posterior nodules, nodules >1 cm, or nodules with >50% cysts are assessed.

FIGURE 7.54. Thyroid scan showing a nodule as a photopenic area (cold or nonfunctioning nodule) in the right lobe of the thyroid.

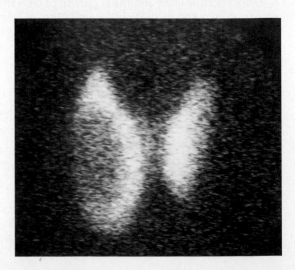

Note: Page numbers in **boldface** indicate the primary entry for the term, which appears in **boldface** on the page indicated and is followed by a definition or explanation; page numbers in *italics* denote figures; those followed by "t" denote tables.

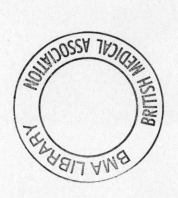